Implant Dentistry: Surgical Principles

Implant Dentistry: Surgical Principles

Edited by Jonathan Lewis

STATES
ACADEMIC PRESS
www.statesacademicpress.com

States Academic Press,
109 South 5th Street,
Brooklyn, NY 11249, USA

Visit us on the World Wide Web at:
www.statesacademicpress.com

ISBN: 978-1-63989-284-6

Cataloging-in-Publication Data

Implant dentistry : surgical principles / edited by Jonathan Lewis.
p. cm.
Includes bibliographical references and index.
ISBN 978-1-63989-284-6
1. Dental implants. 2. Mouth--Surgery. 3. Implants, Artificial. 4. Dentures. 5. Prosthodontics. I. Lewis, Jonathan.
RK667.I45 I46 2022
617.693--dc23

Table of Contents

Preface

Implant dentistry is a procedure in which the roots of the tooth are replaced with metal screwlike posts, and missing or damaged teeth are replaced with artificial teeth that function and look similar to the real ones. The main benefit of the implants is that they provide support for the new teeth during bone healing because it requires time for the bone to heal tightly around the implant. They are surgically placed in the jawbone so that they can serve as the roots of the missing teeth. Titanium is present in the implants that fuses with the jawbone and doesn't let the implant slip. This book is a compilation of chapters that discuss the most vital concepts and emerging trends in the field of implant dentistry. It presents this complex subject in the most comprehensible and easy to understand language. This book attempts to assist those with a goal of delving into this field.

This book is a result of research of several months to collate the most relevant data in the field.

When I was approached with the idea of this book and the proposal to edit it, I was overwhelmed. It gave me an opportunity to reach out to all those who share a common interest with me in this field. I had 3 main parameters for editing this text:

1. Accuracy - The data and information provided in this book should be up-to-date and valuable to the readers.
2. Structure - The data must be presented in a structured format for easy understanding and better grasping of the readers.
3. Universal Approach - This book not only targets students but also experts and innovators in the field, thus my aim was to present topics which are of use to all.

Thus, it took me a couple of months to finish the editing of this book.

I would like to make a special mention of my publisher who considered me worthy of this opportunity and also supported me throughout the editing process. I would also like to thank the editing team at the back-end who extended their help whenever required.

Editor

1

Osseointegration and Bioscience of Implant Surfaces - Current Concepts at Bone-Implant Interface

Mustafa Ramazanoglu[1] and Yoshiki Oshida[2]
[1]*Istanbul University/Department of Oral Surgery*
[2]*Syracuse University/Department of Mechanical and Aerospace Engineering*
[1]*Turkey*
[2]*USA*

1. Introduction

The high success rates for the dental rehabilitation of patients with endosseous implants have resulted from many research approaches with the aim of enhancing and accelerating bone anchorage to the implant, thereby providing optimal support for the intraoral prosthetic devices. This revolutionary breakthrough has first evolved from the research efforts of the Brånemark group in the late 1960s by pioneering the insertion of machined screw-type commercially pure titanium (cpTi) implants with minimum surgical trauma and a consolidation period for the healing of the bone (Albrektsson et al., 1981; Brånemark et al., 1969). This first endosseous titanium implant was produced with an industrial turning process, which led to surfaces with minimally rough topographies at the micron level. The bone bonding ability, termed as "osseointegration" by Brånemark *et al.* (1977), of this machined implant was mainly the result of the proper surgical technique providing macro-stability to the implant and the biocompatible nature of the bulk titanium. In the past three decades, much has been learned about the concept of osseointegration and significant improvements on the design and surface of implants were done to eliminate the important challenges of the implant dentistry.

Osseointegration was first defined as a direct contact between living bone and the surface of a load-carrying implant at the histological level (Brånemark, 1983) and, in clinical terms, as a biomechanical phenomenon whereby clinically asymptomatic rigid fixation of the implant is achieved and maintained in bone during functional loading (Albrektsson & Johansson, 2001). Typically, an implant is considered to be osseointegrated when there is an absence of movement between the implant and bone under normal conditions of loading following a defined healing period. This clinical state is the result of direct bone apposition to an implant surface without formation of a poorly vascularised collagenous capsule, termed as fibrous encapsulation. Although the concept of "osseointegration" was first put forth to define the connection between bone and titanium, it has been shown that bone anchorage can also be achieved with the use of other materials without an adverse tissue reaction (Wenz et al., 2008). Thus, osseointegration is currently accepted as a general term for bone-implant surface contact. However, the quality of the host bone/foreign implant interface is mostly affected by the characteristics of the material. Especially, titanium has been shown to have a closer contact with the calcified tissue and to be covered by a thinner proteoglycan structure compared to zirconium and stainless steel (Albrektsson et al., 1985, 1986). Various studies have also suggested that titanium exhibits a better biocompatible nature and less foreign body reaction compared to other conventional materials (Eisenbarth et al., 2004; Hallab et al., 2003). It has been stated that osseointegration of titanium does not result due to a positive tissue reaction, instead it occurs in the absence of a negative tissue response (Stanford & Keller, 1991). Therefore, the bioinert character of titanium is the main reason of its enhanced bone bonding behaviour. Now, osseointegration of titanium is widely accepted as the prerequisite for dental implant success in dentistry. Although the reported success rates are higher than 90% in controlled clinical trials (Henry et al., 1996; Jemt et al., 1996), important challenges, such as the long latency period between implant placement and loading, remain to be elucidated. Also, achieving high success rates in specific patient groups (e.g. diabetics, oncology patients, smokers) seems to be elusive (Esposito et al., 1998). Over the past two decades, elevating the local quality and quantity of the host tissue for an optimal osseointegration was the major goal of implant dentistry in order to overcome these drawbacks. Therefore, various approaches have focused on finding alternative methods to accelerate and optimize osseointegration, aiming at sufficient mechanical integrity to withstand occlusal forces at an early period (Morton et al., 2010).

During the first 10–20 years of understanding the healing mechanisms of traumatized bone where implants are placed, the concept that successful osseointegration was the result of titanium implant biocompatibility dominated clinical thinking. Subsequently, implant surface modifications encouraged new considerations of improvements in bone formation at the implant surface. Since the biological mechanisms at the bone-implant interface determine the fate of the implant, characteristics of the implant surface play a central role in challenging the process of osseintegration with early loading. Upon insertion, premature loading can disrupt the healing process and may result in early failure of the implant. Enhancing the biological response using a surface science approach therefore has attracted the attention of many research groups (Ramazanoglu et al., 2011; von Wilmowsky et al. 2009). It is well established that characteristics of the implants surface, such as nano- and micro-topography, and physicochemical composition, have a major influence on the outcome of osseointegration, especially at the histological level, aiming at biological and morphological compatibilities (Mendonça et al., 2008).

In general, the implantation of devices for the maintenance or restoration of a body function imposes extraordinary requirements on the materials of construction. Foremost among these is an issue of biocompatibility. It was found, after extensive literature review, that there are three major required compatibilities for placed implants to exhibit biointegration to receiving hard tissue and biofunctionality thereafter. They include biological comatobility (in short, called as biocompatibility), mechanical compatibility, and morphological compatibility to receiving host tissues (Oshida et al., 1994; Oshida, 2000; Oshida et al., 2010). Accordingly, numerous studies have been conducted to meet aforementioned requirements for successful implant systems (i.e., mechanical compatibility, biological compatibility, and morphological compatibility) by altering surface characteristics for overcoming the potential drawbacks of the implant therapy (Oshida, 2007; Oshida et al., 2009). This chapter focuses on essential mechanisms governing the peri-implant healing and surface science approaches for enhancing osseointegration. The future of the implant surface science and prospective tissue engineering attempts for the biological constitution of the peri-implant area are also topics of this chapter for providing ideas for forthcoming studies.

2. Healing around the endosseous implant

Ossification mechanisms that occur following the placement of the implant are very important for understanding the biologic response to endosseous implants. Osborn (1979) categorized this bio-response into the following three groups: (1) biotolerant type, characterized by distance osteogenesis, the implant is not rejected from the tissue, but it is surrounded by a fibrous connective tissue, (2) bioinert type, characterized by contact osteogenesis, the osteogenic cells migrate directly to the surface where they will establish de novo bone formation, and (3) bioreactive type, the implant allows new bone formation around itself, thereby exchanging ions to create a chemical bond with the bone. Upon insertion, various implant materials exhibit different biologic responses. While biotolerant materials, such as gold, cobalt-chromium alloys, stainless steel, polyethylene and polymethylmethacrylate, exhibit distance osteogenesis, titanium and titanium alloys are accepted to be bioinert according to their surface oxides (Kienapfel et al., 1999). Besides, the rutile-type oxide, which is formed on titanium as a titanium dioxide, is described as a stable crystalline form similar to ceramics in its bioreactive behaviour (Zhao et al., 2005). Although titanium has superior characteristics compared to other implant metals, the ostoconductivity of titanium is lower than calcium phosphate (CaP) based bioceramics (Kilpadi et al., 2001). Therefore, CaP based ceramics are referred to be bone-bonding materials, whereas titanium is a nonbonding material to bone (Hench & Wilson, 1984). Therefore, approaches have mainly focused on enhancing the bioactivity of titanium and providing a higher osteoconductivity to the bulk material by altering the surface properties.

The character of the host tissue also plays an important role on the ossification mechanism following implantation. Understanding the different peri-implant healing cascades of the cortical and trabecular bone is crucial for better orientating the osseointegration in poor quality bone (Davies, 1996). Following surgical trauma, the vascular injury of the cortex results in death of the peri-implant cortical bone, and followed by a slow proceeding osteoclastic remodelling. The removal of the injured tissue by osteoclasts and the subsequent formation of the new bone is a long lasting process. Therefore, the healing around the implant in cortical bone results in distance osteogenesis. Although this slow remodelling phase provides early stability in cortical bone leading to low rate of implant failure (Adell et al., 1981), especially in the parasymphyseal mandible, it is a handicap for the surface science approaches for enhancing the osseointegration histologically. On the other hand, the trabecular bone enables the migration of osteogenic cells due to its marrow component. The colonization of differentiating progenitor cells on the implant surface and *de novo* bone formation provides the evidence that peri-implant healing in trabecular bone occurs via contact osteogenesis. Actually, the presence of osteprogenitor populations in the spongious bone, which is characterized to be of poor quality in implant dentistry (Lekholm and Zarb type III and IV bone), favours the migration and bone forming activity of these cells directly on the surface when the implant is considered to be bioinert (Marco et al., 2005). In the recent decades, the development of novel osteoconductive titanium surfaces, that increased the local quantity and quality of osseous tissue at the interface, thereby improved the success of implants, especially in regions of the jaw such as the edentulous posterior maxillae where the cortical thickness is frequently insufficient for the primary stability.

The surgical placement of the implant results in injury of the host bone. If the implant is considered to be bioinert, the body responds to this injury with physiological mechanisms similar to the bone fracture healing. Following implant placement, the implant surface first gets in contact with the blood originating from the injured vessels facing the implant cavity. After several seconds, the surface is completely covered with a thin layer of serum proteins. This protein modification of the surface occurs for all implant materials in the same way. However, the type and surface characteristics of the material have a major influence on the structure and conformation of this protein layer (Dee et al., 2002). Shortly after protein adsorption, the surface becomes associated with thrombocytes. As a result of thrombocyte aggregation and degranulation on the surface, coagulation mechanisms take place and cytokines (e.g. transforming growth factor-β (TGF-β) and platelet derived growth factor (PDGF)) and several vasoactive factors (e.g. serotonin and histamine) are released from cytoplasmic granules of thrombocytes. These chemoattractants stimulate proliferation and migration of various cells, thereby orientating the peri-implant healing mechanisms (Dereka et al., 2006). For example, PDGF has important mitogenic and migrative effects on several cell types, such as inflammatory leukocytes, osteoblasts, smooth muscle cells and fibroblasts (Heldin & Westermark, 1999).

Polymorphonuclear neurophils (PMNs) are also first group of cells that play an important role in the inflammatory response. PMNs dominate the bone-implant interface at the first and second days. The number of PMNs tends to decrease when bacteria and endotoxins are not present at the interface. At the second day of healing, monocyte migration and macrophage accumulation starts to take place (Davies, 2003). PMNs and macrophages remove dead cells, extracellular matrix (ECM) residues and bacteria. Beside their role on the initial inflammatory phase, another mission of macrophages is the expression of cytokines, such as fibroblast growth factor (FGF), PDGF and vascular endothelial growth factor (VEGF). Thus, they provide important signals in order to stimulate the recruitment of osteogenic and endothelial progenitors for the next proliferative phase. The release of vasoactive amines, thrombocyte and leukocyte infiltration, the establishment of the coagulum and fibrin network, macrophage actions are important events that occur at the inflammatory phase. This first phase, which can sometimes extend to five days, is followed by the removal of the coagulum by PMNs and subsequently by monocytes, at the same time angiogenesis starts also to take place (Stanford & Keller, 1991). The growth of new capillaries into the fibrin network is mostly stimulated by the growth factors (primarily FGF and VEGF) expressed by macrophages and endothelial cells as a response to hypoxic and acidic nature of the bone-implant interface (Schliephake, 2002). In this way, the proliferation, maturation and organization of endothelial cells to new capillary tubes take place, thereby providing oxygen and nutrients to the newly formed tissue at the interface.

The behaviour of blood cells inside the fibrin-based structural matrix has a major impact on the healing mechanisms at the bone-implant interface. Besides, the quality of bone healing around an implant is also affected by the capacity of osteogenic cells to proliferate and migrate. Meyer et al. (2004) have demonstrated that the osteoprogenitor cells started to attach the implant surface after one day following insertion. This was a similar finding, as stated by Davies (1996), showing that early recruitment and colonization of mesenchymal stem (MSCs) cells occur on an implant surface in a short time through modulation of white blood cells, fibrin network and thrombocytes (Park & Davies, 2000). The three dimensional structure of fibrin matrix and the migrating effects of growth factors expressed by the first arriving cells play an important role in the establishment of an osteoprogenitor reservoir at the interface. Therefore, the chemistry of the implant material and its surface characteristics are of special interest in implantology, since they initially influence the binding capacity of fibrin and the release of growth factors, thereby affecting the migration of mesenchymal cells directly (Puleo & Nanci, 1999).

Titanium implant materials possess ideal fibrin retention on their surface. Through this fibrin matrix, osteogenic cells having the migration ability arrive the implant surface and start to produce bone directly on the surface. Davies (2003) termed this phenomenon as *de novo* bone formation through contact osteogenesis. Upon arrival to the surface, the differentiated osteogenic cells secrete the collagen-free matrix (cement lines / lamina limitans) for the mineralisation through calcium and phosphate precipitation. This layer, where the initial mineralisation occurs, consists of non-collagenous proteins (mostly osteopontin and bone sialoprotein) and proteoglycans (Klinger et al., 1998). Following calcium phosphate precipitation, the formation and mineralisation of collagen fibers take place. Thus, a non-collagenous tissue is established between the implant surface and the calcified collagen compartment through contact osteogenesis. This intermediary tissue is very important for the understanding the bonding mechanism between bone and a bioinert titanium implant.

Following the establishment of the calcified matrix on the implant surface, woven bone formation and organization of the bone trabeculae start to take place for the reconstitution of the damaged bone at the peri-implant area (Marco et al., 2005). Since the woven bone mostly consists of irregular shaped and loosely packed collagen fibers, it does not provide sufficient mechanical stability compared to the organized the lamellar bone. However, most of woven bone usually remodels in three months and replaced by the lamellar bone. At three months of healing the implant is mostly surrounded by a mixture of woven and lamellar bone (Chappard et al., 1999). The formation and remodeling of the new lamellar bone around the implant occur more rapidly in the regions where there is denser marrow component present. Therefore, the biologic fixation of the implant is achieved faster in the trabecular bone, while a better primary stability is obtained in the cortical bone following implantation.

An implant surface is considered to be clean following fabrication processes. If not stored under special conditions, contaminations (e.g. hydrocarbon, sulphur dioxide and nitric oxide) occur from the atmosphere (Kasemo & Lausmaa, 1988). In order to decrease and eliminate such risk of contamination, commercial implant surfaces are usually subjected to passivation treatments and stored carefully in optimal packages until usage. If such an implant is placed into the bone, its surface first get in contact with the blood, which is mostly composed of water molecules. Differently from the liquid water, the water molecules bind to the surface and form water mono- or bi-layer (Kasemo & Gold, 1999). The organization of water molecules differs according to the wettability characteristics of the surface (Lim & Oshida, 2001). While on hydrophilic surfaces the interaction with water molecules results in the dissociation of molecules and in the formation hydroxyl groups, the water binding capacity of hydrophobic surfaces is very low. Following the establishment of water overlayer, the ions (e.g. Cl^- and Na^+) enter the layer and become hydrated. The characteristics of an implant surface have a major implant on this arrangement of ions and their water shells. After the establishment of an intermediate layer composed of ions and water molecules, the biomolecules arrive at the surface in milliseconds. Proteins absorb first onto the surface, then change their conformation, denaturize and desorb from surface leaving their place to other proteins that have more affinity to the surface. Thus, a biologic layer having a different arrangement and conformation surrounds the surface.

It is well known that surface characteristics have an important effect on the adsorption of biomolecules by changing the arrangement of water molecules and ions (Puleo & Nanci, 1999). While on hydrophobic surfaces proteins bind with their hydrophobic regions, on hydrophilic surfaces the connection is established with the help of hydrophilic regions Kasemo & Gold, 1999). This protein overlayer is never considered to be static. It is subjected to structural and conformational changes in time. Normally the protein, which is found in higher concentration in the biological fluid, reaches and adsorbs to the surface first. Usually, this protein is afterwards replaced with another one that has a more affinity to the surface, although its concentration is low in the biological fluid. As a result of these adsorption and desorption mechanisms, a diverse layer which is composed of different protein is formed and maintained at the surface. The major role of this protein layer is the attachment of functionary cells of the healing process. If a bone implant is planning to be developed, the establishment of a surface, that generates an optimal protein composition and conformation for the attachment of osteogenic cells on itself, is one most important strategies of the production.

Several proteins (e.g. fibronectin, vitronectin, laminin, serum albumin and collagen) facilitate the attachment of osteogenic cells on titanium surfaces (Park et al., 2005; Yang et al., 2003). Therefore, the protein binding capacity of an implant surface is considered to be an important factor for as successful osseointegration, since surface properties, such as micro- and nano-topography (Lee et al. 2010), physicochemical composition (Park et al., 2005) and surface free energy (MacDonald et al., 2004), have an influence on the extend of protein adsorption. It has been documented that osteogenic cells preferably attach to the specific protein sequences, such as the arginine-glycine-aspartic acid (RGD) motif. This motif is found in various ECM proteins, including fibronectin, vitronectin, laminin and osteopontin (Ruoslahti, 1996). Osteogenic cells attach to these binding motifs using their membrane receptors, termed as integrins. Integrin mediated cell attachment is crucial for physiological and pathological mechanisms, such as the embryonic development, maintanance of tissue integrity, circulation, migration and phagocytic activity of leukocytes, wound healing and angiogenesis. Integrins are obligate heterodimers composed of two distinct glycoprotein subunits; α and β subunits (Hynes, 2002). Integrin subunits cross the plasma membrane with a long extracellular ligand, while generally a very short domain remains in the cytoplasm. For the integrin family eighteen α and eight β subunits have been characterized in mammals until now. Through the combination of these different α and β subunits, 24 distinct integrins can be assembled. A cell can modulate more than one integrin receptor and change their location, thereby modifying its capacity to bind to different protein sequences (Dee et al., 2002).

As mentioned before, adhesion-promoting proteins in blood (e.g. fibronectin, vitronectin and various collagen types) bind to integrins through an RGD-dependent pathway (Ruoslahti, 1996). But, there are also different domains within these proteins that have the ability to bind to integrins and provoke integrin-mediated cellular signalling cascades. Briefly, integrin-mediated cell attachment to ECM initiate several intracellular events, including protein kinase C and Na^+/H^+ antiporter, phophoinositide hydrolysis, tyrosine phosphorylation of membrane and intracellular proteins (Plopper et al., 1995). These mechanisms result in mitogen stimulated protein kinase activation by altering the cellular pH and calcium concentration. Thus, intracellular communication is established and the extracellular signal is transmitted to the nucleus. The cell responds to this integrin-mediated signal through migration, proliferation and differentiation (Sawyer et al., 2005). The response of osteogenic cells to the initial protein layer on the implant surface is very important for the activation of osteoblastic pathways through integrin-mediated signalling, thereby for optimal osseointegration. Therefore, the development of an implant surface, that favours an osteogenic protein conformation on itself, has been one of the major areas of implant surface science. In the recent decades, various approaches have focused on understanding the effect of the surface characteristics on the protein dependent mechanisms of cell adhesion, proliferation, differentiation and bone matrix deposition, aiming at the development of novel implant surfaces.

3. Surface treatments for enhanced osseointegration

The surface of a titanium implant plays a crucial role in determining the biological response of the host bone for several reasons (Fig.1.). The surface of titanium is the only region in contact with the bone, and is always different in characteristics from the bulk. Therefore, mainly the characteristics of the surface govern the healing mechanisms at the bone-implant interface. For enhancing the biomechanical anchorage of the implant and for promoting osseointegration at the histological level, the modification of surface topography or the coating of titanium with bioactive materials has captured the interest of many scientists, clinicians, and manufacturers as well (Oshida, 2007). Commonly used techniques to alter surface properties of titanium are as follows: sand-blasting (Rosa &Beloti, 2003), acid-etching (Juodzbalys et al., 2007), alkali-etching (Kim et al., 2000), plasma spraying (Vercaigne et al., 1998), electropolishing (Harris et al., 2007), anodic oxidation (Yamagami et al., 2005), hydroxylapatite (HA) (Dalton & Cook, 1995) and calcium phosphate (CaP) (Liu et al. 2004) coatings, etc. Such modifications have, in general, resulted in several changes in surface properties, including morphology, physicochemical composition and surface energy. Although various studies have shown that surface alterations, such as the resulting roughness, have improved the outcome of osseointegration (Abrahamsson et al., 2001; Buser et al., 1991), it is still poorly understood that either this enhancement was caused due to topographical reasons or fabrication-related changes in surface composition and wettability characteristics. Furthermore, the majority of published papers lack of an adequate surface characterization, as stated in the literature (Wennerberg & Albrektsson, 2009), that makes the evaluation of the effect of unique surface properties on osseointegration. However, general observations using different *in vitro* and *in vivo* studies can be still made to evaluate the effect of surface properties *per se* (topography, composition, crystal structure and wettability) on osseointegration. Commonly, two categories of surface properties are suggested to be the most important aspects for affecting the tissue response to the implant: surface topography and chemical composition. Therefore, this chapter focuses mainly on these two categories.

3.1 Topographical features of titanium surfaces

Any dental implant, once inserted into the host bone, first comes into contact with tissue fluids. The adsorption of biomolecules and the subsequent interactions of cells on an implant surface determine the fate of the implant. For many years, the "machined" surface of the Brånemark implant was the gold standard for implant surfaces. However, the decreased success rates of these smooth textured implants at compromised sites (Jaffin & Berman, 1991), especially at the posterior maxillae, motivated the approaches for finding better implant surfaces promoting bone formation. In the search for methods modifying

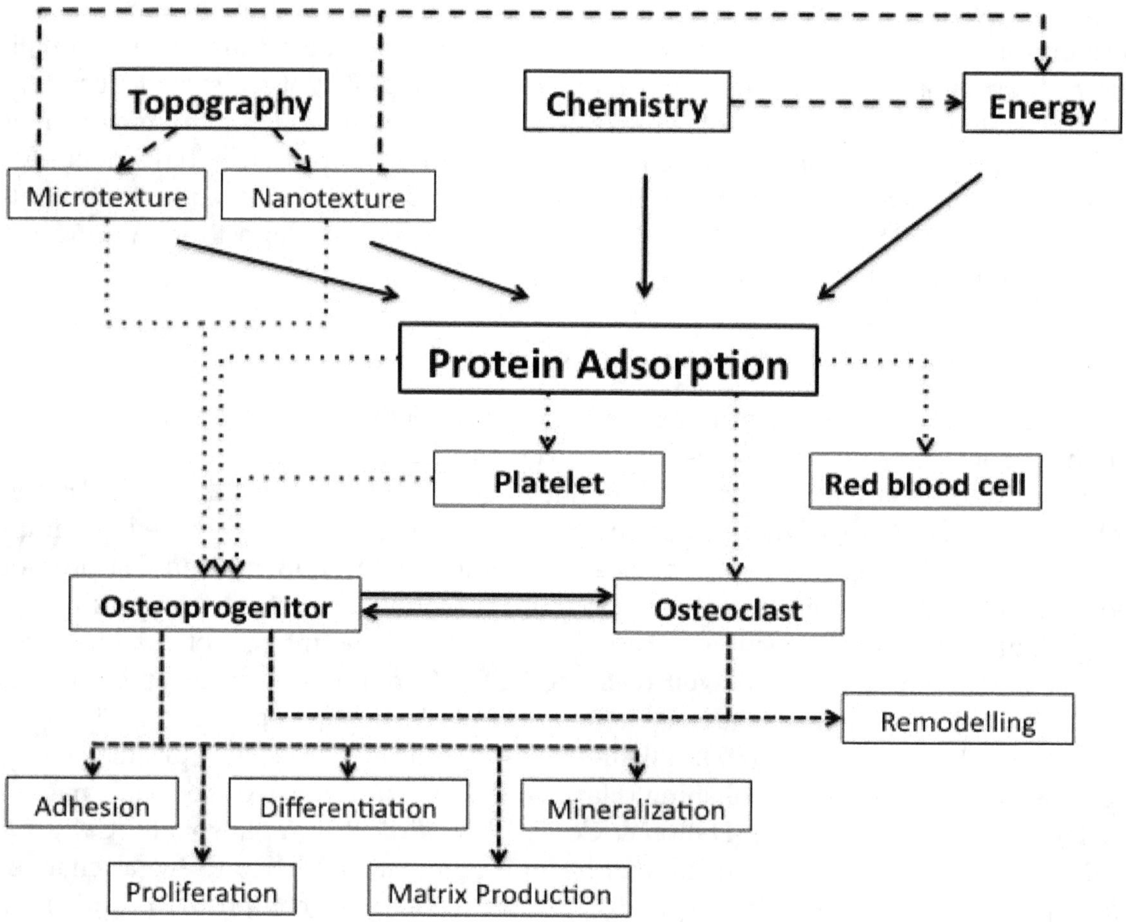

Fig. 1. Effect of submacron surface characteristics of the implant on the osteogenic response

surface properties to achieve better osseointegration, much attention has been focused on increasing the surface roughness for improving the interfacial retaining mechanics. The main idea behind the establishment of such a rough topography was to increase the surface area of the implant adjacent to the bone and to improve the cell adhesion to the surface, thereby achieving higher bone-to-implant contact and better biomechanical integrity (Oshida et al., 1994; Cooper, 2000). Until now, extensive number of papers has been published on this topic. Numerous studies have shown that moderate roughness and complex microtopographies are important for the likely development of bone-implant interfaces and for the enhanced osseointegration of titanium implants (Abrahamsson et al., 2001; Buser et al., 1991). Compared with smooth surfaces, implants with rough surfaces exhibited greater contact with bone (Al-Nawas et al., 2008). However, systematic reviews (Shalabi et al., 2006) and the Cochrane collaboration (Esposito et al., 2007) were not able to find any clinical evidence supporting the positive effect of increasing surface roughness on osseointegration. Although it has been suggested that a moderate rougness value (R_a, between 1 and 2 μm) is optimal for bone-implant interactions (Wennerberg & Albrektsson, 2000), there is still no suitable roughness to specific metallic biomaterials. The effect of surface topography, especially the microroughness, on bone response around dental implants has been reviewed intensively elsewhere (Cooper, 2000; Oshida, 2007; Wennerberg & Albrektsson, 2009).

From an *in vitro* standpoint, the response of cells and tissues at implant interfaces can be affected by the surface topography (Gaydos et al., 2000; Moore et al., 2000). Culture models provide better conditions to test the direct interactions between the implant surfaces and cells. Surface roughness in the range from 1 to 10 μm influences the interface biology, since it is the same order in size of various cell types responsible for bone-implant healing. The literature contains plentiful information about the effects of micro-scale textures on cells and tissues. However, due to multiplicity of roughening protocols and cell culture models in literature, it is difficult to draw an ultimate conclusion about the effect of microroughness on cellular activities. In order to obtain ideal cell colonization on the surface, an increase in cell proliferation is an important parameter when evaluating the effectiveness of surface micro-morphology. There are limited studies that documented better cellular proliferation on surfaces with microrough topography (Deligianni et al., 2001; Marinucci et al., 2006). Mustafa et al. (2001) blasted the machined titanium surfaces with 63-90 μm, 106-180 μm and 180-300 μm TiO2 particles and obtained test models having different microtopographies. They showed that on all microrough surfaces the cell proliferation was better compared with machined surfaces and they found an insignificant increase in cell proliferation parallel to increasing roughness. However, most studies until now argued that surface microroughness influenced cell proliferation negatively (Anselme et al., 2000a; Linez-Bataillon, 2002; Sader et al., 2005). Anselme et al. (2000b) mechanically polished and sand-blasted Ti-6Al-4V surfaces with 500 μm or 3mm alumina particles, so they created surfaces having increased roughness values. They documented that increasing roughness caused a significant decrease in cell proliferation and they based this negative correlation upon the change in surface elemental composition (AlO_x contamination) after blasting with alumina particles. However, there are also studies that didn't found any negative relation between alumina contamination and biological response (Wennerberg et al., 1996).

To evaluate the effect of surface microtopography on osteogenic cell functions, Boyan and her colleagues (Boyan et al., 1998, 2001; Schwartz et al. 2001a) established an experimental study design that consists of pure titanium disks having increased roughness values. They produced dual acid-etched (PT), dual acid–etched and corrundum-blasted (SLA) and titanium plasma sprayed (TPS) test groups. Other researchers (Lossdörfer et al., 2004) that were using the same protocol revealed that on rough surfaces such as SLA and TPS, the cell attachment and ^{3}H-tymidin incorporation, an important finding of cell proliferation, was decreased compared with smoother PT surfaces. Kieswetter et al. (1996) asserted that this decrease in cell proliferation was a sign of a more differentiated cellular phenotype in culture, as described in the theory by Lian and Stein (1992). To test this hypothesis, Boyan et al. (2002) cultured fetal rat calvarial cells on PT, SLA and TPS surfaces and documented that after 14 days of culture on rough surfaces, in spite of decreased cell proliferation, the bone nodule formation and ALP specific activity which is an early marker of osteogenic differentiation was significantly increased. Besides, it has been shown that on surfaces with rough microtopographies, osteoblasts secrete factors, such as osteoprotegerin (OPG), receptor activator of nuclear factor kappa B ligand (RANKL), prostoglandins (PGE_1 and PGE_2) and TGF-β1, that enhance osteoblast differentiation while decreasing osteoclast formation and activity (Lossdörfer et al., 2004). These results indicate that on rough surfaces osteoblasts exhibit a more differentiated phenotype, even though the proliferation is negatively affected.

The mechanism by which topography influences osteoblast differentiation appears to be mediated by integrin signaling (Olivares-Navarrete et al., 2008) and mitogen-activated proteine kinase (MAPK) pathways (Schwartz et al., 2001b). The topography has also an effect on subsequent expression of transcription factors, ECM protein genes and cytokines

(Balloni et al., 2009; Marinucci et al., 2006). However, the *in vivo* interaction of osteogenic cells with an implant surface is different from the *in vitro* culture studies. Therefore, two essential aspects should also be taken into consideration when testing titanium surfaces under *in vitro* conditions. First, the osteoblast-surface interaction studies do not provide information about the role of surface topography on the initial platelet activation within the associated blood clot. The platelet adhesion on the surface and the subsequent release of platelet-derived growth factors is critical for the recruitment of bone-forming cells into the interface. Park et al. (2001) have demonstrated, that platelet adherence, platelet-derived microparticle (MP) formation and P-selectin expression were enhanced on microrough surfaces, and suggested that this increased activation of platelets may be the reason for up-regulation of osteogenic responses during bone healing. Second, the initial adsorption of blood-derived molecular factors influences the attachment of osteogenic cells on titanium implants. The plasma protein adsorption behaviour is also affected by the surface topography. The effect of surface roughness on protein adsorption was investigated by determining the adsorption of bovine serum albumin (BSA) and fibronectin, from single protein solutions on rough and smooth Ti-6Al-4V surfaces (Deligianni et al, 2001). It was reported that the rough substratum bound a higher amount of total protein (from culture medium supplied with 15% serum) and fibronectin (10-fold) than did the smooth one. Sela et al. (2007) showed that the increase of the 3D surface area through acid-etching and blasting of titanium has resulted in increased adsorption of plasma proteins.

In general, a huge number of animal investigations also agree on the positive effect of surface roughening protocols on osseointegration. Numerous animal models and surgical protocols were performed to evaluate the bone response around dental implants. Until now, the majority of the studies have focused on commercially available implant surface designs and compared them mostly with machined controls. Various microrough profiles established by different surface methodologies, such as blasting, etching, blasting/etching, plasma spraying and oxidation, were found to be stronger integrated in bone when compared with machined surfaces (Wennerberg & Albrektsson, 2009). Unfortunately, it is very difficult to compare different studies, because wound healing conditions and kinetics differ between animal models. Also, the topographical parameters vary between different microrough surfaces among previously published studies; therefore, it is impossible to obtain and establish an appropriate roughness profile of titanium for better osseointegration. Besides, it should be not neglected that procedures for the establishment of microroughness also result in changes in the surface chemistry and hence it makes the evaluation of the unique effect of roughness on the bone response (Wennerberg & Albrektsson, 2009).

3.2 Physicochemical composition of titanium surfaces

Beside topographical features of titanium surfaces, the chemistry, wettability and charges are also important parameters affecting the extent of bone response (Elias et al., 2008). If a titanium implant is inserted into the host bone, titanium dioxide should be considered as an interacting surface, rather than its bulk. Due to high affinity to oxygen, a very thin oxide film is formed on titanium when exposed to air (Kasemo & Gold, 1999). Titanium dioxides are different from the metallic Ti and have properties similar to ceramics. The biocompatibility of titanium is therefore the result of the chemical stability and corrosion resistance of its dense and protective oxide film (Healy & Ducheyne, 1992). The crystal structure of this film is believed to be important for the success of implant integration.

Although marketed biomedical titanium implants mostly exhibit anatase or rutile type crystal phase, amorphous structure can be also formed on titanium following electrochemical procedures. For example, Sul et al. (2001, 2005) investigated several microarc oxidized implant surfaces having different crystal structures (amorphous, anatase, anatase-rutile mixture) in rabbit tibia model. Both anatase and anatase/rutile surfaces exhibited better torque resistance values compared with amourphous ones. It has been stated that, beside the titania crystal structure, also the microporous topography and oxide thickness has a positive effect on the positive outcome of bone response. These results were also confirmed by other *in vitro* studies. Anatase or rutile surfaces showed better cellular responses, such as increased adhesion, proliferation, expression of osteoblastic markers (procollagen type I peptide, osteocalcin and alkaline phosphatase) and mineralized nodule formation, compared with amorphous ones (Li et al., 2004; Saldana et al., 2005).
While the crystal structure of titanium can be changed following various thermal and non-thermal treatments, the wettability characteristics of the surface is also altered with respect to this modification. Also, various attempts have tried to find an optimal surface wettability profile for achieving better bone response. According to the literature, highly hydrophilic surfaces are proposed to be more desirable than hydrophobic ones (Junker et al., 2009; Schwarz et al., 2009). Preliminary *in vitro* studies indicated the hydrophilic nature of titanium surfaces significantly influences the cell differentiation and growth factor production positively (Rausch-Fan et al., 2008; Zhao et al., 2007). Besides, animal studies also shown that on hydrophilic surfaces osseointegration can be established at an early period (Bornstein et al., 2008; Buser at al., 2004; Schwarz et al., 2007). However, there are also contradictory results from other *in vitro* studies. For example, Kern et al. (2005) sintered titanium surfaces at 750° C for 90 min to transform amorphous crystal structure into anatase and found no significant differences in osteoblast adhesion despite of changes in hydrophilicity and oxide structure. Le Guehennec et al. (2008) cultured MC3T3-E1 cells on alumina blasted, biphasic calcium phosphate blasted (BCP-Ti) and commercial SLA surfaces and were not able to demonstrate any significant differences between hydrophobic SLA and hydrophilic BCP-Ti surfaces in their MTS and ALP assays. Bauer et al. (2008) cultured rat MSCs on nanotubular titanium surfaces having different wettability characteristics and found an increased cell attachment on super-hydrophobic surfaces compared with super-hydrophilic ones. Due to the ambiguous results in the literature, it is difficult to state that the hydrophilicity of surface is the only reason for enhanced outcomes. The microtopography, chemistry and wettability must be taken together into consideration.

4. Novel trends at the bone-implant interface

4.1. Biomimetic coating of titanium surfaces with calcium phosphates

Beside its excellent biocompatibility and biomechanics, titanium itself is not bioactive. To overcome the limited bioactivity of titanium and to improve the *de novo* bone formation around these implants, research was focused on preparing calcium phosphate (Ca-P) coatings on titanium and its alloys. It has been well established that the Ca-P based coating of titanium favours the bone response compared with the uncoated titanium (Chang et al., 1999a; Wheeler, 1996). Additionally, Ca-P based surfaces bind more attachment proteins, such as fibronectin and vitronectin, for the integrin mediated binding action of osteoprogenitors compared to titanium surfaces (Kilpadi et al., 2001). Several techniques were described for the deposition of Ca-P coatings on titanium implants, including ion beam deposition, plasma spraying, sol-gel methods, laser deposition, radiofrequency sputtering, biomimetic deposition and electrostatic spray deposition (Ong & Chan 2000). Among these procedures, plasma spraying is the most popular method for the deposition of Ca-P coatings on titanium implants. But this technique has some drawbacks, including the difficulty in controlling the coating structure, the weakening of the coating-implant interface and the high temparature of the deposition process (Cofino et al., 2004; Dalton & Cook, 1995)

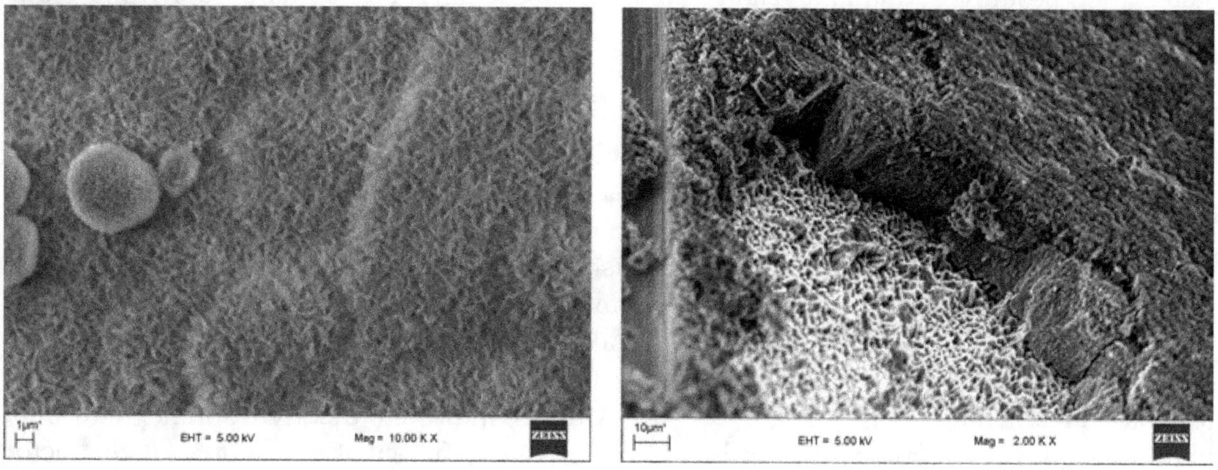

Fig. 2. Top and cross sectional SEM images of biomimetic Ca-P coatings

Biomimetic calcium Ca-P coating procedure, first introduced by Kokubo et al. (1990), is one of the novel approaches for preparing bioactive calcium phosphate layers on titanium surface. This technique involves the precipitation of bone like apatite crystals from a simulated body fluid (SBF) onto titanium surfaces under physiological temperature (37°C) and pH (7.4) that mimics the normal conditions in human blood plasma. To shorten the immersion period of the substrate within calcium phosphate containing solution, the method was further revised by a group of investigators (Barrere et al., 2001; Liu et al., 2004) Thus, a calcium phosphate lattice can be formed on titanium surfaces in order to provide osteoconductive properties to the substrate (Fig. 2.). Another advantage of this simple and economical procedure is that the biomimetic surface acts as a tissue-engineering scaffold and this process can be combined with deposition of signalling molecules, like growth factors and bone morphogenetic proteins (Liu et al., 2004, 2007; Ramazanoglu et al., 2011).

4.2 Biomolecular coatings of titanium surfaces

Beside the topographical and physicochemical modifications, biochemical approaches to immobilize different bioactive molecules, peptides, proteins and others on dental implants attracted the interest of many scientists. The main idea behind these methodologies was as follows: (1) to eliminate the adsorption of proteins that would result in the adhesion of unspecific cells leading to fibrous integration; (2) to enhance the specific attachment of osteogenic cells for the establishment of a tight bone-implant interface; (3) to provide integrin-mediated signals for provoking the bone healing mechanisms. For this purpose, various immobilization methods were utilized, including physical adsorption (Wikesjö et al., 2008), incorporation into Ca-P lattice (Liu et al., 2004, 2007; Ramazanoglu et al., 2011), covalent attachment (Bagno et al., 2007), self-assembly of monolayers (Heijink et al., 2008) and electrochemical methods (Beutner et al., 2010). Complete description of these methods is beyond the scope of this chapter and reviewed intensively elsewhere (Beutner et al., 2010).

However, the organic molecules used for bio-functionalization of titanium-based materials are of importance for orientating the tissue response. Especially, extensive studies have been performed on binding ECM proteins and their peptide sequences to titanium to promote osteogenic cell adhesion. Although the coating of titanium with a single protein has resulted in enhancement of cellular adhesion (MacDonald et al., 2004), research has mainly focused on immobilizing short cell binding motifs within these ECM molecules due to their structural integrity (Morra, 2006). In particular, the RGD motif, as discussed before, is one of the most studied protein sequence capable of promoting cell adhesion and thereby initiating intracellular signalling cascades through multiple integrins including $\alpha_v\beta_3$ and $\alpha_5\beta_1$ (Ruoslahti, 1996). This motif is usually covalently attached to titanium using silanization (Bagno et al., 2007) or functionalized using polymer chemistry (Tosatti et al., 2004), and has been reported to increase osteoblast attachment and proliferation (Schuler et al., 2006). While several *in vivo* studies (Elmengaard et al., 2005; Kroese-Deutman et al., 2005) demonstrated better osseointegration results, others did not find any significant enhancement for the RGD functionalization (Petrie et al., 2008; Schliephake et al., 2009).
Another approach for enhancing the osseointegration is the delivery signalling molecules, especially the osteogenic growth factors. The concept of coating implant surfaces with osteogenic growth factors, such as bone morphogenic proteins (BMPs), to enhance osseointegration has been documented in several studies using different delivery strategies (Becker et al. 2006; Sykaras et al. 2004; Wikesjö et al. 2008). The bone forming potential of BMPs around implants have been shown in an experimental study using an atelopeptide type-I collagen carrier as a coating (Bessho et al. 1999). However, other studies utilizing a collagen/chondroitin sulphate (CS) carrier system on titanium found an enhancement of bone volume density (BVD) and bone-implant contact (BIC) around coated implants, but they were not able to show any significant difference between bare collagen/CS and BMP integrated coatings (Schliephake et al. 2005; Stadlinger et al. 2007). Due to the variation of findings between different studies, it can be stated that there is still a need for an optimal 3D carrier on the implant surface to provide sufficient retention of BMPs at the repair site. As mentioned before, the biomimetic coating method has been shown to have the potential of being an appropriate BMP carrier on the titanium surface. It has been demonstrated that BMP-2 incorporated in calcium phosphate coatings can induce bone formation at an ectopic site and the sustained release of BMP-2 from this coating has an important effect on the osteoinductivity of the material (Liu et al. 2005). However, studies using this methodology failed to show a significant effect of biomimetic coated implants with incorporated BMP-2, VEGF or their combination on osseointegration, and it has been stated that an ideal dose of BMP-2 or VEGF, which resembles the growth factor release from natural bone matrix should be achieved for enhancing the osseointegration (Liu et al. 2007; Ramazanoglu et al., 2011).

4.3 Nanotopographical modification of titanium surfaces

The structures encountered by osteoblasts in the human body are not only in micrometer scale, since bone is made up by nanostructures. Thus, there is a need to produce better implant materials having also nanometer roughness. Several studies have suggested that nanophase materials produced from various chemistries, such as metals, polymers, composites and ceramics, improved cellular activities when compared with conventional microrough materials (Gutwein & Webster, 2004; Webster & Ejiofor, 2004). Nanobiomaterials have an increased percentage of atoms and crystal structures, and also provide a higher surface area than the conventional ones. Thus, nanoscale surfaces possess high surface energy leading to increasing initial protein adsorption that is very important in regulating the cellular interactions on the implant surface. Webster et al. (2001) suggested increased osteoblast adhesion on nanophase materials. Numerous studies have shown that osteoblasts cultured on nanophase biomaterials exhibited better osteogenic behaviour, including adhesion, ECM production and mineralization, than on conventional materials (Elias et al., 2002; Price et al., 2003).

In recent years, several methods have been also developed to produce nanoscale structures on titanium surface. While irregular nanomorphologies can be established using solution chemistry (Mendonça et al., 2010), the electrochemical anodization of titanium is the most popular and novel strategy to produce controlled structures (including nanotubes, pillar-like nanostructures, and nanodots) on implant surfaces for load bearing approaches (Oh et al., 2006; Sjöström et al., 2009). Especially, the titania nanotube arrays are one of the most promising candidate of titanium nanosurfaces for dental implantology (Fig. 3.). Several *in vitro* studies have demonstrated that cells cultured on these nanotubular surfaces showed higher adhesion, proliferation, ALP activity and bone matrix deposition (Oh et al., 2006; Popat et al., 2007a).

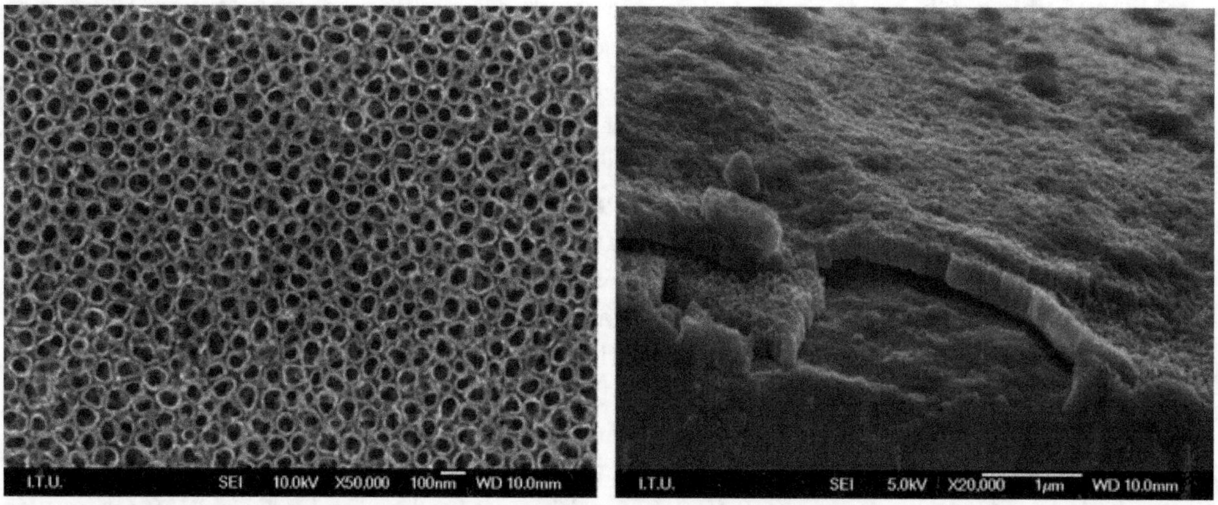

Fig. 3. Top and cross sectional SEM images of titania nanotubes

These increased *in vitro* cellular activities for titania nanotubes also translated to *in vivo* bone bonding. Nanotubular surfaces significantly improved bone bonding strength by as much as nine-fold compared with gritblasted surfaces, and histological analysis revealed greater bone-implant contact and collagen type I expression confirming the better *in vivo* behaviour of titania nanotubes (Bjursten et al., 2008; von Wilmowsky et al., 2008). It has been also shown that various nanomorphological features of titania nanotubes, such as length, diameter, wall thickness, have a major impact on the cellular reponses, providing the evidence that cells are susceptible to nanoscale dimesions (Brammer et al., 2009; Park et al., 2009). Besides, nanotubular structures on titanium provide a suitable infrastructure for loading and subsequent releasing of antibiotics (Aninwene et al., 2008; Popat et al., 2007b) or for immobilizing biosignalling molecules for better osseointegration (Balasundaram et al., 2007). However, there is still a need for additional studies that would optimize the fabrication of nanotubes for better bioactivity.

5. Future trends and concluding remarks

Nowadays, patients can be treated dental implants with a success rate above 97 %. Although novel approaches were able to accelerate and enhance the osseointegration, the healing limits of the body, which make the immediate loading challenging, should not be neglected. Osseointegrated or ankylotic titanium implants don't behave like natural teeth. Since they lack a periodontal ligament, they only had tenth of the mobility of the natural teeth (Schulte, 1995). Axial and horizontal loads bellow a subjective tolerance limit can be compensated by the natural periodontium, but such loads on osseointegrated implants would lead to local disruption of the bony interface. Additionally, it has been reported that the defensive capacity of the peri-implant tissue against bacterial invasion is inferior to that of the natural tooth, that make them more prone to bone loss (Chang et al., 1999b). A third disadvantage of the osseointegrated implant is the absence of a periodontal neurophysiological mechanoreceptive system for the biocybernetic control of the stomatognatic system (Jacobs & Van Steenberghe, 2006).

Considering these drawbacks, establishment of a periodontal ligament surrounding an implant, termed as bio-root, would provide the ideal condition for implant-supported treatments in future. To overcome the above mentioned disadvantages of the dental implants, several *in vivo* experiments attempted to create a periodontal ligament around these implants by placing them adjacent to retained tooth roots (Urabe et al., 2000; Warrer et al., 1993). Although they were able to partially regenerate the periodontal ligament consisting of cementum, periodontal ligament and alveolar bone, the application of these methods in patients seems to be impossible due to technical and physical factors. Furthermore, several studies have reported that periodontal ligament cells cultured on titanium implants can produce a periodontal ligament-like tissue when placed in the jaws of animals (Choi, 2000; Gault et al., 2010; Lin et al., 2011). Although it has been shown that generating a periodontal-like tissue around implants may be experimentally possible, also in human trials (Gault et al., 2010), approaches until now were not able to innovate a predictable and feasible method for producing dental implants with periodontal-like ligament.

Furthermore, gradient functional concept (GFC) on materials and structures has been receiving special attention not only in industrial applications, but in dental as well as medical fields. Particularly, when such structures and concepts are about to be applied to implants, its importance becomes more clinically crucial. For example, the majority of implant mass (implant core portion) should be strong and tough, so that occlusal force can be smoothly transferred from the placed implant to the receiving hard tissue. However, the surface (implant case portion) needs to be engineered to exhibit some extent of roughness. From such macro-structural changes from bulk core to the porous case, again the structural integrity should be maintained. The GFC can also be applied for the purpose of having a chemical (compositional) gradient. Ca-, P-enrichment is not needed in the interior materials of the implants. Some other modifications related to chemical dressing or conditioning can also be utilized for achieving gradient functionality on chemical alternations on surfaces as well as near-surface zones (Oshida, Y.; 2007).

6. Acknowledgment

This chapter is dedicated to Prof. Dr. Harzem Özger, a well of wisdom in the reconstructive orthopaedic oncology.

7. References

Abrahamsson, I.; Zitzmann, N.U.; Berglundh, T.; Wennerberg, A. & Lindhe, J. (2001). Bone and soft tissue integration to titanium implants with different surface topography: an experimental study in the dog. The *International Journal of Oral and Maxillofacial Implants*, Vol.16, No.3, pp. 323-332, ISSN 0882-2786

Adell, R.; Lekholm, U.; Rockler, B. & Branemark, P.I. (1981). A 15-year study of osseointegrated implants in the treatment of the edentulous jaw, *International Journal of Oral Surgery*, Vol.10, No.6, pp. 387–416, ISSN 0300-9785

Albrektsson, T.; Brånemark, P.I.; Hansson, H.A. & Lindström, J. (1981). Osseointegrated titanium implants. Requirements for ensuring a long-lasting, direct bone-to-implant anchorage in man. *Acta Orthopaedica Scandinavica,* Vol.52, No.2, pp. 155-170, ISSN 0001-6470

Albrektsson, T.; Hansson, H.A. & Ivarsson, B. (1985). Interface analysis of titanium and zirconium bone implants. *Biomaterials,* Vol.6, No.2, pp. 97-101, ISSN 0142-9612

Albrektsson, T.; Jansson, T. & Lekholm, U. (1986). Osseointegrated dental implants. *Dental Clinics of North America,* Vol.30, No.1, pp. 151-174, ISSN 0011-8532

Albrektsson, T. & Johansson, C. (2001). Osteoinduction, osteoconduction and osseointegration. *European Spine Journal,* Vol.10, Suppl.2, pp. 96-101, ISSN 0940-6719

Al-Nawas,B.; Groetz, K.A.; Goetz, H.; Duschner, H. & Wagner, W. (2008). Comparative histomorphometry and resonance frequency analysis of implants with moderately rough surfaces in a loaded animal model. *Clinical Oral Implants Research,* Vol.19, No.1, pp. 1-8, ISSN 0905-7161

Aninwene, G.E.; Yao, C. & Webster, T.J. (2008). Enhanced osteoblast adhesion to drug-coated anodized nanotubular titanium surfaces. *International Journal of Nanomedicine,* Vol.3, No.2, pp. 257-264, ISSN 1176-9114

Anselme, K.; Bigerelle, M.; Noel, B.; Dufresne, E.; Judas, D.; Iost, A. & Hardouin, P. (2000a) Qualitative and quantitative study of human osteoblast adhesion on materials with various surface roughnesses. *Journal of Biomedical Materials Research,* Vol.49, No.2, pp. 155-166, ISSN 0021-9304

Anselme, K.; Linez, P.; Bigerelle, M.; Le Maguer, D.; Le Maguer, A.; Hardouin, P.; Hildebrand, H.F.; Iost, A. & Leroy, J.M. (2000b). The relative influence of the topography and chemistry of TiAl6V4 surfaces on osteoblastic cell behaviour. *Biomaterials,* Vol.21, No.15, pp. 1567-1577, ISSN 0142-9612

Bagno, A.; Piovan, A.; Dettin, M.; Chiarion, A.; Brun, P.; Gambaretto, R.; Fontana, G.; Di Bello, C.; Palù, G. & Castagliuolo, I. (2007). Human osteoblast-like cell adhesion on titanium substrates covalently functionalized with synthetic peptides. *Bone,* Vol.40, No.3, pp. 693-699, ISSN 8756-3282

Balasundaram, G.; Yao, C. & Webster, T.J. (2008). TiO2 nanotubes functionalized with regions of bone morphogenetic protein-2 increases osteoblast adhesion. *Journal of Biomedical Materials Resarch Part A,* Vol.84, No.2, pp. 447-453, ISSN 1549-3296

Balloni, S.; Calvi, E.M.; Damiani, F.; Bistoni, G.; Calvitti, M.; Locci, P.; Becchetti, E. & Marinucci, L. (2009). Effects of titanium surface roughness on mesenchymal stem cell commitment and differentiation signaling. *The International Journal of Oral and Maxillofacial Implants,* Vol.24, No.4, pp. 627-635, ISSN 0882-2786

Barrere, F.; Layrolle, P.; Van Blitterswijk, C.A. & De Groot, K. (2001). Biomimetic coatings on titanium: a crystal growth study of octacalcium phosphate. *Journal of Materials Science. Materials in Medicine,* Vol.12, No.6, pp. 529-534, ISSN 0957-4530

Bauer, S.; Park, J.; Mark ,K.V. & Schmuki, P. (2008). Improved attachment of mesenchymal stem cells on super-hydrophobic TiO(2) nanotubes. *Acta Biomaterialia*, Vol.4, No.3, pp. 1576-1582, ISSN 1742-7061

Becker, J.; Kirsch, A.; Schwarz, F.; Chatzinikolaidou, M.; Rothamel, D.; Lekovic, V.; Laub, M. & Jennissen, H.P. (2006). Bone apposition to titanium implants biocoated with recombinant human bone morphogenetic protein-2 (rhBMP-2). A pilot study in dogs. *Clinical Oral Investigations*, Vol.10, No.3, pp. 217-224, ISSN 1432-6981

Bessho, K.; Carnes, D.L.; Cavin, R.; Chen, H.Y. & Ong, J.L. (1999). BMP stimulation of bone response adjacent to titanium implants in vivo. *Clinical Oral Implants Research*, Vol.10, No.3, pp. 212-218, ISSN 0905-7161

Beutner, R.; Michael, J.; Schwenzer, B. & Scharnweber, D. (2010). Biological nano-functionalization of titanium-based biomaterial surfaces: a flexible toolbox. *Journal of the Royal Society, Inetrface*, Vol.7, Suppl.1, pp. 93-105, ISSN 1742-5662

Bjursten, L.M.; Rasmusson, L.; Oh, S.; Smith, G.C.; Brammer, K.S. & Jin, S. (2010) .Titanium dioxide nanotubes enhance bone bonding in vivo. *Journal of Biomedical Materials Research Part A*, Vol.92, No.3, pp. 1218-1224, ISSN 1549-3296

Bornstein, M.M.; Valderrama, P.; Jones, A.A.; Wilson, T.G.; Seibl, R. & Cochran, D.L. (2008). Bone apposition around two different sandblasted and acid-etched titanium implant surfaces: a histomorphometric study in canine mandibles. *Clinical Oral Implants Research*, Vol.19, No.3, pp. 233–241, ISSN 0905-7161

Boyan, B.D.; Batzer, R.; Kieswetter, K.; Liu, Y.; Cochran, D.L.; Szmuckler-Moncler, S.; Dean, D.D. & Schwartz, Z. (1998). Titanium surface roughness alters responsiveness of MG63 osteoblast-like cells to 1 alpha,25-(OH)2D3. *Journal of Biomedical Materials Research*, Vol.39, No.1, pp. 77-85, ISSN 0021-9304

Boyan, B.D.; Lohmann, C.H.; Sisk, M.; Liu, Y.; Sylvia, V.L.; Cochran, D.L.; Dean, D.D. & Schwartz, Z. (2001). Both cyclooxygenase-1 and cyclooxygenase-2 mediate osteoblast response to titanium surface roughness. *Journal of Biomedical Materials Research*, Vol.55, No.3, pp.350-359, ISSN 0021-9304

Boyan, B.D.; Bonewald, L.F.; Paschalis, E.P.; Lohmann, C.H.; Rosser, J.; Cochran, D.L.; Dean, D.D.; Schwartz, Z. & Boskey, A.L. (2002). Osteoblast-mediated mineral deposition in culture is dependent on surface microtopography. *Calcified Tissue International*, Vol.71, No.6, pp. 519-529, ISSN 0171-967X

Brånemark, P.I.; Adell, R.; Breine, U.; Hansson, B.O.; Lindström, J. & Ohlsson, A. (1969). Intra-osseous anchorage of dental prostheses. I. Experimental studies. *Scandinavian Journal of Plastic and Reconstructive Surgery*, Vol.3, No.2, pp. 81-100, ISSN 0036-5556

Brånemark, P.I.; Hansson, B.O.; Adell, R.; Breine, U.; Lindström, J.; Hallén, O. & Ohman, A. (1977). Osseointegrated implants in the treatment of the edentulous jaw. Experience from a 10-year period. *Scandinavian Journal of Plastic and Reconstructive Surgery Supplementum*, Vol.16, pp. 1-132, ISSN 0581-9474

Brånemark, P.I. (1983). Osseointegration and its experimental background. *Journal of Prosthetic Dentistry*, Vol.50, No.3, pp. 399-410, ISSN 0022-3913

Brammer, K.S.; Oh, S.; Cobb, C.J.; Bjursten, L.M.; van der Heyde, H. & Jin, S. (2009). Improved bone-forming functionality on diameter-controlled TiO(2) nanotube surface. *Acta Biomaterialia*, Vol.5, No.8, pp. 3215-3223, ISSN 1742-7061

Buser, D.; Schenk, R.K.; Steinemann, S.; Fiorellini, J.P.; Fox, C.H. & Stich, H. (1991). Influence of surface characteristics on bone integration of titanium implants. A histomorphometric study in miniature pigs. *Journal of Biomedical Materials Research*, Vol.25, No.7, pp. 889-902, ISSN 0021-9304

Buser, D.; Broggini, N.; Wieland, M.; Schenk, R.K.; Denzer, A.J.; Cochran, D.L.; Hoffmann, B.; Lussi, A. & Steinemann, S.G. (2004). Enhanced bone apposition to a chemically modified SLA titanium surface. *Journal of Dental Research*, Vol.83, No.7, pp. 529-533, ISSN 0022-0345

Chang, Y.L.; Lew, D.; Park, J.B. & Keller, J.C. (1999a). Biomechanical and morphometric analysis of hydroxyapatite-coated implants with varying crystallinity. *Journal of Oral and Maxillofacial Surgery*, Vol.57, No.9, pp. 1096-1108, ISSN 0278-2391

Chang, M.; Wennström, J.L.; Odman, P. & Andersson, B. (1999b). Implant supported single-tooth replacements compared to contralateral natural teeth. Crown and soft tissue dimensions. *Clinical Oral Implants Research*, Vol.10, No. 3, pp. 185-194, ISSN 0905-7161

Chappard, D.; Aguado, E.; Huré, G.; Grizon, F. & Basle, M.F. (1999). The early remodeling phases around titanium implants: a histomorphometric assessment of bone quality in a 3- and 6-month study in sheep. *The International Journal of Oral and Maxillofacial Implants*, Vol.14, No.2, pp. 189-196, ISSN 0882-2786

Choi, B.H. (2000). Periodontal ligament formation around titanium implants using cultured periodontal ligament cells: a pilot study. *The International Journal of Oral and Maxillofacial Implants*, Vol.15, No.2, pp. 193-196, ISSN 0882-2786

Cofino, B.; Fogarassy, P.; Millet, P. & Lodini, A. (2004). Thermal residual stresses near the interface between plasma-sprayed hydroxyapatite coating and titanium substrate: finite element analysis and synchrotron radiation measurements. *Journal of Biomedical Materials Research Part A*, Vol.70, No.1, pp. 20-27, ISSN 1549-3296

Cooper, L.F. (2000). A role for surface topography in creating and maintaining bone at titanium endosseous implants. *The Journal of Prosthetic Dentistry*, Vol.84, No.5, pp. 522-534, ISSN 0022-3913

Dalton, J.E. & Cook, S.D. (1995). In vivo mechanical and histological characteristics of HA-coated implants vary with coating vendor. *Journal of Biomedical Materials Research*, Vol.29, No.2, pp. 239-245, ISSN 0021-9304

Davies, J.E. (1996). In vitro modeling of the bone/implant interface. *The Anatomical Record*, Vol.245, No.2, pp. 426-445, ISSN 0003-276X

Davies, J.E. (2003). Understanding peri-implant endosseous healing. *Journal of Dental Education* Vol.67, No.8, pp. 932-949, ISSN 0022-0337

Dee, K.C.; Puleo, D.A. & Bizios, R. (2002). *An Introduction To Tissue-Biomaterial Interactions.* John Wiley&Sons, ISBN 9780471253945, New Jersey, US

Dereka, X.E.; Markopoulou, C.E. & Vrotsos, I.A. (2006). Role of growth factors on periodontal repair. *Growth Factors*, Vol.24, No.4, pp. 260-267, ISSN 0897-7194

Deligianni, D.D.; Katsala, N.; Ladas, S.; Sotiropoulou, D.; Amedee, J. & Missirlis, Y.F. (2001). Effect of surface roughness of the titanium alloy Ti-6Al-4V on human bone marrow cell response and on protein adsorption. *Biomaterials*, Vol.22, No.11, pp. 1241-1251, ISSN 0142-9612

Eisenbarth, E.; Velten, D.; Müller, M.; Thull, R. & Breme, J. (2004). Biocompatibility of beta-stabilizing elements of titanium alloys. *Biomaterials*, Vol.25, No.26, pp. 5705-5713, ISSN 0142-9612

Elias, C.N.; Oshida, Y.; Lima, J.H.C. & Muller, C.A. (2008). Relationship between surface properties (roughness, wettability and morphology) of titanium and dental implant torque. *Journal of Mechanical Behavior of Biomedical Materials,* Vol.1, No.3, pp.234-242, ISSN 1878-0180

Elias, K.L.; Price, R.L. & Webster, T.J. (2002). Enhanced functions of osteoblasts on nanometer diameter carbon fibers. *Biomaterials,* Vol.23, No.15, pp. 3279-3287, ISSN 0142-9612

Elmengaard, B.; Bechtold, J.E. & Søballe, K. (2005). In vivo study of the effect of RGD treatment on bone ongrowth on press-fit titanium alloy implants. *Biomaterials,* Vol.26, No.17, pp. 3521-3526, ISSN 0142-9612

Esposito, M.; Hirsch, J.M.; Lekholm, U. & Thomsen, P. (1998). Biological factors contributing to failures of osseointegrated oral implants. (II). Etiopathogenesis. *European Journal of Oral Sciences,* Vol.106, No.3, pp. 721-764, ISSN 0909-8836

Esposito, M.; Murray-Curtis, L.; Grusovin, M.G.; Coulthard, P. & Worthington, H.V. (2007). Interventions for replacing missing teeth: different types of dental implants. *Cochrane Database of Systematic Reviews,* Vol.17, No.4, CD003815, ISSN 1469-493X

Gault, P.; Black, A.; Romette, J.L.; Fuente, F., Schroeder, K.; Thillou, F.; Brune, T.; Berdal, A. & Wurtz, T. (2010). Tissue-engineering ligament: implant constructs for tooth replacement. *Journal of Clinical Periodontology,* Vol.37, No.8, pp. 750-758, ISSN 1600-051X

Gaydos, J.M.; Moore, M.A.; Garetto, L.P.; Oshida, Y. & Kowolik, M.J. (2000). Bisphosphonate effect on neutrophil activation by titanium and hydroxyapatite implants, *Journal of Dental Research,* Vol. 79, Suppl.1, pp. 336, ISSN 0022-0345

Gutwein, L.G. & Webster, T.J. (2004). Increased viable osteoblast density in the presence of nanophase compared to conventional alumina and titania particles. *Biomaterials,* Vol.25, No.18; pp. 4175-4183, ISSN 0142-9612

Hallab, N.J.; Skipor, A. & Jacobs, J.J. (2003). Interfacial kinetics of titanium- and cobalt-based implant alloys in human serum: metal release and biofilm formation. *Journal of Biomedical Materials Research Part A,* Vol.65, No.3, pp. 311-318, ISSN 1549-3296

Harris, L.G.; Meredith, D.O.; Eschbach, L. & Richards, R.G. (2007). Staphylococcus aureus adhesion to standard micro-rough and electropolished implant materials. *Journal of Materials Science. Materials in Medicine,* Vol.18, No.6, pp. 1151-1156, ISSN 0957-4530

Healy, K.E. & Ducheyne, P. (1992). The mechanisms of passive dissolution of titanium in a model physiological environment. *Journal of Biomedical Materials Research,* Vol.26, No.3, pp. 319-338, ISSN 0021-9304

Heijink, A.; Schwartz, J.; Zobitz, M.E.; Nicole Crowder, K.; Lutz, G.E. & Sibonga, J.D. (2008). Self-assembled monolayer films of phosphonates for bonding RGD to titanium. *Clinical Orthopaedics and Related Research,* Vol.466, No.4, pp. 977-984, ISSN 0009-921X

Heldin, C.H. & Westermark, B. (1999). Mechanism of action and in vivo role of platelet-derived growth factor. *Physiological Reviews,* Vol.79, No.4, pp. 1283-1316, ISSN 0031-9333

Hench, L.L. & Wilson, J. (1984). Surface-active biomaterials. *Science,* Vol.226, No.4675, pp. 630-636, ISSN 0036-8075

Henry, P.J.; Laney, W.R.; Jemt, T.; Harris, D.; Krogh, P.H.; Polizzi, G.; Zarb, G.A. & Herrmann, I. (1996). Osseointegrated implants for single-tooth replacement: A prospective 5-year multicenter study. *International Journal of Oral Maxillofacial Implants,* Vol.11, No.4, pp. 450–455, ISSN 0882-2786

Hynes, R.O. (2002). Integrins: bidirectional, allosteric signaling machines. *Cell*, Vol.110, No.6, pp. 673-687, ISSN 0092-8674

Jacobs, R. & Van Steenberghe, D. (2006). From osseoperception to implant-mediated sensory-motor interactions and related clinical implications. *Journal of Oral Rehabilitation*, Vol.33, No.4, pp. 282-292, ISSN 0305-182X

Jaffin, R.A. & Berman, C.L. (1991). The excessive loss of Branemark fixtures in type IV bone: a 5-year analysis. *Journal of Periodontology*, Vol.62, No.1, pp. 2-4, ISSN 0022-3492

Jemt, T.; Chai, J.; Harnett, J.; Heath, M.R.; Hutton, J.E.; Johns, R.B.; McKenna, S.; McNamara, D.C.; van Steenberghe, D.; Taylor, R.; Watson, R.M. & Herrmann, I. (1996). A 5-year prospective multicenter follow-up report on overdentures supported by osseointegrated implants. *International Journal of Oral Maxillofacial Implants,* Vol.11, No.3, pp. 291–298, ISSN 0882-2786

Junker, R.; Dimakis, A.; Thoneick, M. & Jansen, J.A. (2009). Effects of implant surface coatings and composition on bone integration: a systematic review. *Clinical Oral Implants Research*, Vol.20, Suppl. 4, pp. 185-206, ISSN 0905-7161

Juodzbalys, G.; Sapragoniene, M.; Wennerberg, A. & Baltrukonis, T. (2007) Titanium dental implant surface micromorphology optimization. *Journal of Oral Implantology*, Vol.33, No.4, pp. 177-185, ISSN 0160-6972

Kasemo, B. & Lausmaa J. (1988). Biomaterial and implant surfaces: on the role of cleanliness, contamination, and preparation procedures. *Journal of Biomedical Materials Research,* Vol.22, No.A2 Suppl, pp. 145-158, ISSN 0021-9304

Kasemo, B. & Gold, J. (1999). Implant surfaces and interface processes. *Advances in Dental Research*, Vol.13, pp. 8-20, ISSN 0895-9374

Kern, T.; Yang, Y.; Glover, R. & Ong, J.L. (2005). Effect of heat-treated titanium surfaces on protein adsorption and osteoblast precursor cell initial attachment. *Implant Dentistry*, Vol.14, No.1, pp. 70-76, ISSN 1056-6163

Kienapfel ,H.; Sprey, C.; Wilke, A. & Griss, P. (1999). Implant fixation by bone ingrowth. *The Journal of Arthroplasty* Vol.14, No.3, pp. 355-368, ISSN 0883-5403

Kieswetter, K.; Schwartz, Z.; Dean, D.D. & Boyan, B.D. (1996). The role of implant surface characteristics in the healing of bone. *Critical Reviews in Oral Biology and Medicine,* Vol.7, No.4, pp. 329-345, ISSN 1045-4411

Kilpadi, K.L.; Chang, P.L. & Bellis, S.L. (2001). Hydroxylapatite binds more serum proteins, purified integrins, and osteoblast precursor cells than titanium or steel. *Journal of Biomedical Materials Research*, Vol.57, No.2, pp. 258-267, ISSN 0021-9304

Kim, H.M.; Kokubo, T.; Fujibayashi, S.; Nishiguchi, S. & Nakamura, T. (2000). Bioactive macroporous titanium surface layer on titanium substrate. *Journal of Biomedical Materials Research*, Vol.52, No.3, pp. 553-557, ISSN 0021-9304

Klinger, M.M.; Rahemtulla, F.; Prince, C.W.; Lucas, L.C. & Lemons, J.E. (1998). Proteoglycans at the bone-implant interface. *Critical Reviews in Oral Biology and Medicine,* Vol.9, No.4, pp. 449-463, ISSN 1045-4411

Kokubo, T.; Kushitani, H.; Sakka, S.; Kitsugi, T. & Yamamuro, T. (1990). Solutions able to reproduce in vivo surface-structure changes in bioactive glass-ceramic A-W. *Journal of Biomedical Materials Research*, Vol.24, No.6, pp. 721-734, ISSN 0021-9304

Kroese-Deutman, H.C.; van den Dolder, J.; Spauwen, P.H. & Jansen, J.A. (2005). Influence of RGD-loaded titanium implants on bone formation in vivo. *Tissue Engineering,* Vol.11, No.11-12, pp. 1867-1875, ISSN 1076-3279

Lee, M.H.; Oh, N.; Lee, S.W.; Leesungbok, R.; Kim, S.E.; Yun, Y.P. & Kang, J.H. (2010). Factors influencing osteoblast maturation on microgrooved titanium substrata. *Biomaterials*, Vol.31, No.14, pp. 3804-3815, ISSN 0142-9612

Le Guehennec, L; Lopez-Heredia, M.A.; Enkel, B.; Weiss, P.; Amouriq, Y. & Layrolle, P. (2008). Osteoblastic cell behaviour on different titanium implant surfaces. *Acta Biomaterialia*, Vol.4, No.3, pp. 535-543, ISSN 1742-7061

Li, L.H.; Kong, Y.M.; Kim, H.W.; Kim, Y.W.; Kim, H.E.; Heo, S.J. & Koak, J.Y. (2004). Improved biological performance of Ti implants due to surface modification by micro-arc oxidation. *Biomaterials*, Vol.25, No.14, pp. 2867-2875, ISSN 0142-9612

Lian, J.B. & Stein, G.S. (1992). Concepts of osteoblast growth and differentiation: basis for modulation of bone cell development and tissue formation. *Critical Reviews in Oral Biology and Medicine*, Vol.3, No.3, pp. 269-305, ISSN 1045-4411

Lim, Y.J. & Oshida, Y. (2001). Initial contact angle measurements on variously treated dental/medical titanium materials. *Biomedical Materials and Engineering*, Vol.11, No.4, pp. 325-341, ISSN 0959-2989

Lin, Y.; Galluci, G.O.; Buser, D.; Bosshardt, D.; Belser, U.C. & Yelick, P.C. (2011). Bioengineered periodontal tissue formed on titanium dental implants. *Journal of Dental Research*, Vol.90, No.2, pp. 251-256, ISSN 1544-0591

Linez-Bataillon, P.; Monchau, F.; Bigerelle, M. & Hildebrand, H.F. (2002). In vitro MC3T3 osteoblast adhesion with respect to surface roughness of Ti6Al4V substrates. *Biomolecular Engineering*, Vol.19, No.2-6, pp. 133-141, ISSN 1389-0344

Liu, Y.; de Groot, K. & Hunziker, E.B. (2004). Osteoinductive implants: the mise-en-scene for drug-bearing biomimetic coatings. *Annals of Biomedical Engineering*, Vol.32, No.3, pp. 398-406, pp. 0090-6964

Liu, Y.; de Groot, K. & Hunziker, E.B. (2005). BMP-2 liberated from biomimetic implant coatings induces and sustains direct ossification in an ectopic rat model. *Bone*, Vol.36, No.5, pp. 745-757, ISSN 8756-3282

Liu, Y.; Enggist, L.; Kuffer, A.F.; Buser, D. & Hunziker, E.B. (2007). The influence of BMP-2 and its mode of delivery on the osteoconductivity of implant surfaces during the early phase of osseointegration. *Biomaterials*, Vol.28, No.16, pp. 2677-2686, ISSN 0142-9612

Lossdorfer, S.; Schwartz, Z.; Wang, L.; Lohmann, C.H.; Turner, J.D.; Wieland, M.; Cochran, D.L. & Boyan, B.D. (2004). Microrough implant surface topographies increase osteogenesis by reducing osteoclast formation and activity. *Journal of Biomedical Materials Research Part A*, Vol.70, No.3, pp. 361-369, ISSN 1549-3296

MacDonald, D.E.; Deo, N.; Markovic, B.; Stranick, M. & Somasundaran P. (2004). Thermal and chemical modification of titanium-aluminum-vanadium implant materials: effects on surface properties, glycoprotein adsorption, and MG63 cell attachment. *Biomaterials*, Vol.25, No.16, pp. 3135-3146, ISSN 0142-3835

Marco, F.; Milena, F.; Gianluca, G. & Vittoria, O. (2005). Peri-implant osteogenesis in health and osteoporosis. *Micron*, Vol.36, No.7-8, pp. 630-644 ISSN 0968-4328

Marinucci, L.; Balloni, S.; Becchetti, E.; Belcastro, S.; Guerra, M.; Calvitti, M.; Lilli, C.; Calvi, E.M. & Locci, P.(2006). Effect of titanium surface roughness on human osteoblast proliferation and gene expression in vitro. *The International Journal of Oral and Maxillofacial Implants*, Vol.21, No.5, pp. 719-725, ISSN 0882-2786

Mendonça, G.; Mendonça, D.B.; Aragão, F.J. & Cooper, L.F. (2008). Advancing dental implant surface technology--from micron- to nanotopography. *Biomaterials* Vol.29, No.28, pp. 3822-3835, ISSN 0142-9612

Mendonça, G.; Mendonça, D.B.; Aragão, F.J. & Cooper, L.F. (2010). The combination of micron and nanotopography by H(2)SO(4)/H(2)O(2) treatment and its effects on osteoblast-specific gene expression of hMSCs. *Journal of Biomedical Materials Research Part A*, Vol.94, No.1, pp. 169-179, ISSN 1549-3296

Meyer, U.; Joos, U.; Mythili, J.; Stamm, T.; Hohoff, A.; Fillies, T.; Stratmann, U. & Wiesmann, H.P. (2004). Ultrastructural characterization of the implant/bone interface of immediately loaded dental implants. *Biomaterials* Vol.25, No.10, pp. 1959-1967, ISSN 0142-9612

Moore, M.A.; Oshida, Y.; Garetto, L.P. & Kowolik, M.J. (2000). Neutrophil response to titanium materials - microcompatibility following various surface treatments. *Journal of Dental Research*, Vol.79, Suppl.1, pp. 421, ISSN 0022-0345

Morra, M. (2006). Biochemical modification of titanium surfaces: peptides and ECM proteins. *European Cells and Materials*, Vol.12, pp. 1-15, ISSN 1473-2262

Morton, D.; Bornstein, M.M.; Wittneben, J.G.; Martin, W.C.; Ruskin, J.D.; Hart, C.N. & Buser, D. (2010). Early loading after 21 days of healing of nonsubmerged titanium implants with a chemically modified sandblasted and acid-etched surface: two-year results of a prospective two-center study. *Clinical Implant Dentistry and Related Research*, Vol.12, No.1, pp. 9-17, ISSN 1708-8208

Mustafa, K.; Wennerberg, A.; Wroblewski, J.; Hultenby, K.; Lopez, B.S. & Arvidson, K. (2001) Determining optimal surface roughness of TiO(2) blasted titanium implant material for attachment, proliferation and differentiation of cells derived from human mandibular alveolar bone. *Clinical Oral Implants Research*, Vol.12, No.5, pp. 515-525, ISSN 0905-7161

Oh, S.; Daraio, C.; Chen, L.H.; Pisanic, T.R.; Fiñones, R.R. & Jin, S. (2006). Significantly accelerated osteoblast cell growth on aligned TiO2 nanotubes. *Journal of Biomedical Materials Research Part A*, Vol.78, No.1, pp. 97-103, ISSN 1549-3296

Olivares-Navarrete, R.; Raz, P.; Zhao, G.; Chen, J.; Wieland, M.; Cochran, D.L.; Chaudhri, R.A.; Ornoy, A.; Boyan, B.D. & Schwartz, Z. (2008). Integrin alpha2beta1 plays a critical role in osteoblast response to micron-scale surface structure and surface energy of titanium substrates. *Proceedings of the National Academy of Sciences of the United States of America*, Vol.105, No.41, pp. 15767-15772, ISSN 1091-6490

Ong, J.L. & Chan D.C. (2000). Hydroxyapatite and their use as coatings in dental implants: a review. *Critical Reviews in Biomedical Engineering*, . Vol.28, No.5-6, pp. 667-707, ISSN 0278-940X

Osborn, J.F. (1979). Biomaterials and their application to implantation. *SSO Schweizerische Monatsschrift für Zahnheilkunde* Vol.89, No.11, pp. 1138-1139, ISSN 0036-7702

Oshida, Y.; Hashem, A.; Nishihara, T. & Yapchulay, M.V. (1994). Fractal dimension analysis of mandibular bones; toward a morphological compatibility of implants. *Biomedical Materials and Engineering*, Vol.4, No.3, pp.397-407, ISSN 0959-2989

Oshida, Y. (2000). Requirements for successful biofunctional implants. *International Symposium on Advanced Biomaterials*. p.5

Oshida, Y.; (2007). *Bioscience and Bioengineering of Titanium Materials*, Elsevier, ISBN 0-08-045142-X, Oxford UK

Oshida, Y. & Tuna, E.B. (2009). Science and Technology Integrated Titanium Dental Implant Systems, In: *Advanced Biomaterials*, Basu, B.; Katti, D.S.; Kumar, A. ed., pp. 143-177, A John Wiley & Sons.

Oshida, Y.; Tuna, E.B.; Aktoren, A. & Gencay, K. (2010). Dental Implant Systems. *International Journal of Molecular Sciences*, Vol.11 No.4, pp.1580-1678, ISSN 1422-0067

Park, J.Y. & Davies, J.E. (2000). Red blood cell and platelet interactions with titanium implant surfaces. *Clinical Oral Implants Research*, Vol.11, No.6, pp. 530-539, ISSN 0905-7161

Park, J.Y.; Gemmell, C.H. & Davies, J.E. (2001). Platelet interactions with titanium: modulation of platelet activity by surface topography. *Biomaterials*, Vol.22, No.19, pp. 2671-2682, ISSN 0142-9612

Park, B.S.; Heo, S.J.; Kim, C.S.; Oh, J.E.; Kim, J.M.; Lee, G.; Park, W.H.; Chung, C.P. & Min, B.M. (2005). Effects of adhesion molecules on the behavior of osteoblast-like cells and normal human fibroblasts on different titanium surfaces. *Journal of Biomedical Materials Research Part A*, Vol.74, No.4, pp. 640-651, ISSN 1549-3296

Park, J.; Bauer, S.; Schlegel, K.A.; Neukam, F.W.; von der Mark, K. & Schmuki, P. (2009). TiO2 nanotube surfaces: 15 nm--an optimal length scale of surface topography for cell adhesion and differentiation. *Small*, Vol.5, No.6, pp. 666-671, ISSN 1613-6829

Petrie, T.A.; Raynor, J.E.; Reyes, C.D.; Burns, K.L.; Collard, D.M. & García, A.J. (2008). The effect of integrin-specific bioactive coatings on tissue healing and implant osseointegration. *Biomaterials*, Vol.29, No.19, pp. 2849-2857, ISSN 0142-9612

Plopper, G.E.; McNamee, H.P.; Dike, L.E.; Bojanowski, K. & Ingber D.E. (1995). Convergence of integrin and growth factor receptor signalling patways within focal adhesion complex. *Molecular Biology of the Cell*, Vol.6, No.10, pp. 1349-1365, ISSN 1059-1524

Popat, K.C.; Leoni, L.; Grimes, C.A. & Desai, T.A. (2007a). Influence of engineered titania nanotubular surfaces on bone cells. *Biomaterials*, Vol.28, No.21, pp. 3188-3197, ISSN 0142-9612

Popat, K.C.; Eltgroth, M.; Latempa, T.J.; Grimes, C.A. & Desai, T.A. (2007b). Decreased Staphylococcus epidermis adhesion and increased osteoblast functionality on antibiotic-loaded titania nanotubes. *Biomaterials*, Vol.28, No.32, pp. 4880-4888, ISSN 0142-9612

Price, R.L.; Gutwein, L.G.; Kaledin, L.; Tepper, F. & Webster, T.J. (2003). Osteoblast function on nanophase alumina materials: Influence of chemistry, phase, and topography. *Journal of Biomedical Materials Research Part A*, Vol.67, No.4, pp. 1284-1293, ISSN 1549-3296

Puleo, D.A. & Nanci, A. (1999). Understanding and controlling the bone-implant interface. *Biomaterials*, Vol.20, No. 23-24, pp. 2311-2321, ISSN 0142-9612

Ramazanoglu, M.; Lutz, R.; Ergun, C.; von Wilmowsky, C.; Nkenke, E. & Schlegel, K.A. (2011). The effect of combined delivery of rhBMP-2 and rhVEGF165 from biomimetic Ca-P coated implants on osseointegration. *Clinical Oral Implants Research* xx, 2010; 000–000. doi: 10.1111/j.1600-0501.2010.02133.x

Rausch-fan, X.; Qu, Z.; Wieland, M.; Matejka, M. & Schedle, A. (2008). Differentiation and cytokine synthesis of human alveolar osteoblasts compared to osteoblast-like cells (MG63) in response to titanium surfaces. *Dental Materials*, Vol.24, No.1, pp. 102-110, ISSN 0109-5641

Rosa, A.L. & Beloti, M.M. (2003). Rat bone marrow cell response to titanium and titanium alloy with different surface roughness. *Clinical Oral Implants Research*, Vol.14, No.1, pp. 43-48, ISSN 0905-7161

Ruoslahti, E. (1996). Rgd and other recognition sequences for integrins. *Annual Review of Cell and Developmental Biology*, Vol.12, pp. 697-715, ISSN 1081-0706

Sader, M.S.; Balduino, A.; Soares Gde, A. & Borojevic, R. (2005). Effect of three distinct treatments of titanium surface on osteoblast attachment, proliferation, and differentiation. *Clinical Oral Implants Research*, Vol.16, No.6, pp. 667-675, ISSN 0905-7161

Saldaña, L.; Vilaboa, N.; Vallés, G.; González-Cabrero, J. & Munuera, L. (2005). Osteoblast response to thermally oxidized Ti6Al4V alloy. *Journal of Biomedical Materials Research Part A*, Vol.73, No.1, pp. 97-107, ISSN 1549-3296

Sawyer, A.A.; Hennessy, K.M. & Bellis, S.L. (2005). Regulation of mesenchymal stem cell attachment and spreading on hydroxyapatite by RGD peptides and adsorbed serum proteins. *Biomaterials*, Vol.26, No.13, pp. 1467-1475, ISSN 0142-9612

Schliephake, H. (2002). Bone growth factors in maxillofacial skeletal reconstruction. *International Journal of Oral Maxillofacial Surgery* Vol.31, No.5, pp. 469-484, ISSN 0901-5027

Schliephake, H.; Aref, A.; Scharnweber, D.; Bierbaum, S.; Roessler, S. & Sewing, A. (2005). Effect of immobilized bone morphogenic protein 2 coating of titanium implants on peri-implant bone formation. *Clinical Oral Implants Research,* Vol.16, No.5, pp. 563-569, ISSN 0905-7161

Schliephake, H.; Aref, A.; Scharnweber, D.; Bierbaum, S. & Sewing, A. (2009). Effect of modifications of dual acid-etched implant surfaces on peri-implant bone formation. Part I: organic coatings. *Clinical Oral Implants Research,* Vol.20, No.1, pp. 31-37, ISSN 0905-7161

Schuler, M.; Owen, G.R.; Hamilton, D.W.; de Wild, M.; Textor, M.; Brunette, D.M.; Tosatti, S.G. (2006). Biomimetic modification of titanium dental implant model surfaces using the RGDSP-peptide sequence: a cell morphology study. *Biomaterials*, Vol.27, No.21, pp. 4003-4015, ISSN 0142-9612

Schulte, W. (1995). Implants and the periodontium. *International Dental Journal*, Vol.45, No.1, pp. 16-26, ISSN 0020-6539

Schwartz, Z.; Lohmann, C.H.; Sisk, M.; Cochran, D.L.; Sylvia, V.L.; Simpson, J.; Dean, D.D. & Boyan, B.D. (2001a). Local factor production by MG63 osteoblast-like cells in response to surface roughness and 1,25-(OH)2D3 is mediated via protein kinase C- and protein kinase A-dependent pathways. *Biomaterials*, Vol.22, No.7, pp. 731-741, ISSN 0142-9612

Schwartz, Z.; Lohmann, C.H.; Vocke, A.K.; Sylvia, V.L.; Cochran, D.L.; Dean, D.D. & Boyan, B.D. (2001b). Osteoblast response to titanium surface roughness and 1alpha,25-(OH)(2)D(3) is mediated through the mitogen-activated protein kinase (MAPK) pathway. *Journal of Biomedical Materials Research*, Vol.56, No.3, pp. 417-426, ISSN 0021-9304

Schwarz, F.; Ferrari, D.; Herten, M.; Mihatovic, I.; Wieland, M.; Sager, M. & Becker, J. (2007). Effects of surface hydrophilicity and microtopography on early stages of soft and hard tissue integration at nonsubmerged titanium implants: an immunohistochemical study in dogs. *Journal of Periodontology*, Vol.78, No.11, pp. 2171–2184, ISSN 0022-3492

Schwarz, F.; Wieland, M.; Schwartz, Z.; Zhao, G., Rupp, F.; Geis-Gerstorfer, J.; Schedle, A.; Broggini, N.; Bornstein, M.M.; Buser, D.; Ferguson, S.J.; Becker, J.; Boyan, B.D. & Cochran, D.L. (2009). Potential of chemically modified hydrophilic surface characteristics to support tissue integration of titanium dental implants. *Journal of Biomedical Materials Research Part B Applied Biomaterials*, Vol.88, No.2, pp. 544-557, ISSN 1552-4981

Sela, M.N.; Badihi, L.; Rosen, G.; Steinberg, D. & Kohavi, D. (2007). Adsorption of human plasma proteins to modified titanium surfaces. *Clinical Oral Implants Research*, Vol.18, No.5, pp. 630-638, ISSN 0905-7161

Shalabi, M.M.; Gortemaker, A.; Van't Hof, M.A.; Jansen, J.A. & Creugers, N.H. (2006). Implant surface roughness and bone healing: a systematic review. *Journal of Dental Research*, Vol.85, No.6, pp. 496-500, ISSN 0022-0345

Sjöström, T.; Dalby, M.J.; Hart, A.; Tare, R.; Oreffo, R.O. & Su, B. (2009). Fabrication of pillar-like titania nanostructures on titanium and their interactions with human skeletal stem cells. *Acta Biomaterialia*, Vol.5, No.5, pp. 1433-1441, ISSN 1742-7061

Stadlinger, B.; Pilling, E.; Huhle, M.; Mai, R.; Bierbaum, S.; Bernhardt, R.; Scharnweber, D.; Kuhlisch, E.; Hempel, U. & Eckelt, U. (2007). Influence of extracellular matrix coatings on implant stability and osseointegration: an animal study. *Journal of Biomedical Materials Research Part B, Applied Biomaterials*, Vol.83, No.1, pp. 222-231, ISSN 1552-4981

Stanford, C.M. & Keller, J.C. (1991). The concept of osseointegration and bone matrix expression. *Critical Reviews in Oral Biology and Medicine* Vol.2, No.1, pp.83-101, ISSN 1045-4411

Sul, Y.T.; Johansson, C.B.; Jeong, Y.; Röser, K.; Wennerberg, A. & Albrektsson, T. (2001). Oxidized implants and their influence on the bone response. *Journal of Materials Science. Materials in Medicine*, Vol.12, No.10-12, pp. 1025-31, ISSN 0957-4530

Sul, Y.T.; Johansson, C.; Wennerberg, A.; Cho, L.R.; Chang, B.S. & Albrektsson, T. (2005). Optimum surface properties of oxidized implants for reinforcement of osseointegration: surface chemistry, oxide thickness, porosity, roughness, and crystal structure. *The International Journal of Oral and Maxillofacial Implants*, Vol.20, No.3, pp. 349-359, ISSN 0882-2786

Sykaras, N.; Woody, R.D.; Lacopino, A.M.; Triplett, R.G. & Nunn, M.E. (2004). Osseointegration of dental implants complexed with rhBMP-2: a comparative histomorphometric and radiographic evaluation. *The International Journal of Oral and Maxillofacial Implants*, Vol.19, No.5, pp. 667-678, ISSN 0882-2786

Tosatti, S.; Schwartz, Z.; Campbell, C.; Cochran, D.L.; VandeVondele, S.; Hubbell, J.A.; Denzer, A.; Simpson, J.; Wieland, M.; Lohmann, C.H.; Textor, M. & Boyan, B.D. (2004). RGD-containing peptide GCRGYGRGDSPG reduces enhancement of osteoblast differentiation by poly(L-lysine)-graft-poly(ethylene glycol)-coated titanium surfaces. *Journal of Biomedical Materials Research Part A*, Vol.68, No.3, pp. 458-472, ISSN 1549-3296

Urabe, M.; Hosokawa, R.; Chiba, D., Sato, Y. & Akagawa, Y. (2000). Morphogenetic behavior of periodontium on inorganic implant materials: an experimental study of canines. *Journal of Biomedical Material Research*, Vol.49, No.1, pp. 17-24, ISSN 0021-9304

Vercaigne, S.; Wolke, J.G.; Naert, I. & Jansen, J.A. (1998) Bone healing capacity of titanium plasma-sprayed and hydroxylapatite-coated oral implants. *Clinical Oral Implants Research*, Vol.9, No.4, pp. 261-271, ISSN 0905-7161 von Wilmowsky, C.; Bauer, S.; Lutz, R.; Meisel, M.; Neukam, F.W.; Toyoshima, T.; Schmuki, P.; Nkenke, E. & Schlegel, K.A. (2009). In vivo evaluation of anodic TiO2 nanotubes: an experimental study in the pig. *Journal of Biomedical Materials Res Part B: Applied Biomaterials* Vol.89, No.1, pp. 165-171, ISSN 1552-4981

Warrer, K.; Karring, T. & Gotfredsen, K. (1993). Periodontal ligament formation around different types of dental titanium implants. I. The self-tapping screw type implant system. *Journal of Periodontology*, Vol.64, No.1, pp. 29-34, ISSN 0022-3492

Webster, T.J. & Ejiofor, J.U. (2004). Increased osteoblast adhesion on nanophase metals: Ti, Ti6Al4V, and CoCrMo. *Biomaterials*, Vol.25, No.19, pp. 4731-4739, ISSN 0142-9612

Webster, T.J.; Schadler, L.S.; Siegel, R.W. & Bizios, R. (2001). Mechanisms of enhanced osteoblast adhesion on nanophase alumina involve vitronectin. *Tissue Engineering*, Vol.7, No.3, pp. 291-301, ISSN 1076-3279

Wennerberg, A.; Albrektsson, T.; Johansson, C. & Andersson, B. (1996). Experimental study of turned and grit-blasted screw-shaped implants with special emphasis on effects of blasting material and surface topography. *Biomaterials*, Vol.17, No.1, pp.15-22, ISSN 0142-9612

Wennerberg, A. & Albrektsson, T. (2000) Suggested guidelines for the topographic evaluation of implant surfaces. *International Journal of Oral and Maxillofacial Implants*, Vol.15, No.3, pp. 331-344, ISSN 0882-2786

Wennerberg, A. & Albrektsson, T. (2009). Effects of titanium surface topography on bone integration: a systematic review. *Clinical Oral Implants Research*, Vol.20, Suppl.4, pp. 172-184, ISSN 1600-0501

Wenz, H.J.; Bartsch, J.; Wolfart, S. & Kern, M. (2008). Osseointegration and clinical success of zirconia dental implants: a systematic review. *International Journal of Prosthodontics* Vol.21, No.1, pp. 27-36, ISSN 0893-2174

Wheeler, S.L. (1996). Eight-year clinical retrospective study of titanium plasma-sprayed and hydroxyapatite-coated cylinder implants. *The International Journal of Oral and Maxillofacial Implants*, Vol.11, No.3, pp. 340-350, ISSN 0882-2786

Wikesjö, U.M.; Qahash, M.; Polimeni, G.; Susin, C.; Shanaman, R.H.; Rohrer, M.D.; Wozney, J.M. & Hall, J. (2008). Alveolar ridge augmentation using implants coated with recombinant human bone morphogenetic protein-2: histologic observations. *Journal of Clinical Periodontology*, Vol.35, No.11, pp. 1001-1010, ISSN 1600-051X

Yamagami, A.; Yoshihara, Y. & Suwa, F. (2005). Mechanical and histologic examination of titanium alloy material treated by sandblasting and anodic oxidization. *The International Journal of Oral Maxillofacial Implants*, Vol.20, No.1, pp. 48-53, ISSN 0882-2786

Yang, Y.; Cavin, R. & Ong, J.L. (2003). Protein adsorption on titanium surfaces and their effect on osteoblast attachment. *Journal of Biomedical Materials Research Part A*, Vol.67, No.1, pp. 344-349, ISSN 1549-3296

Zhao, X.; Liu, X. & Ding, C. (2005). Acid-induced bioactive titania surface. *Journal of Biomedical Materials Research Part A* Vol.75, No.4, pp. 888-894, ISSN 1549-3296

Zhao, G.; Raines, A.L.; Wieland, M.; Schwartz, Z. & Boyan, B.D. (2007). Requirement for both micron- and submicron scale structure for synergistic responses of osteoblasts to substrate surface energy and topography. *Biomaterials*, Vol.28, No.18, pp. 2821-2829, ISSN 0142-9612

2

State-of-the-Art Technology in Implant Dentistry: CAD/CAM

Ilser Turkyilmaz and Roxanna J. Nicoll
Department of Comprehensive Dentistry
University of Texas Health Science Center
San Antonio, Texas
United States of America

1. Introduction

Implant dentistry has come a long way since 1982 when Per-Ingvar Branemark first presented his work on osseointegration of endosseous dental implants (Branemark & Albrektsson, 1982). In the last three decades, the use of dental implants has increased exponentially (Friberg B & Jemt T, 2010; Turkyilmaz et al., 2010). Initially, very few specialists were trained in surgical placement and subsequent restoration. As the treatment became more predictable, the benefits of therapy became evident. The tremendous demand for implants has fueled a rapid expansion of the market. Presently, general dentists and multiple specialists offer implants as a solution to partial and complete edentulism. The field is evolving and expanding, from surgical techniques to types of restorations available. Whereas early implant restorations were primarily indicated for rehabilitation of function, increasing consideration is being placed on esthetics in modern implant dentistry.

1.1 Role of CAD/CAM in dental technology

Presently, there is a trend toward decreasing numbers of dental laboratory technicians in the United States. The number of dental technology programs in the U.S. has decreased by half since 1990 (Christensen, 2005). Conventional implant restorations are time and labor intensive, due to the multiple steps in fabrication, such as casting and fitting. Simultaneously, there is an increasing demand for efficient treatment that can be completed in minimal time— the "drive-thru" mentality of modern society. Fortunately, technology has kept up with this demand, and the application of CAD/CAM in implant dentistry is a promising solution (Valente et al., 2009; Van Assche et al., 2010).

Computer-aided design and computer-aided manufacturing (CAD/CAM) is being utilized in many fields besides dentistry. In the manufacturing industry, rapid prototyping using SLA modeling, which is a crisp, highly detailed CAM method, is used to produce prototypes (Jacobs, 1992; Ozan et al., 2009). Frequent applications of SLA technology are highly detailed and accurate medical models, master patterns for casting and even soft tissue facial prostheses. Several authors have suggested that CAD/CAM may improve the accuracy of dental implant planning and placement (Sarment, 2003; Tardieu, 2003; Van Assche et al., 2010; Arisan et al.,2010; Mandelaris et al., 2010). An extension of this application is the ability to prefabricate dental prosthesis prior to the implant surgery.

1.2 Range of implant-supported restorations

Dental implants can support many types of dental restorations, ranging from a single tooth to a full-arch fixed bridge. The prosthetic design must take into consideration many factors, including number of teeth to be replaced, biomechnical considerations regarding how many implants are necessary to support the restoration, functional considerations such as the occlusal scheme and opposing dentition or restoration, and relative cost of the restorative materials. Implant based restorations can be either fixed or removable, depending on the patient's desires, ability to perform adequate hygiene, and whether adequate support can be achieved by the implants alone, without additional support of the soft tissue. The final prosthetic design must account for all the individual patient variables, take into consideration the best available evidence regarding long-term prognosis, and ideally meet the patient's expectations for both esthetics and function.

1.3 Edentulism and role of implant-based restorations

Considering the range or restorations available, implants can serve the greatest utility when considering complete dentures. Conventional dentures have significant functional limitations when compared to natural teeth. Masticatory performance of people wearing complete dentures is less than 20% of those with natural dentition (Kapur & Soman, 1964). Patients commonly report pain, areas of discomfort, poor denture stability and difficulties eating as reasons for dissatisfaction with conventional dentures (Allen & McMillan, 2003). However, there are many clinical factors that may affect the overall function and patient satisfaction with conventional complete dentures, such as residual ridge height, salivary flow, and technical quality of the dentures (Turkyilmaz et al., 2010). It is therefore essential that a thorough clinical examination of the patient and any existing prostheses be coupled with a detailed patient interview about masticatory performance of the existing prostheses and impact on quality of life. This information is vital to proper treatment planning and consideration of one of the many possible implant-based restorations including a two-implant overdenture with ball or locator attachments, a bar overdenture supported by two or four implants, or a completely implant supported fixed hybrid denture.

Many authors have investigated the impact of implant supported dentures compared to conventional dentures. A clinical study by Awad et. al.(2003), included 104 edentulous adults, aged 35 to 65 years. Patients were randomly assigned to one of two groups that received either a mandibular conventional denture or a two-implant bar overdenture. Patients rated their general satisfaction and specific factors of both their previous dentures, as well as their new prosthesis at 2 months post-delivery. Oral health-related quality of life was also evaluated pre- and post-treatment. The mean general satisfaction of the implant-overdenture group was significantly higher than the conventional denture group. The implant-overdenture group also rated comfort, stability, and ease of chewing better than the conventional group. The conclusion of this study was that a mandibular implant-supported overdenture opposing a maxillary complete denture was more satisfactory than conventional dentures.

Heydecke et al.(2005), studies the impact of mandibular two-implant overdentures compared to conventional complete dentures on leisure and sexual activities. This study of 102 patients found social activity was improved with implant-supported overdentures compared to conventional dentures. Implant-supported dentures including either complete overdentures or a hybrid prosthesis significantly improve the quality of life for edentulous patients compared with conventional complete removable complete dentures.

It is true that people are keeping their teeth longer than in the past. Measures such as oral hygiene, access to care and water fluoridation are having a positive impact on oral health in this country. The decrease in percentage of edentulous adults over the past 20 years has prompted some educators to propose that complete dentures be removed from the dental curriculum (Turkyilmaz et al., 2010). However, it appears that the decrease in rates of edentulism among older adults is insufficient to offset the growing US population.

Several trends are apparent when relating the US Census data from 1991-2020. The population projections from the 1996 Statistical Abstracts of the United States illustrate these trends. The total adult population will increase significantly from 187,020,000 to 245,139,000 people. The number of adults aged from 55 to 74 years will increase by 86%. The number of adults aged 75 and older will increase by 61%. Thus the US population of older adults will grow dramatically over the next 12 years. Estimated decreases in the percentage of edentulism for maxillary and mandibular arches for each age group of 10% for year 2000, 20% for year 2010, and 30% for year 2020 (Weintraub & Burt, 1985). Even if a decrease in edentulism is assumed, an increase in the actual number of adults will result in an increase in the number of dentures needed over the next 12 years. Actually, the 2010 US Census reported 308,745,538 residents, which indicates a significant increase compared to the predicted number (245,139,000).

We can conclude that there will be a significant need for denture therapy, and that implant dentistry has the potential to dramatically improve the quality of life for those edentulous patients. Further, a range of treatment is available for improving the function, from two-implant overdenture with mechanical attachments to a fully fixed-detachable hybrid prosthesis.

1.4 Patient demand and knowledge regarding implant therapy

The number of implants placed has been increasing significantly each year, (about 18% in the USA) (Turkyilmaz et al., 2010). Improved implant surfaces and surgical techniques have led to a marked increase in predictability. This has resulted in a tremendous demand. The demand for implant therapy has fueled growth of the industry, and now many clinicians offer implant therapy, not just specialists. Problems with implants have been raising as more clinicians who do not have advanced training and skills have been involved in implant placement. Unfortunately, little quantitative data regarding implant complications related to level of training are available.

Consecutive surveys of the Australian population showed that patient awareness of implant dentistry is increasing (Pommer et al., 2011). Most patient's trust their general dentist for information regarding implant therapy, while one quarter turn to the media. Overall, the level of knowledge is satisfactory. The exception is patient's unrealistic expectations. Patient's demand for high-quality restorations has increased, and the majority felt that practice of implant dentistry should be limited to specialists.

Similar trends regarding increasing patient awareness in the United States have been observed. However, due to the increasing prevalence of direct marketing, more patients are relying on media and internet sources for information regarding implant therapy. Advertisement has contributed to patient's unrealistic expectations regarding treatment times, and led to significant confusion regarding the range of treatment options available. Few resources are available to assist patient's in understanding of the variety of implant restorations along with the advantages and disadvantages of each.

1.5 Success criteria for implant therapy

Objective evaluation of the treatment outcome is paramount in order to ensure predictability and excellent long-term prognosis. The first criteria for success were proposed by Albrektsson et. al., in 1986. However, success and failure lie at opposite ends of a spectrum. In order to better elucidate the actual condition of an implant, not just it's presence in the mouth, the Health Scale for Dental Implants was developed (Misch et al., 2008). This scale consists of four categories: success with optimum health, satisfactory survival, compromised survival, and failure. The clinical indices evaluated in this scale include pain, mobility, radiographic bone loss, probing depths, and peri-implant disease. Optimum health is defined as the absence of pain or tenderness on function, zero mobility, less than 2 mm of radiographic bone loss from time of placement, and no history of exudate. At the other end of the spectrum is absolute or clinical failure, in which any of the following are present: pain on function, mobility, radiographic bone loss greater than 1/2 the length of the implant, uncontrolled exudate, or the implant is no longer in the mouth.

1.6 Treatment planning for implant-based restorations

The first phase of implant dentistry is planning. It is insufficient to identify an edentulous space, or missing tooth, and simply initiate surgery. First, a diagnostic wax-up of the proposed tooth form and ideal location must be achieved. From this, a radiographic guide is fabricated that simulates the wax-up. Next, diagnostic imaging must be done in order to determine the alveolar bone available for implant placement. Traditional radiographs including periapical films and panoramic films are helpful, but limited in application due their two dimensional nature and potential distortion. In 1972, the invention of computed tomography revolutionized medical and dental imaging. It became possible to obtain 3-dimensional digital images, thus an accurate assessment of the height and width of alveolar bone available for implant placement.

This 3-dimensional image is the basis of establishing the treatment plan. It allows a practitioner to identify potential implant sites, measure the height and width of the available bone, and the necessary restorative space for the planned prosthesis and the components. If bone grafting, such as sinus augmentation, is necessary in order to position implants properly for a given prosthetic design, the necessary procedures can be incorporated into the treatment plan. Basically, this 3-dimensional image gives both the clinician and the patient a better idea of the limitations that will be encountered at the time of surgery, ensuring better predictability of both the surgery and the final prosthetic outcome.

2. CAD/CAM technology- surgical guides

CAD/CAM technology takes implant planning a step further, and enables fabrication of a surgical guide (Figure 1). The surgical guide directs the surgeon in the exact location and angulation to place the implant. There is a growing number of software programs that allow viewing and analysis of the 3D images and subsequent fabrication of a surgical guide.

In the youth of implant dentistry, the treatment was surgically driven, meaning that the implant was placed according to the bone available at the time of surgery. This approach eventually proved erroneous, because many implants were placed in locations and angulations that made them difficult or impossible to restore. The evolution of the field has led to a restoratively-driven approach, where the restorative dentist communicates the desired position and angulation via a surgical guide. Conventional surgical guides, however, have some significant limitations.

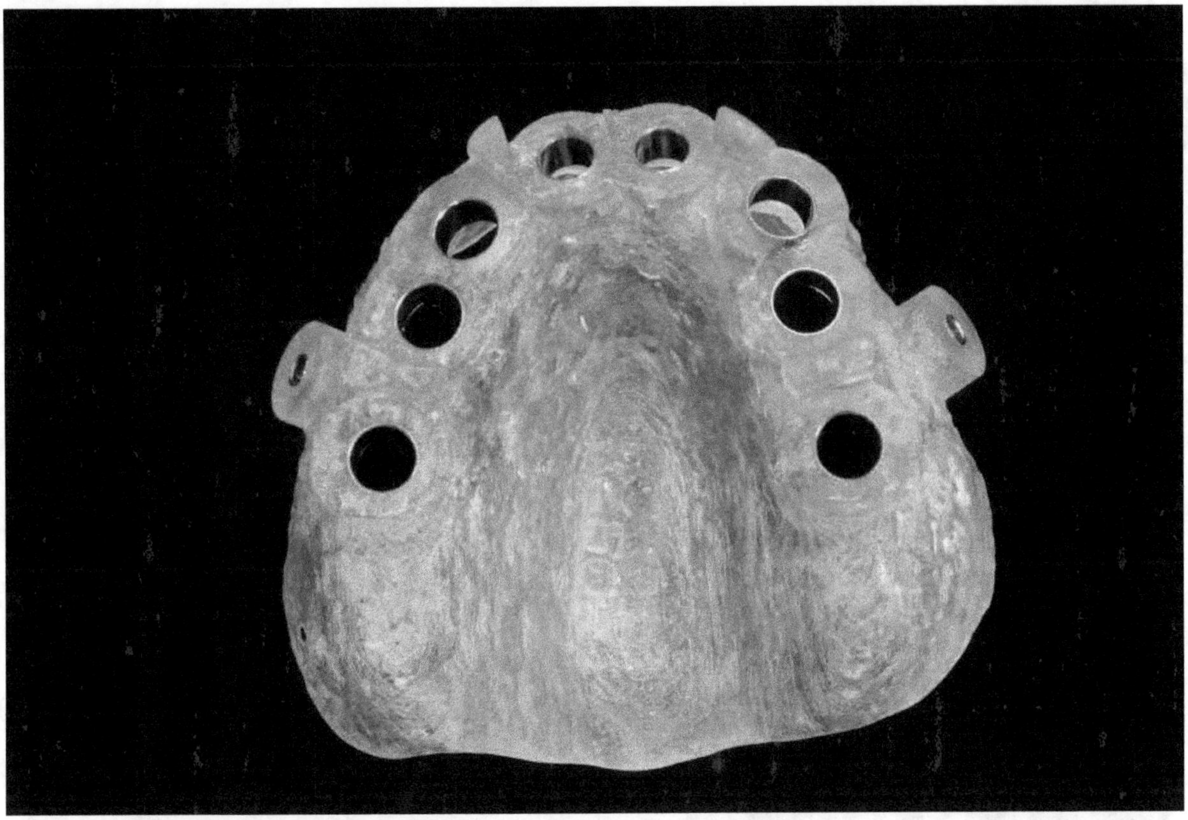

Fig. 1. Example of CAD/CAM surgical guide for implant placement.

2.1 Surgical guides for implant placement

Computer-assisted planning and use of CAM surgical guides dramatically increases the accuracy of implant placement, which directly improves the outcome of the final restoration. These surgical guides help the surgeon avoid vital structures, and may decrease the length of the surgery. Furthermore, it assures the restorative dentist and dental technician a functional, esthetic, and predictable outcome. Equally important, CAD/CAM design and fabrication of guides improves the patient's experience with implants. CAD/CAM allows the possibility of flapless surgery, which entails less bleeding, less swelling, decreased healing time and post-operative pain (Fortin et al., 2006).

There are three broad categories of surgical guides: conventional, SLA fabricated, and cast-fabricated. Conventional implies it was the method employed prior to CAD/CAM, but with the rapid evolution of the field, the term conventional is unclear, and encompasses a large variety of techniques. One specific conventional technique for surgical guide fabrication entails fabricating a scanning template or radiographic guide, usually tooth-borne. Then, according to the findings of the CBCT, identifying reference points that allow orientation of the radiographic guide on a surveyor table in conjunction with a drill press to create the pilot hole that will guide the surgeon. This technique, since it is the opposite of digital, is coined "analog".

The major distinction between the two types of CAD/CAM surgical guides lies in the fabrication. SLA guides are purely CAD/CAM, whereas cast-fabricated are initially made on a stone model, then a computerized version of the surveyor and drill press create the pilot holes based on the digitally planned implant placement. Each has its advantages and disadvantages. The SLA process leaves topographic seams, which may not fit the occlusal and axial anatomy of a tooth. If the surgical guide does not fit precisely and accurately, the surgical result may be compromised. A surgical guide that is fabricated on a stone model, however, can be tried in intra-orally and verified prior to the CBCT scan and subsequent conversion into a surgical guide.

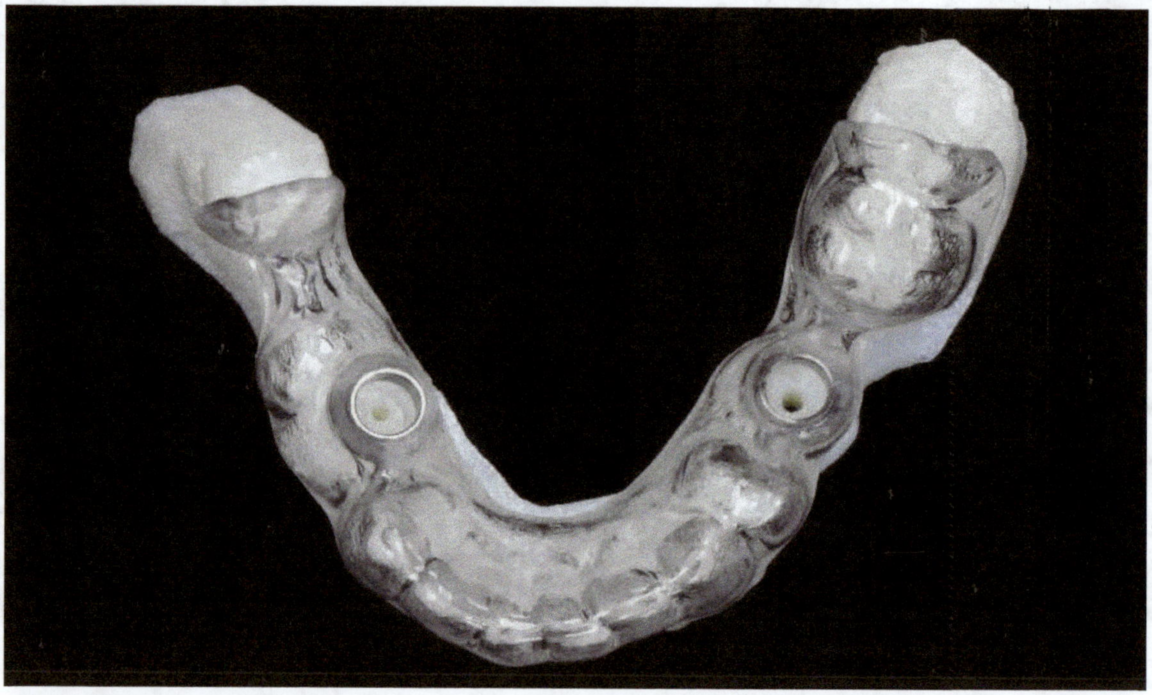

Fig. 2. A tooth-supported CAD/CAM surgical guide on the cast.

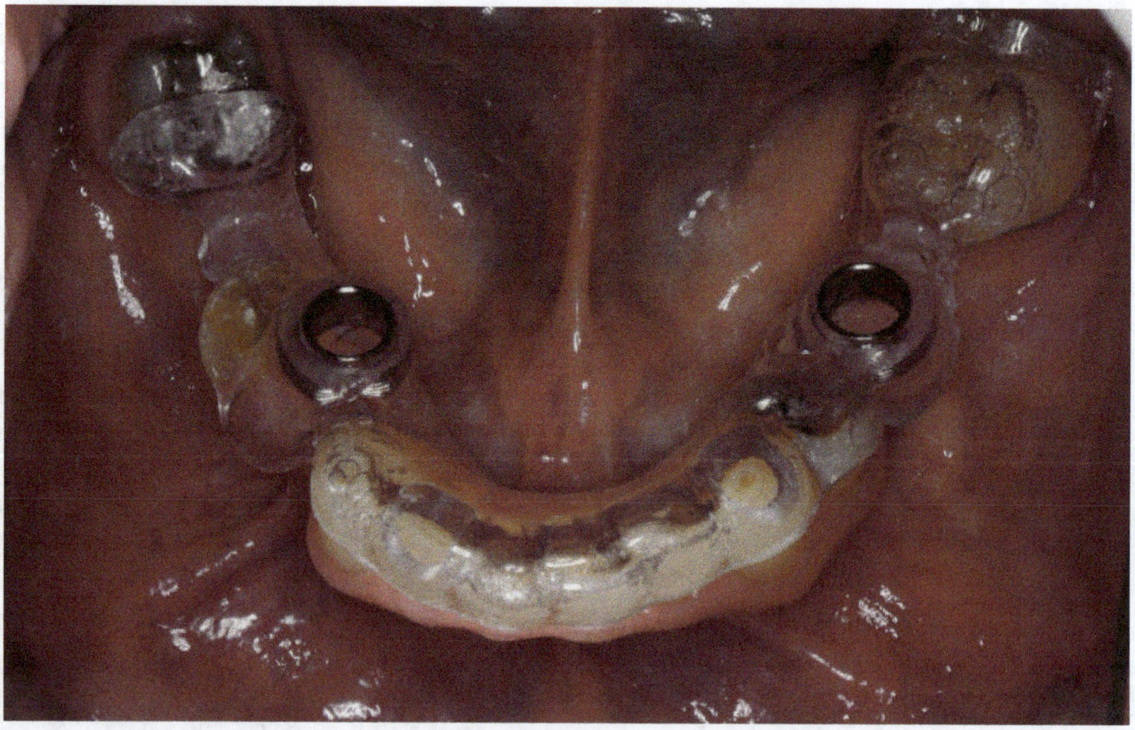

Fig. 3. A tooth-supported CAD/CAM surgical guide seated on the teeth.

2.2 Type of support for implant surgical guides

Surgical guides can also be classified according to the type of support: bone, mucosa, tooth (Figures 2,3), or combination tooth-mucosa. The choice of which type of support depends on many factors, such as the number of teeth remaining in the arch, whether the mandibular or maxillary arch is being treated, and the anatomy of the edentulous or partially edentulous ridge. Teeth offer a very stable support for a surgical guide, but the complex topography of the occlusal surface may make increase the time required to fit the surgical guide to the mouth. Soft tissue, is by definition compressible and displaceable to varying degrees. Extra measures must be taken to ensure that a mucosa-supported surgical guide is positioned accurately to ensure surgical success.

2.3 Software for implant planning and surgical guide fabrication

Presently, there are a multitude of software programs for virtual placement of implants and subsequent fabrication of surgical guides. The most well-known are Procera from Nobel Biocare and Simplant by Materialise, but many more have recently been introduced to the market. Each software platform varies in the types of guides available and which implant system it is compatible with. Procera NobelGuide includes mucosa and tooth based guides and is strictly compatible with Nobel Biocare implants. Simplant offers bone, tooth, or mucosa based guides and is can be employed with virtually any implant system. Each software presents it's own limitations and challenges; cost is also a consideration for the clinician. All of the current software programs are based on algorithms for medical CT, not CBCT, which may influence interpretation of the data. In addition, the corresponding surgical kit for each implant system may or may not offer depth control, which will ultimately influence the surgical outcome.

2.4 Accuracy of guided implant surgery

The accuracy of CAD/CAM surgical guides has been investigated with in vitro, human cadaver, and clinical studies. The available research supports the hypothesis that guided surgery is accurate, with certain limitations. Ersoy et. al.(2008), placed 94 implants using SLA surgical guides generated from CT. CT images were obtained with radiographic templates in place, and implants were placed virtually. SLA surgical guides including bone-based, mucosa-support, and tooth-support were then fabricated and used for implant surgery. Following implant placement, a new CT scan was taken. Special software was employed to overlay the planned placement with the post-surgical outcome, matching anatomical markers. This allows analysis of the outcome in three dimensions. The mean linear deviation was 1.22 ± 0.85 mm at the implant neck and 1.51 ± 1 mm at the implant apex. In general, a greater distance between simulated and actual implants was observed at the implant apex than at the implant neck. The mean angular deviation in long axis between the planned and placed implants was 4.9 ± 2.36 degrees.

Careful consideration must be given to the mean error, versus actual error for an individual patient. In the previous study, the mean angular deviation was 4.9 degrees, but the actual error for one patient was 9 degrees. Depending on the available height and width of the alveolus, this error could result in dehiscence of the bone and eventual failure of the implant.

In vitro studies such as Besimo et al. (2005), aimed to determine the magnitude of error in transferring the planned position of implants from CT scans to a surgical guide. The deviation between the positions of the apex of the proposed implants in cross-sectional CT images and on the corresponding study cast was measured in 77 prospective sites in five maxillae and nine mandibles. The transfer error was 0.6 ± 0.4 mm in the maxilla and 0.3 ± 0.4 mm in the mandible. However, they concluded that the transfer errors found in their study were not clinically relevant as their study was an in vitro study. They also stated that other factors involved in transferring positional and angular measurements from CT images to the surgical area may result in greater errors.

Little evidence is available regarding the accuracy of guided surgery compared to conventional implant placement, using the analog technique for guide fabrication. Sarment et al.(2003), placed 50 implants into five epoxy edentulous mandibles. Each epoxy mandible received five implants in each side. On the right side, five implants were placed using a conventional surgical guide (control side), while on the left side, five implant were placed using a stereolithographic surgical guide (test side). They found a statistically significant improvement in all measurements when SLA surgical guides were used compared to conventional guides and suggested that the clinical significance of this result may be relevant when multiple parallel distant implants are placed, and where the degree of accuracy is critical to obtain a single prosthetic path of insertion. They also reported, when the control surgical guide was used, the center of the osteotomy was 1.5 ± 0.7 mm away from the center of the planned implant at coronal end and 2.1 ± 0.97 mm at the apex. When the test appliance was used, these distances were 0.9 ± 0.5 mm at the implant head and 1 ± 0.6 mm at the apex.

The available evidence suggests that CAD/CAM surgical guides are relatively accurate, but more research is needed in this area. Better data on the possible error will ultimately improve clinical judgement and case selection. This could potentially reduce or even eliminate error.

2.5 Guidelines for CAD/CAM guided surgery

Currently there are no published guidelines regarding indications for flapless surgery versus a conventional open-flap surgery. It is clear from Sarment's study (2003) that the use of a CAD/CAM guide can increase the accuracy of implant placement, and when used in an open-flap surgery, the surgeon has the capacity to intercept potential error by visualizing the bone and implant directly. Thus, in an open-flap surgery, CAD/CAM surgical guides are superior to conventional guides.

The decision of whether to perform a flapless surgery depends on many factors. Patient comfort, decreased healing time, maintenance of blood supply, and decreased surgical time are all advantages of flapless surgery. The accuracy of implant placement required depends in large part on the type of restoration planned. For example, an implant-overdenture has a medium level of accuracy necessary, in that linear and angular deviations can be accommodated by the attachment system. A fixed restoration, on the other hand, has a significantly lower degree of freedom, and may indicate CAD/CAM guided surgery in order to maximize the precision of implant placement.

The type of template support is also an important consideration. Flapless surgery can be accomplished with a tooth-born guide, a tooth-tissue born guide, or a purely tissue-supported guide. The number of teeth, condition of the tissue, and morphology of the residual ridge will all affect the overall stability of the guide and the accuracy of placement, which directly impact the accuracy of implant placement. A good rule of thumb for an edentulous arch is if the denture has reasonable stability and resistance to lateral dislodging forces, a tissue-supported surgical guide will have the same degree of stability. In general, a maxillary denture is more stable than a mandibular denture. In addition, the opposing dentition or prosthesis can aid in predictable placement which will increase the accuracy.

It is reasonable to incorporate the mean accuracy of guided systems into a set of guidelines, particularly for flapless surgery. For example, if the average linear deviation is 1.22-1.51 mm, and 1 mm of bone is necessary buccal and lingual to the implant, one can conclude that the alveolar ridge must be wide enough to accommodate both the implant and the potential error. This window of safety may vary based on the stability of surgical guide, which relates back to the type of support and the stability of the scanned template from which the surgical guide is patterned. Establishing guidelines based on the available is imperative, but ultimately clinical judgement must be the final determinate.

Immediate loading and pre-fabricated provisional restorations are other advantages of CAD/CAM surgical guides. By using a CAD/CAM surgical guide, a pre-fabricated provisional restoration can be delievered immediately after implant placement, which increases the patients' self-confidence dramatically. The pictures of one of our patients using NobelGuide and a maxillary provisonal restoration (screw-retained fixed dental prosthesis) have been presented below (Figures 4-13).

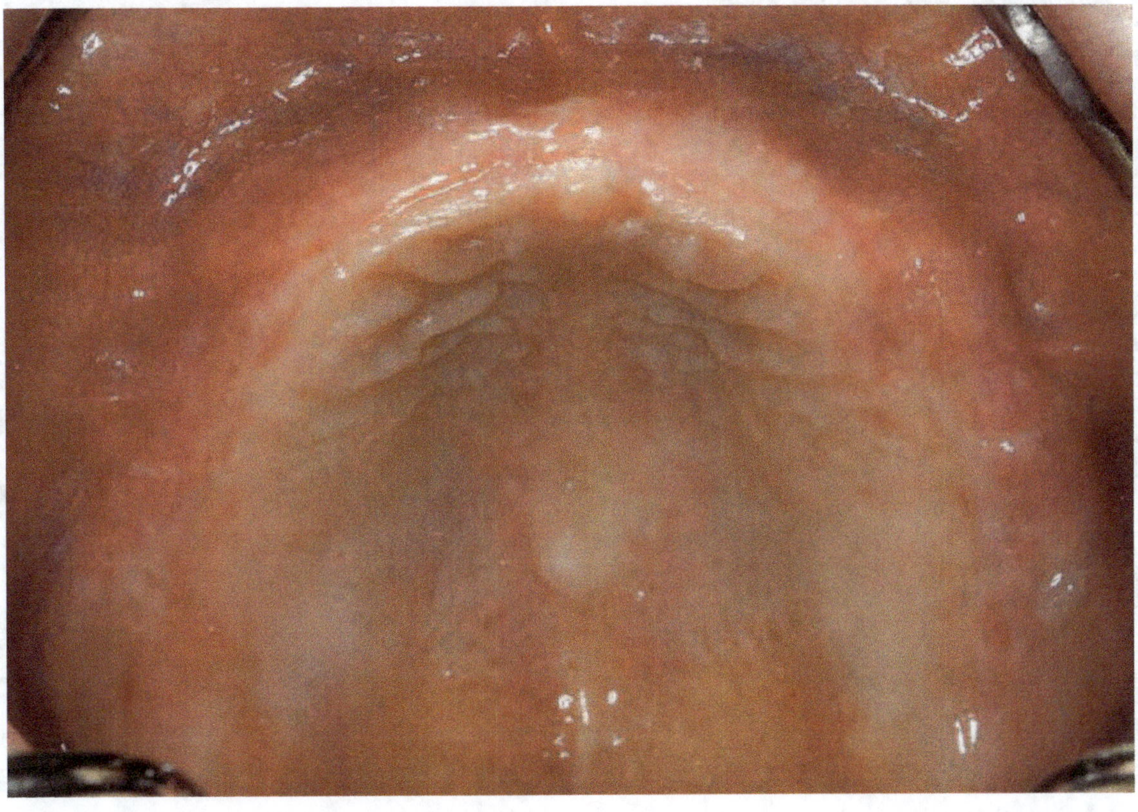

Fig. 4. Occlusal view of edentulous maxilla.

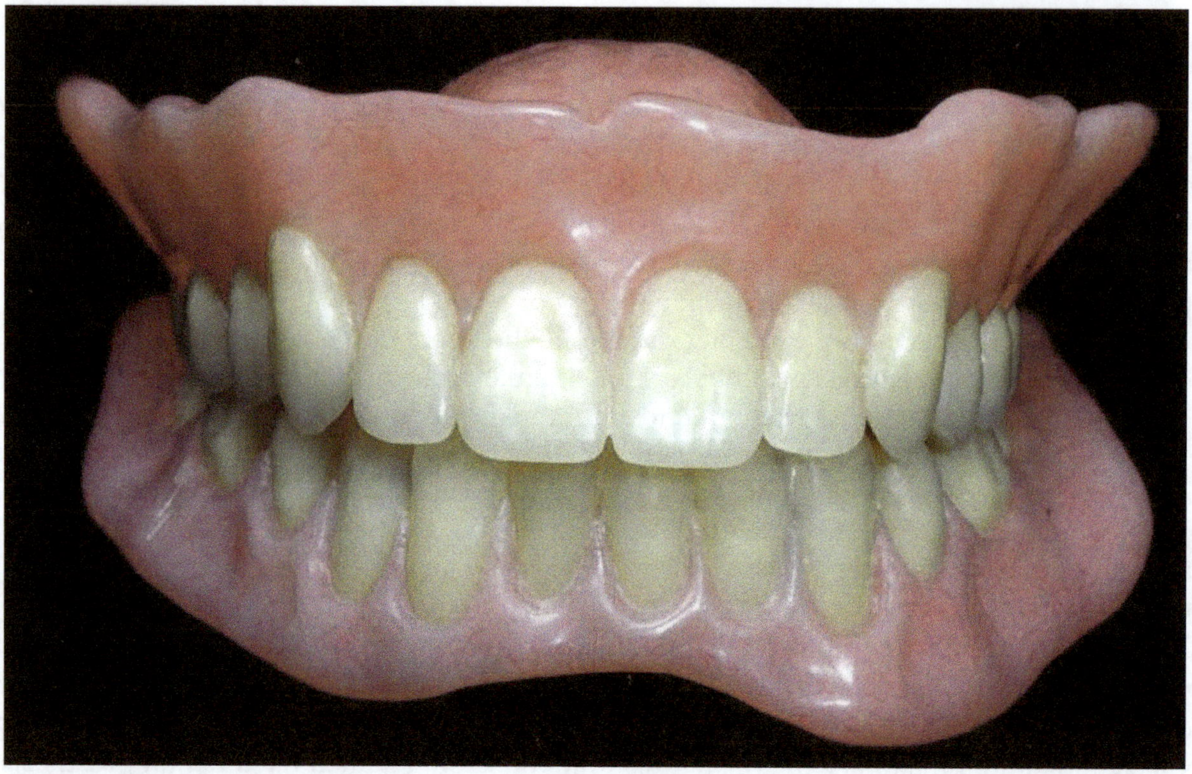

Fig. 5. Implant diagnostic dentures to serve as radiographic template for implant planning and surgical guide fabrication.

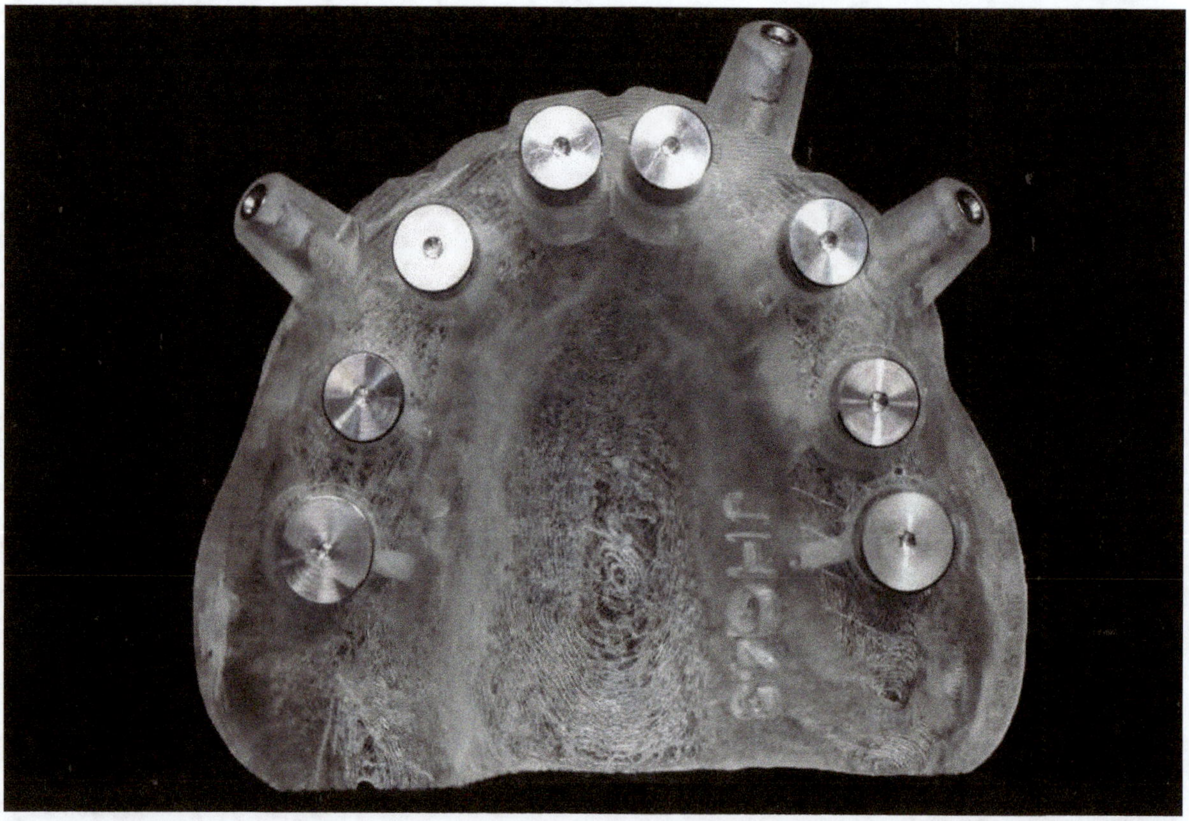

Fig. 6. NobelGuide: steriolithographic surgical guide for flapless implant placement.

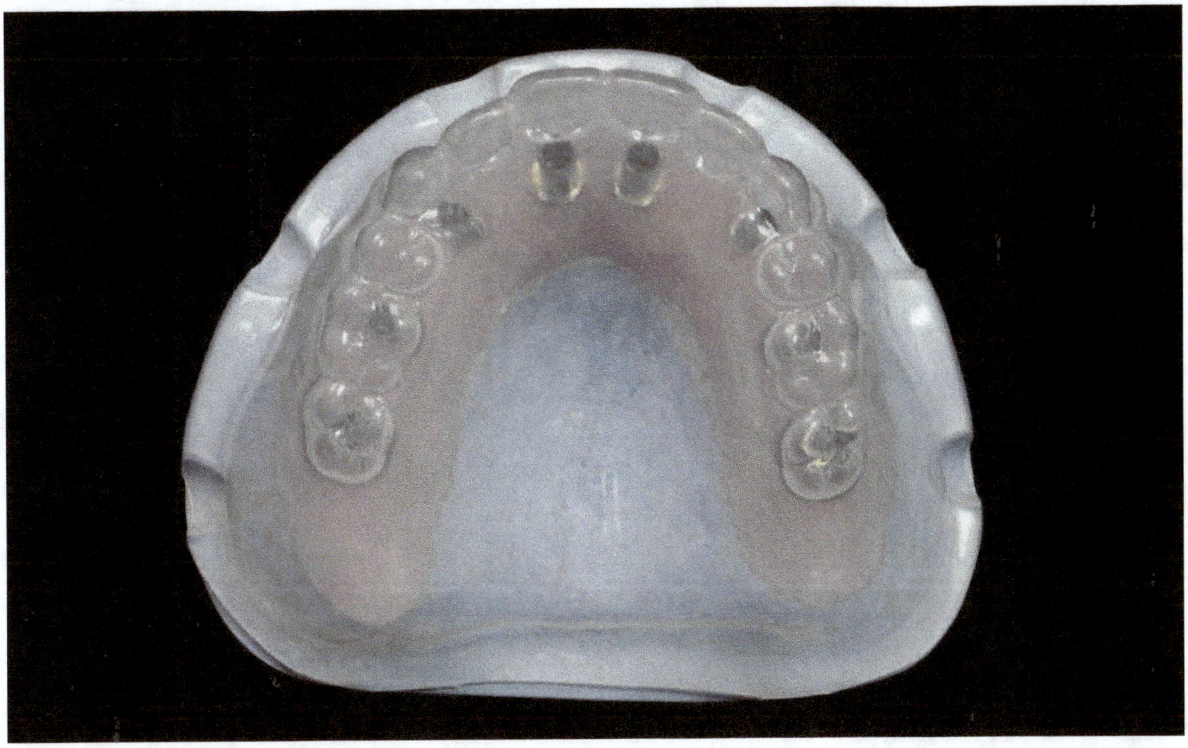

Fig. 7. Pre-surgical fabrication of cast with implant analogs, temporary abutments, and clear matrix of diagnostic tooth arrangement.

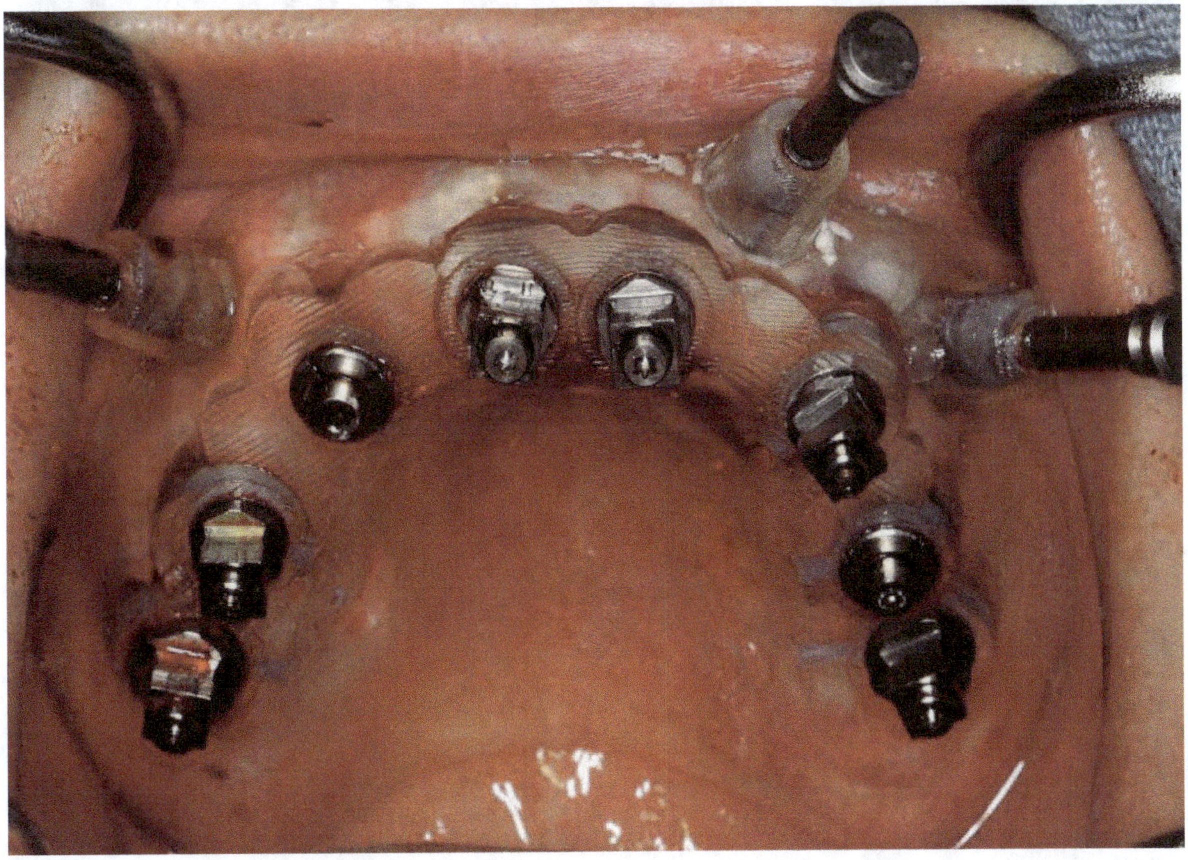

Fig. 8. NobelGuide and fixation pins at time of surgery.

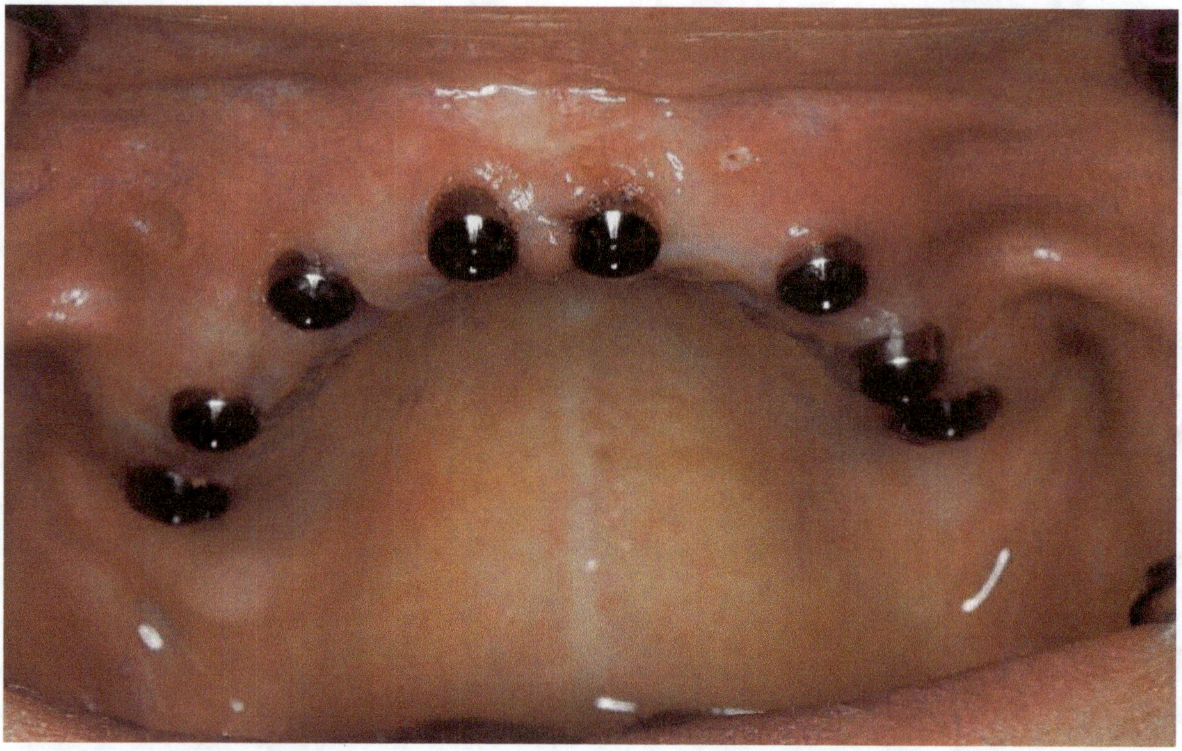

Fig. 9. Immediately post-op following flapless guided implant placement using NobelGuide.

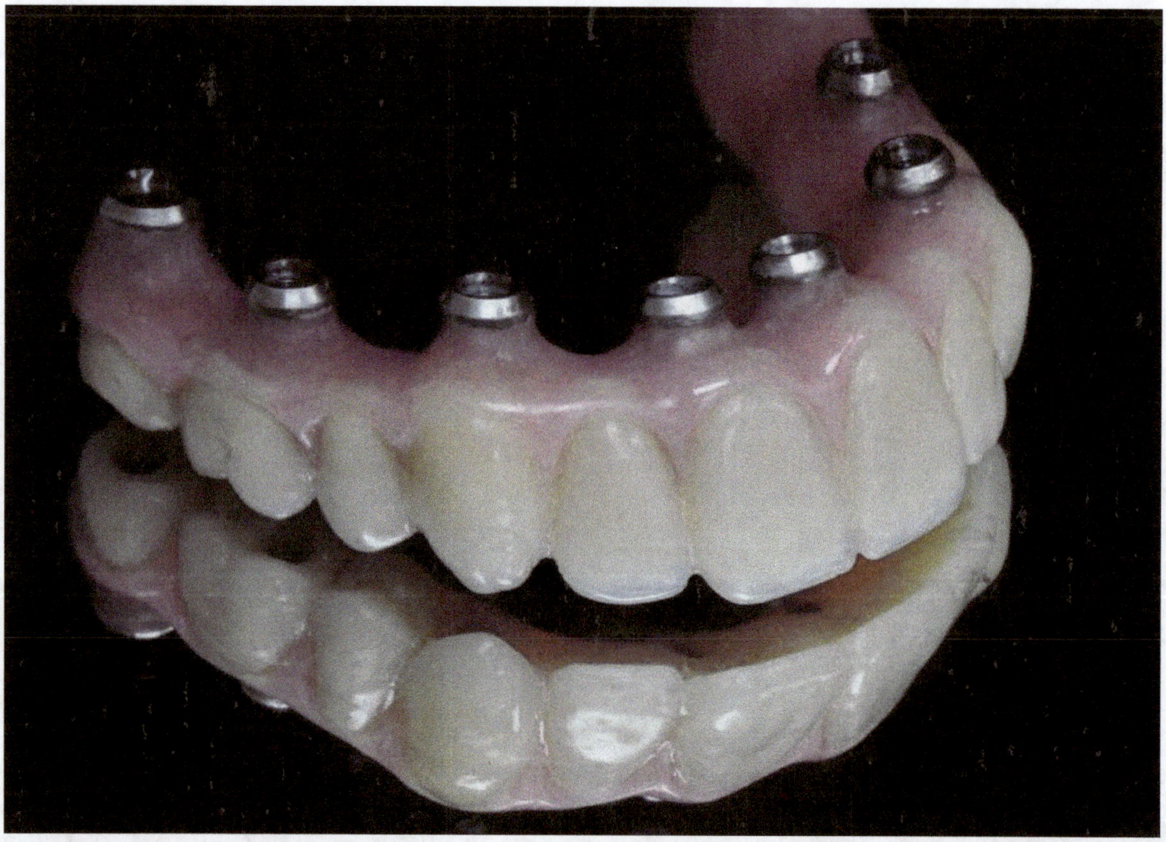

Fig. 10. Diagnostic denture converted into immediate fixed provisional for immediate loading.

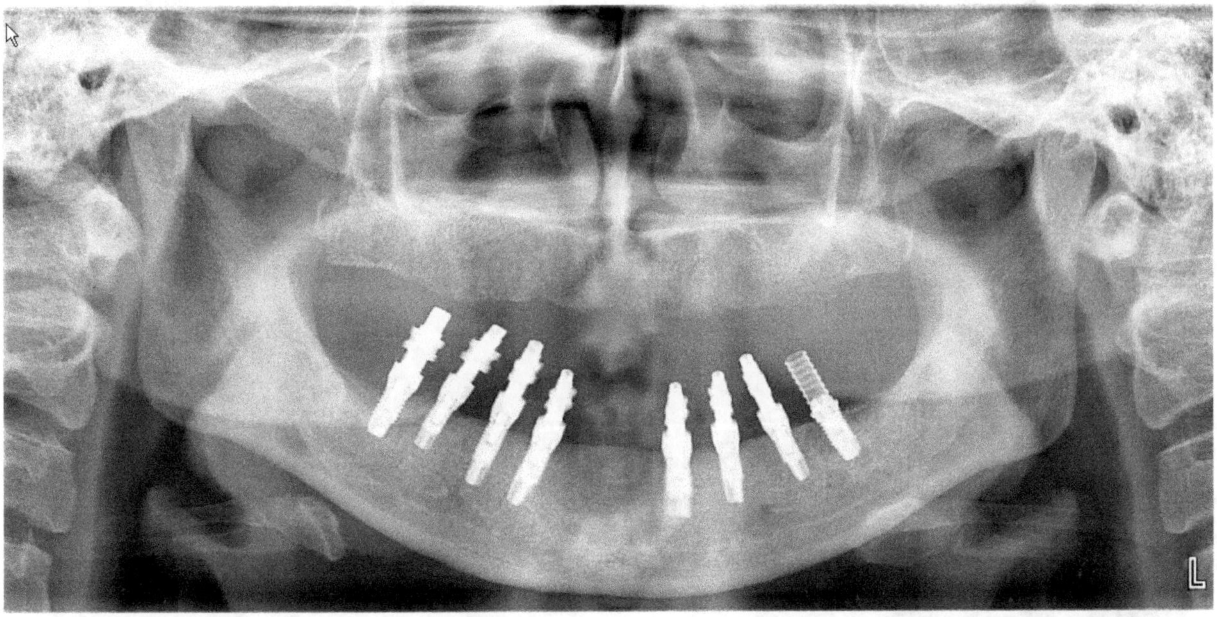

Fig. 11. Pre-operative panoramic image of edentulous maxilla.

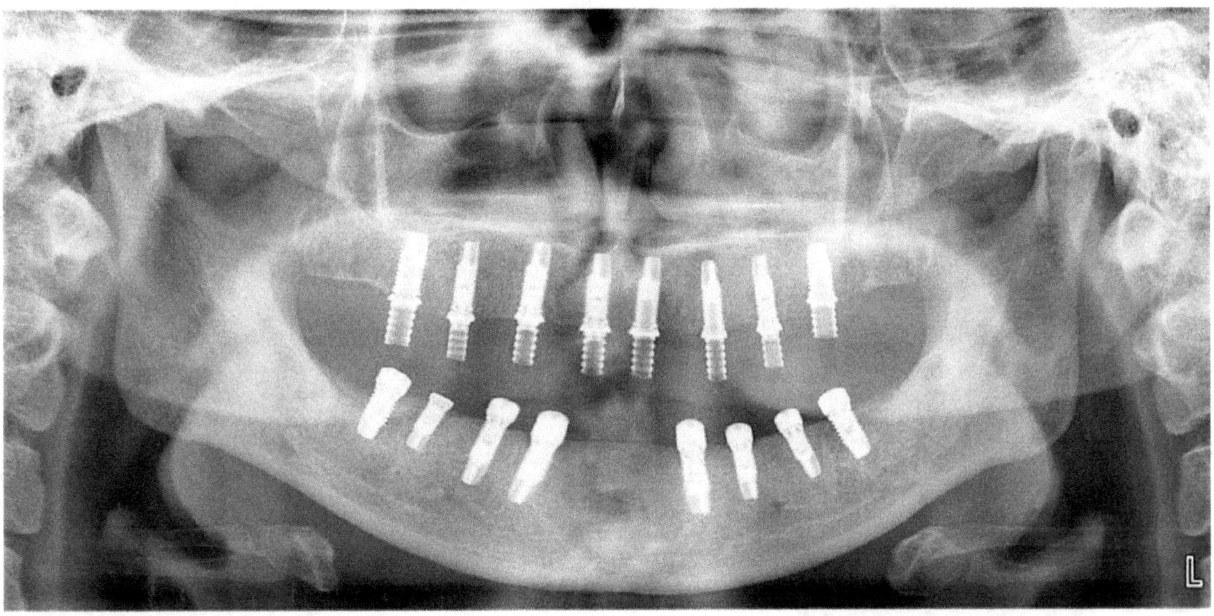

Fig. 12. Post-operative panoramic image following guided implant placement and immediate provisionalization.

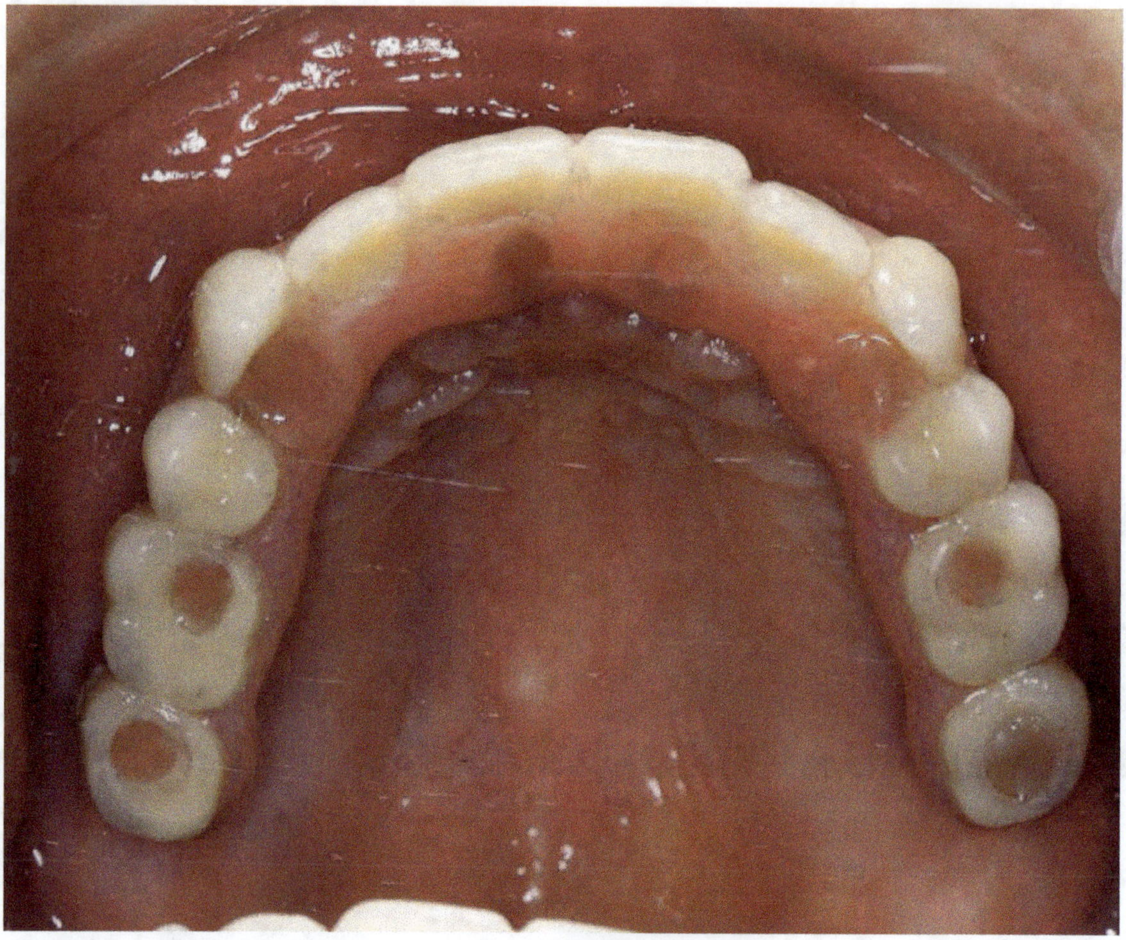

Fig. 13. Occlusal view of immediately loaded maxillary implants.

3. CAD/CAM technology- bars & frameworks

CAD/CAM technology has significantly improved the restorative aspects of implant dentistry as well. Implant restorations can be supported or retained by individual attachments, splinted with a bar for an overdenture, or splinted by a framework that supports a fixed restoration such as a hybrid. Prior to CAD/CAM, bars and frameworks had to be cast from gold alloy.

3.1 Conventional framework fabrication

Traditional castings have a major limitation inherent in the process, which is distortion of the casting with increasing size of the pattern (Takahashi & Gunne, 2003; Al-Fadda et al., 2007). Osseointegrated implants lack a periodontal ligament, thus tolerance of fit is greatly reduced when comparing tooth-supported cast restorations to implant-supported restorations. Single and two implant restorations can be cast within this tolerance, because the distortion is limited based on size. Full arch restorations, however, are difficult to cast successfully. Over the years, a multitude of casting corrective procedures have been employed, including sectioning and soldering, laser welding, and electric discharge machining.

CAD/CAM fabrication of bars and frameworks has resulted in elimination of distortion, better fit, fewer fabrication steps, and faster turn-around (Ortorp & Jemt, 2000; Takahashi &

Gunne, 2003; Al-Fadda et al., 2007). The workflow for creating a CAD/CAM bar starts with an accurate impression and model including the implant analogs. The model containing the implant analogs is then scanned, and then the CAD portion begins. Currently, bars and frameworks can be milled from titanium or zirconium. Titanium is abundant on Earth and offers a significant cost savings relative to gold.

3.2 Prosthetic designs and space allocation

There are several prosthetics designs with dental implants (Figure 14). Overdentures, whether supported by a conventional cast gold bar or a CAD/CAM titanium bar, are space intensive, due to the multiple components involved. Careful planning is necessary to ensure that the implants are placed in the correct position, and there is adequate restorative space for the soft tissue, the implant-supported bar, attachment system, overcasting or prosthetic framework, artificial teeth and pink acrylic base.

The exact amount of restorative space depends on the specific prosthetic design and the restorative materials employed. The issue of space allocation can be addressed in the planning stage for implant placement, utilizing the scan template in order to calculate the distance between the alveolar crest and the occlusal surface. Some authors have advocated 8-12 mm of crown-height space for fixed restorations and greater than 12 mm for removable prostheses (Misch et al., 2005). More specific recommendations based on the specific prosthetic design are 6-8 mm for single implant crown, 8-12 mm for locator retained overdentures, 10-14 mm for acrylic hybrid restoration, and 12-14 mm for a bar-supported overdenture. In actuality, the various prosthetic components exist in three-dimensions, thus linear measurements can only serve as guidelines to ensure adequate restorative space.

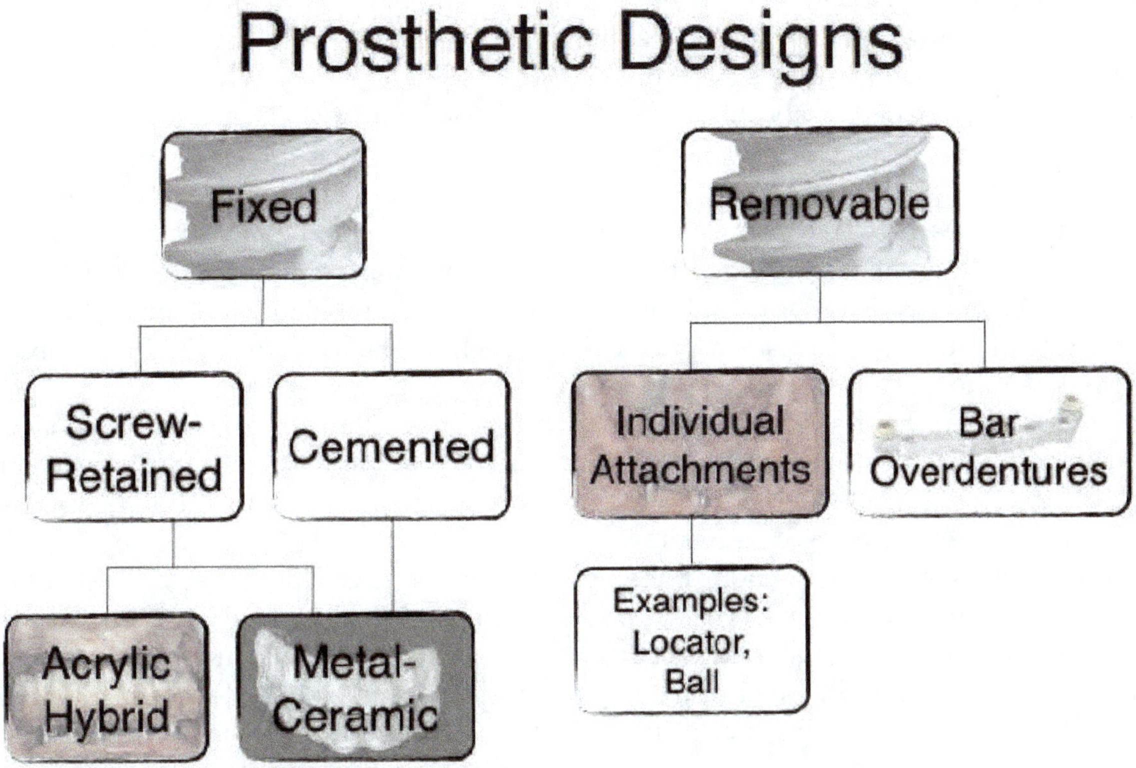

Fig. 14. Classification of prosthetic designs.

Many of the newer software platforms are incorporating virtual abutments so that components can be pre-selected and ordered at the same time as the surgical guide.
Prosthetic design is also influenced by material compatibility. Certain materials are conducive to CAD/CAM while others are not. Titanium and zirconia are well suited for CAM techniques, whereas gold is not. Conversely, porcelain systems developed for gold alloys have been used for many years with a high degree of success, whereas the newer porcelain systems developed for veneering titanium and zirconia lack long term clinical data. For example, a 6 year follow-up on porcelain fused to titanium fixed dental prostheses revealed that titanium PFMs had a 84% survival after six years, compared to a 98% survival for gold alloy PFMs (Walter et al.,1999). As porcelain systems continue to be improved, the applicability of CAD/CAM in implant dentistry will increase.

3.3 Passive fit

Critical to the long term success of implant based restorations is careful consideration of the biomechanics involved. Following osseointegration and placement of a final restoration, both functional and parafunctional loads can be transfered to the implants that may affect remodeling of the bone-implant interface. In the case of splinted implant restorations, it is possible that the restoration itself may transmit strain to the bone-implant interface. Ideally, the restoration would fit passively on the supporting implants, thus minimizing strain and the concomitant biological response.
The concept of passive fit was considered even in early applications of implant-based restorations. The original Branemark design consisted of five implants placed in the anterior mandible, a cast framework supported by five standard abutments and acrylic resin teeth and gingiva processed onto the framework (Figure 15). Branemark considered passive fit to exist when the gap between the framework and the abutment was 10 microns (Abduo et al., 2010). Several authors have proposed definitions of passive fit, however all definitions are theoretical, and difficult to assess clinically.
It has been suggested that absolute passive fit cannot be achieved, nor is there concrete evidence that passive fit ensures the long term prognosis of the implants and restoration (Sahin & Cehreli, 2001). It is, however, reasonable to expect fewer mechanical complications, such as screw loosening and porcelain fracture, when the components fit more accurately. The concept of clinically acceptable fit incorporates the goal of minimizing both biologic complications and mechanical complications. Clinically acceptable fit in combination with control over the occlusal forces is a practical approach to ensuring success of the implants and the restoration.
Framework fit can be assessed by a variety of methods. Clinical methods for assessing framework fit include finger pressure, visual inspection, radiographs, tactile sensation, Sheffield test, disclosing materials, and the screw resistance test (Abduo et al., 2010). Each method has both advantages, disadvantages, and relative accuracy. In general, the intra-oral methods such as visual inspection, finger pressure, and disclosing agents are of limited value with subgingival margins. The screw resistance test (Jorneus et al., 1992) is based on the thread pitch of the original gold prosthetic screws, thus has limited application to newer systems and alloys. The Sheffield test, also known as the single screw test, combined with radiographic evaluation, is an efficient technique, especially for long span frameworks. If a single screw placed in a distal abutment does not create a vertical gap on the opposite end of the framework, the framework is said to have clinically acceptable fit.

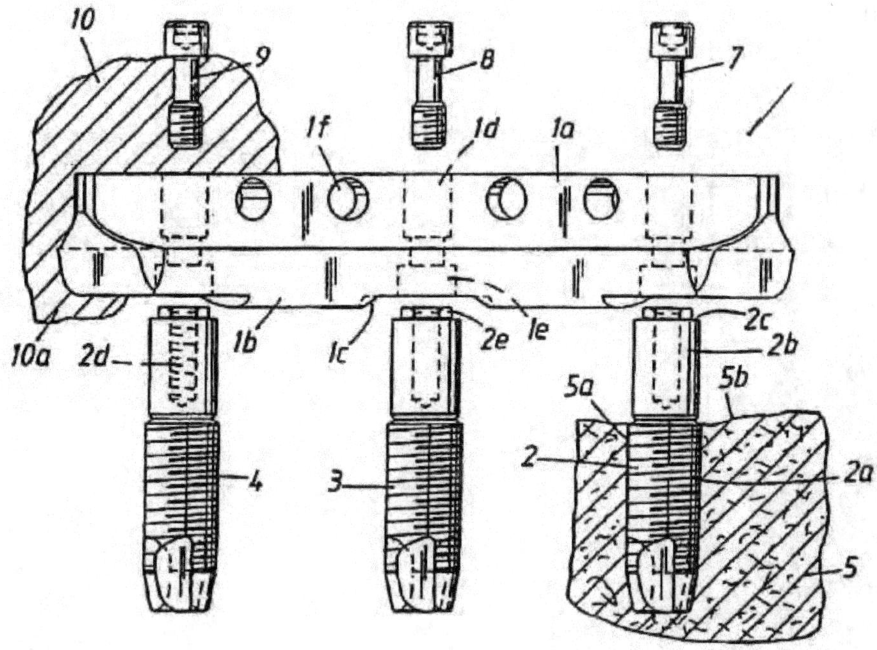

Fig. 15. Illustration of Branemark's original design for restoration of the completely edentulous mandible. (1) Cast gold framework. (2b) Standard Abutment. (2d) Abutment screw. (4) Implant fixture. (9) Prosthetic Screw. (10) Acrylic teeth and gingiva.

Multiple in vitro methods to assess framework fit can be utilized to compare the relative accuracy of various methods of fabrication. In vitro methods include photoelastic, strain gauge analysis, finite element analysis, microscopic, photogrammetric, and coordinate measuring machine (Abduo et al., 2010). These methods can be qualitative, quantitative, 2-dimensional or 3-dimensional. For example, strain gauge analysis is both quantitative and 2-dimensional, yet depends on the location of the strain gauge, and the ability of the material to mimic natural tissues. At this time, none of the available methods for assessing accuracy of fit have been validated with clinically relevant parameters.

3.4 CAD/CAM Framework and bar fabrication

CAD/CAM applications have surged in the market over recent years. There are now multiple commercial sources that can produce purely CAD/CAM bars and frameworks, or copy-milled CAM structures for implant prostheses. Procera from Nobel Biocare, CAMStructure from Biomet 3i, and Vericore from Whip Mix are just a few examples. Most companies offer stock designs such as a Dolder bar or Hader bar that can be masked on a virtual master cast of the implant analogs and soft tissue contour. The stock design is then contoured to the arch form, and modifications can be made to idealize the bar design. A second scan of the wax denture can be overlaid in order to allocate adequate space for attachments and adequate thickness of the resin denture base. For ceramic frameworks, a scan of the full-contour wax-up can be matched to the virtual master cast, and a virtual cutback can be performed to allow adequate thickness for veneering porcelain. By using CAD/CAM frameworks, fixed partial (Figures 16-24) or full-arch (Figures 25-38) dental prostheses can be fabricated.

For more complicated designs, a resin pattern of the desired framework can be scanned and the structure can be CAMed via a process known as copy-milling. Zirkonzahn, for example, utilizes a optical scanner with computerized 5-axis copy-milling technology that allows fabrication of highly detailed zirconia frameworks.

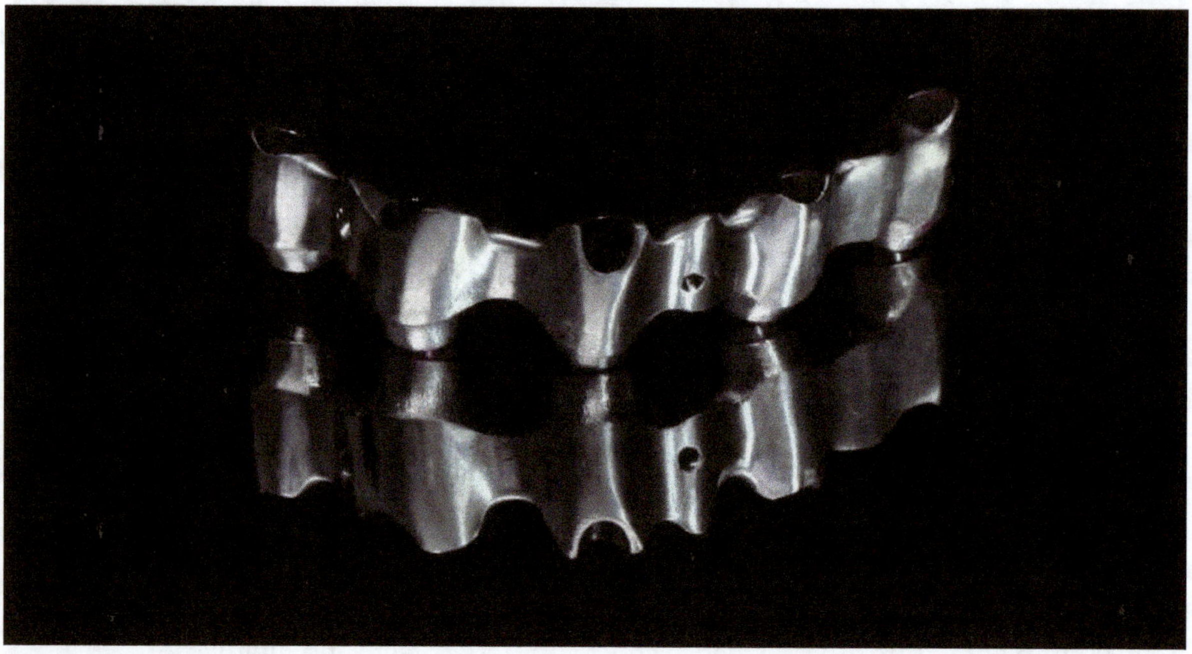

Fig. 16. Procera copy-milled titanium framework from Nobel Biocare.

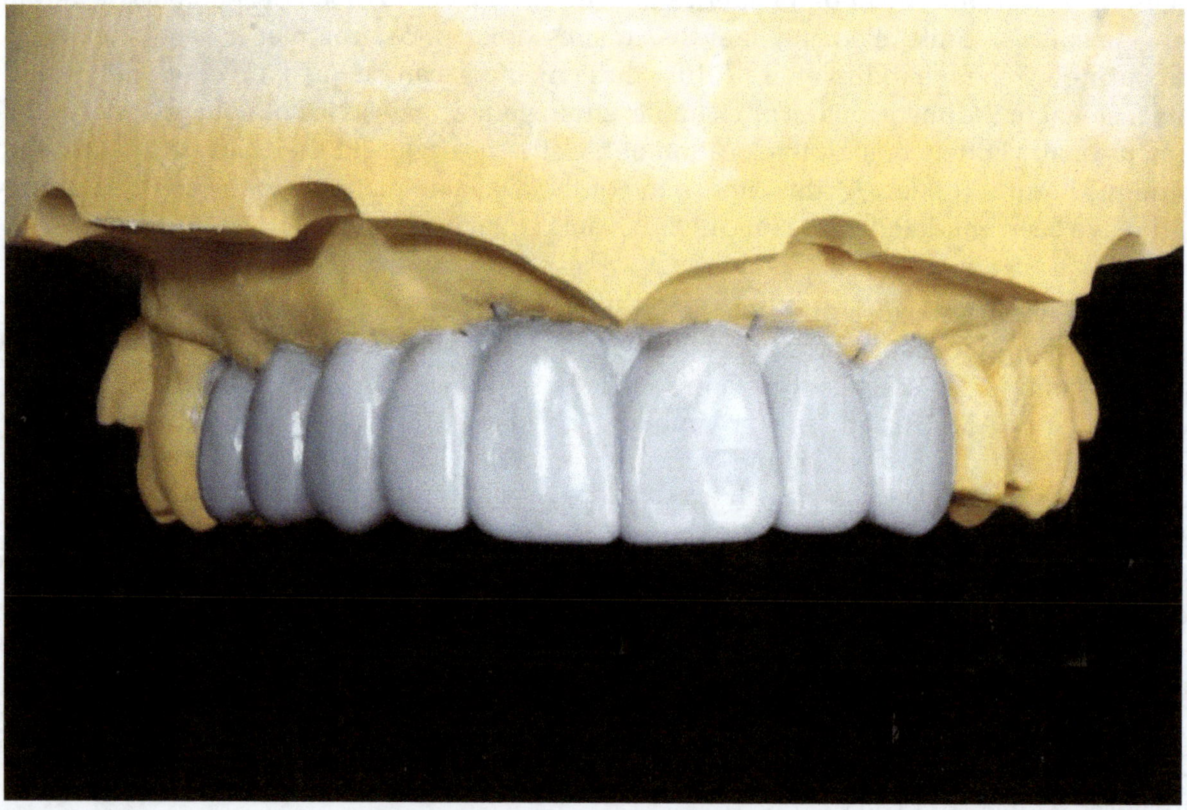

Fig. 17. Diagnostic wax-up for planning implant placement, prosthetic design, and space allocation.

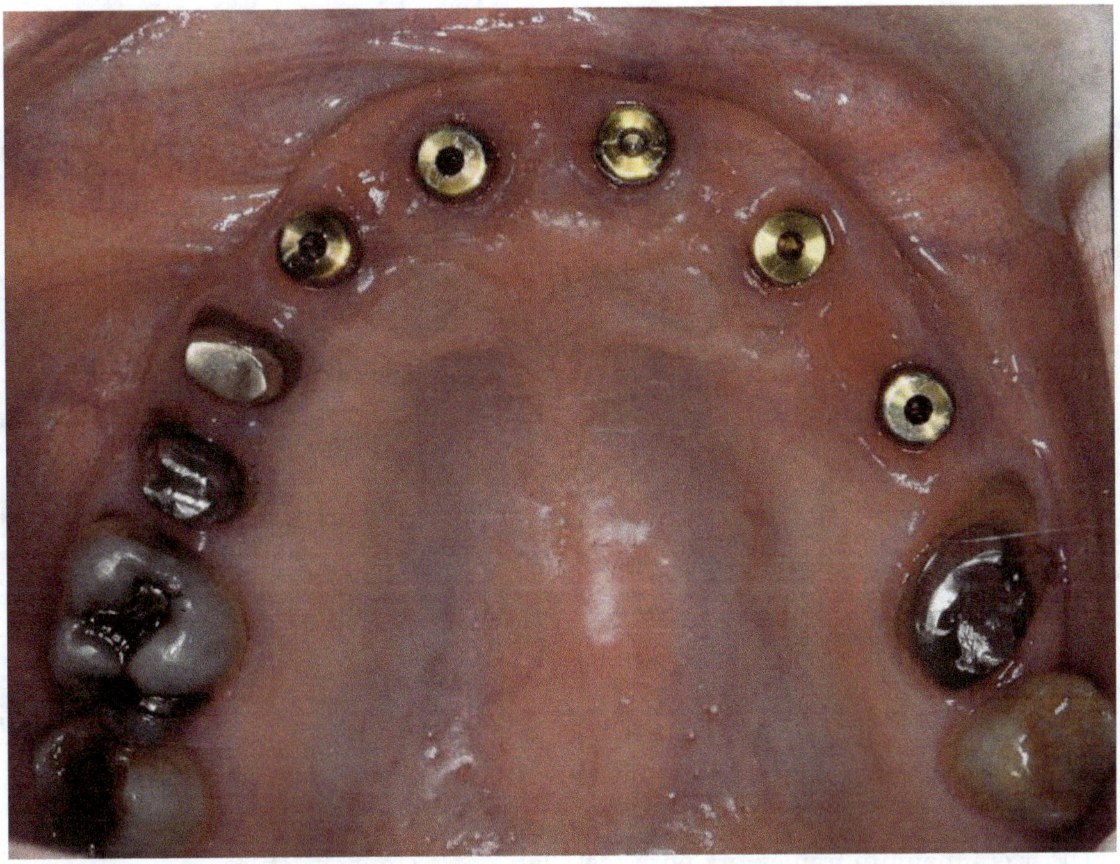

Fig. 18. Occlusal view of implants with healing abutments and tooth preparations.

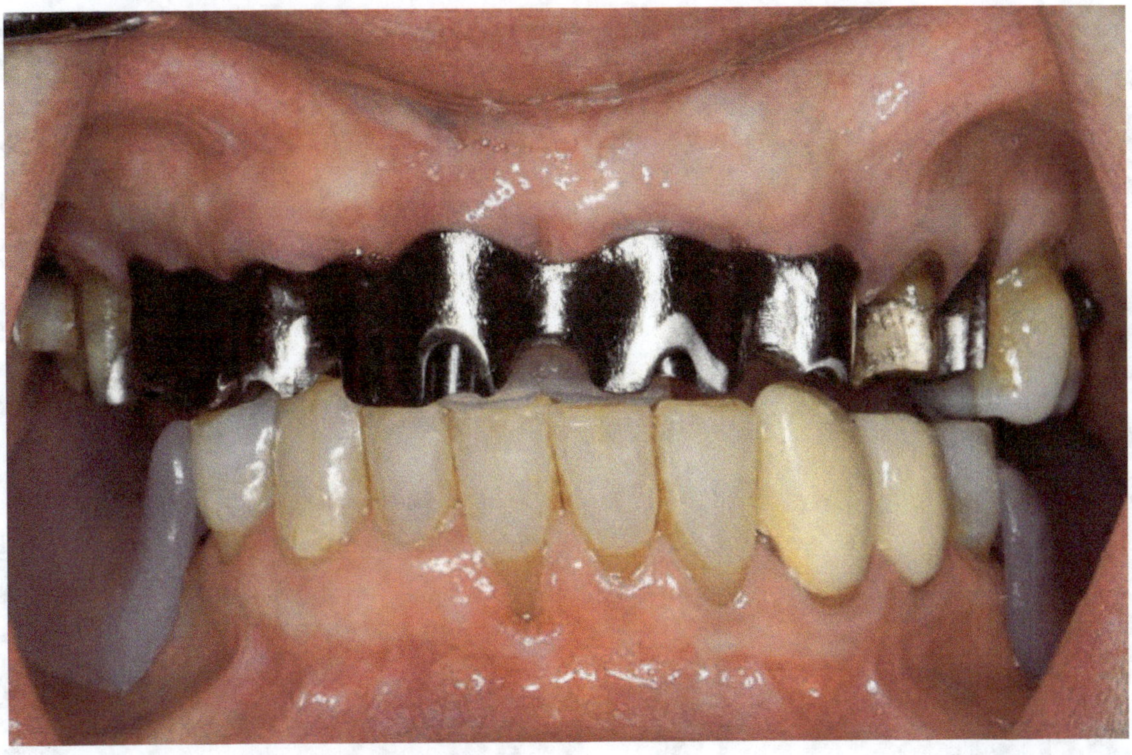

Fig. 19. Nobel Procera copy-milled titanium framework at time of try-in and making inter-occlusal records.

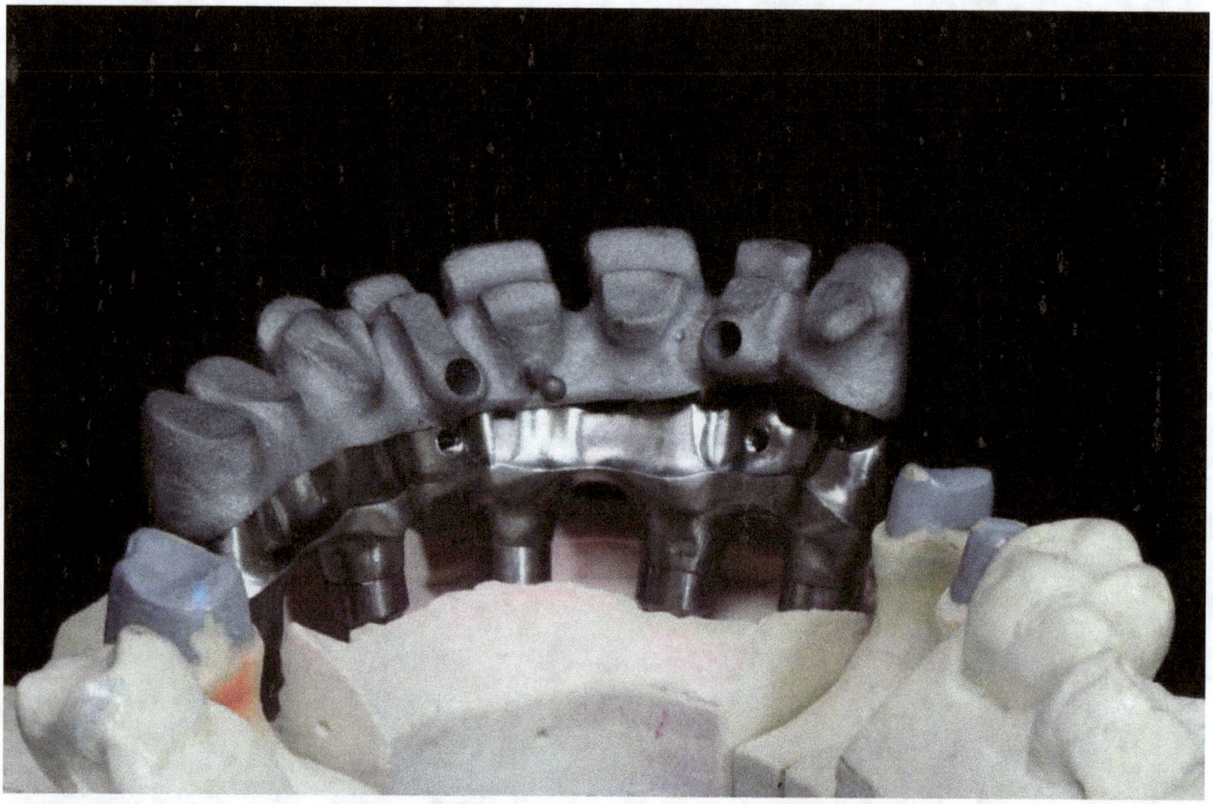

Fig. 20. Procera titanium framework with cast high-noble superstructure.

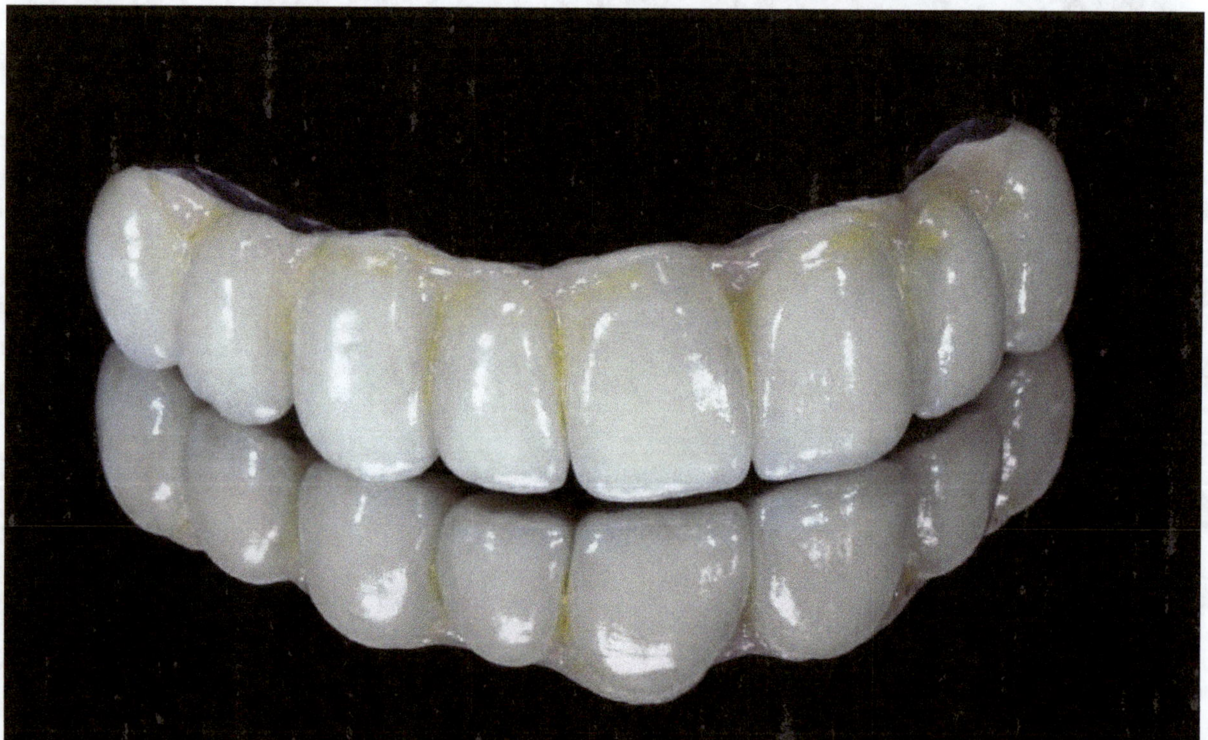

Fig. 21. Cast high-noble superstructure after porcelain application and firing.

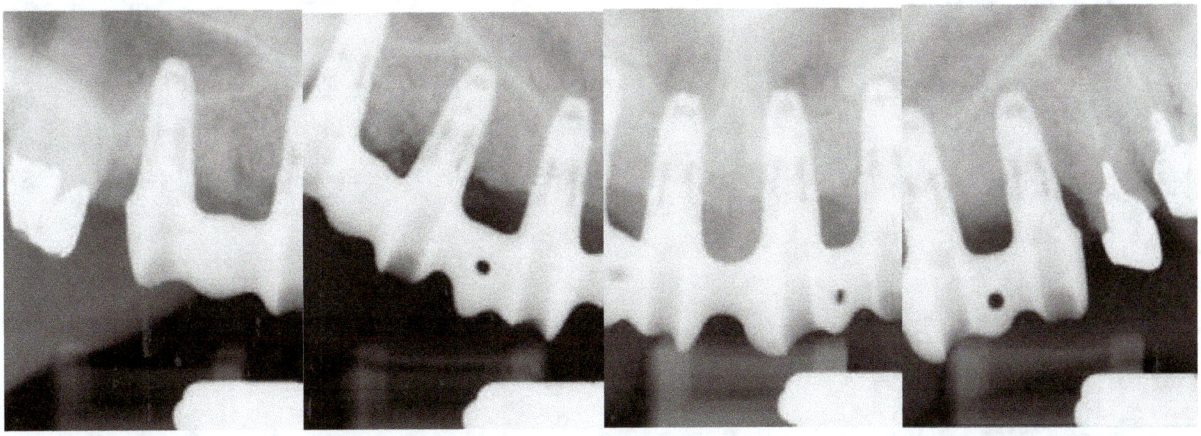

Fig. 22. Radiographic verification of framework fit prior to placement of superstructure.

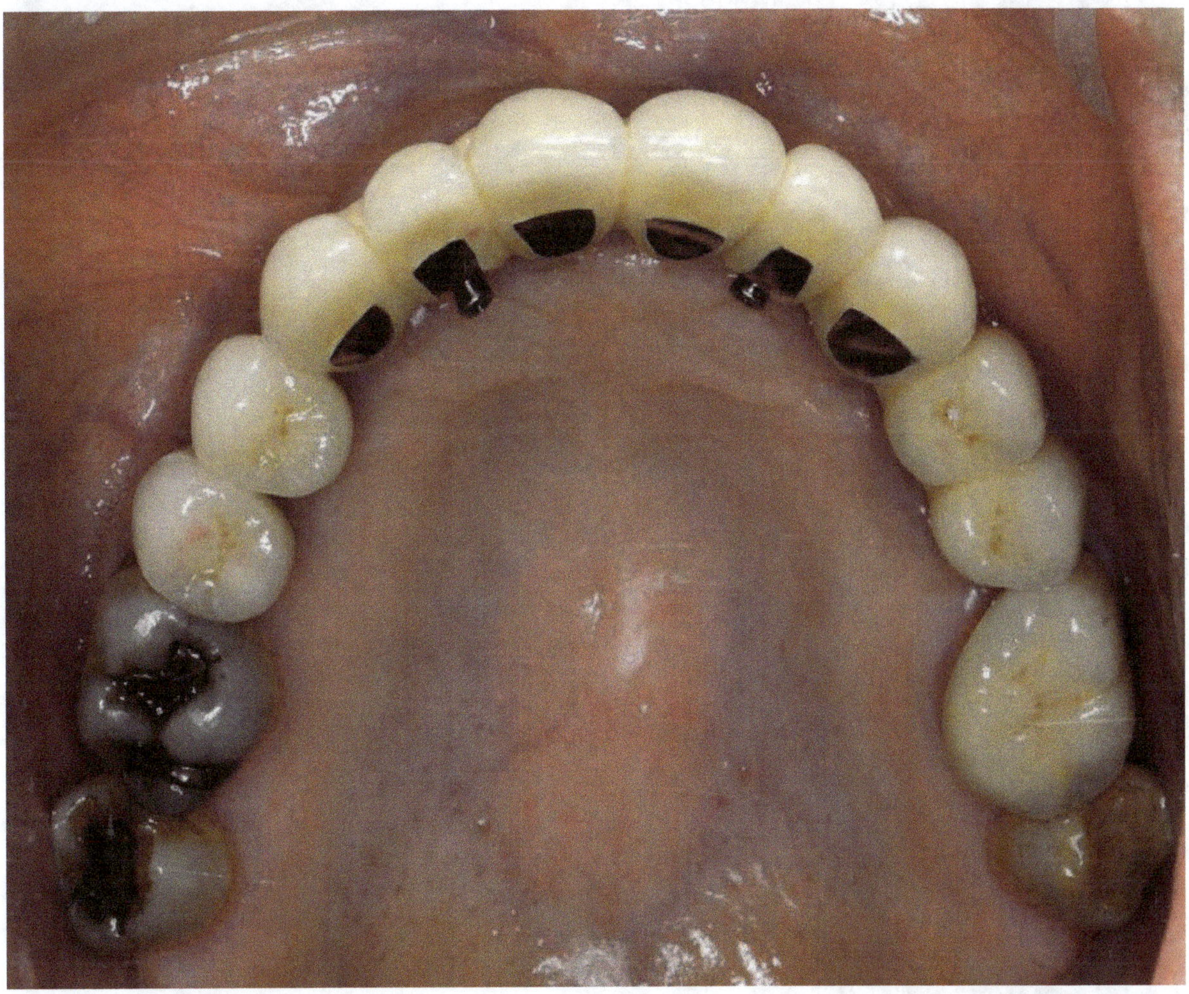

Fig. 23. Occlusal view of lingual set screws retaining metal-ceramic superstructure to CAM framework.

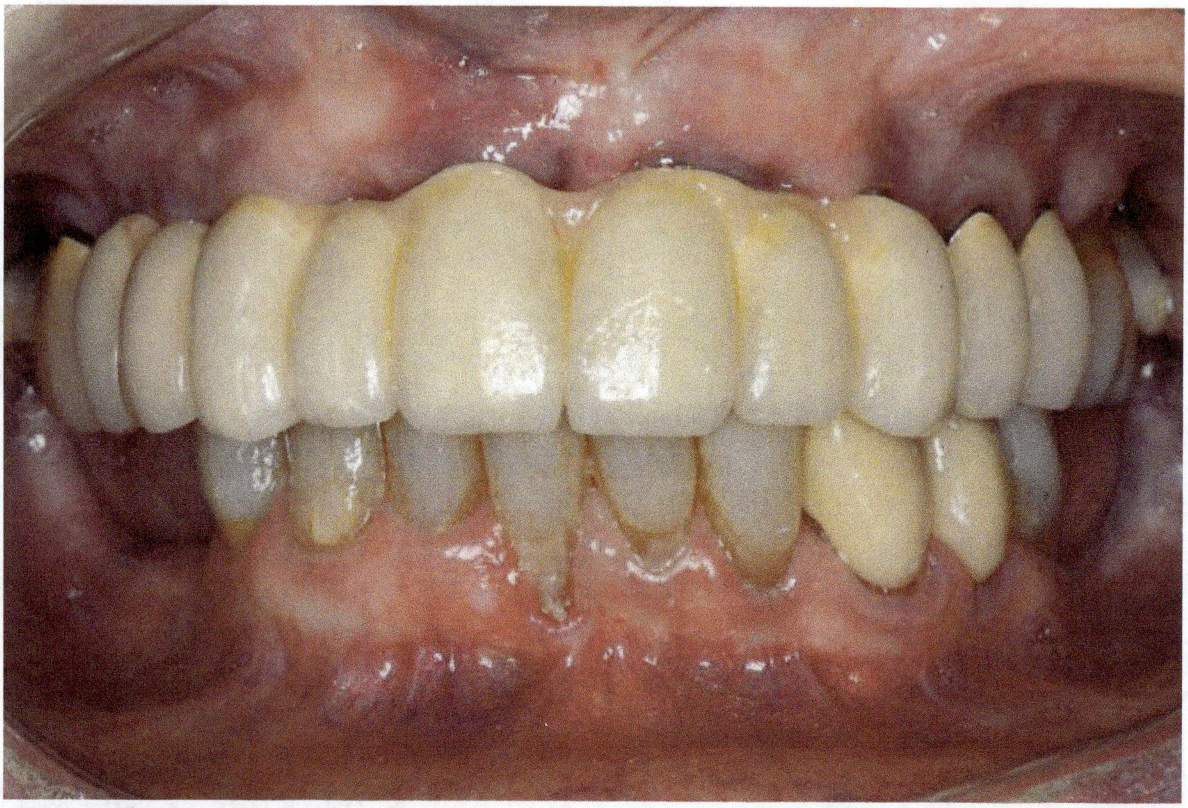

Fig. 24. Frontal view of completed prosthesis.

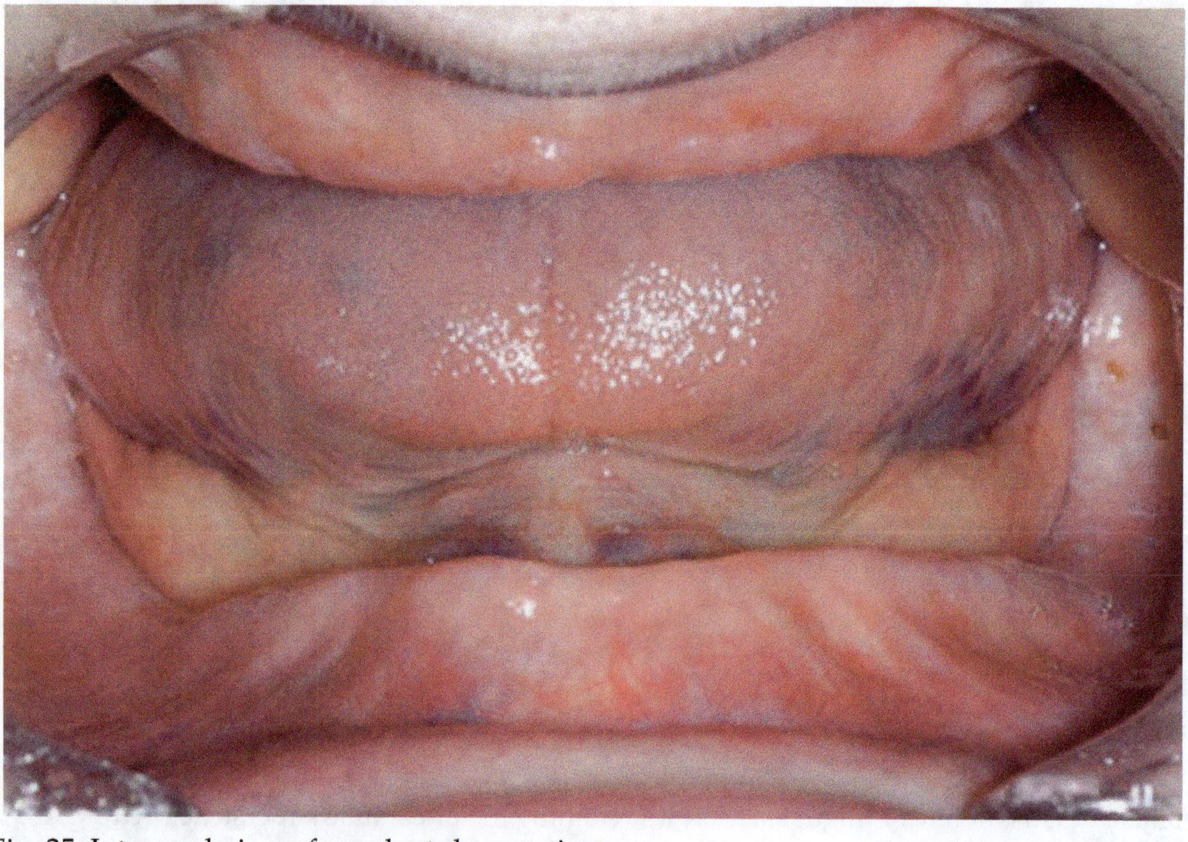

Fig. 25. Intra-oral view of an edentulous patient.

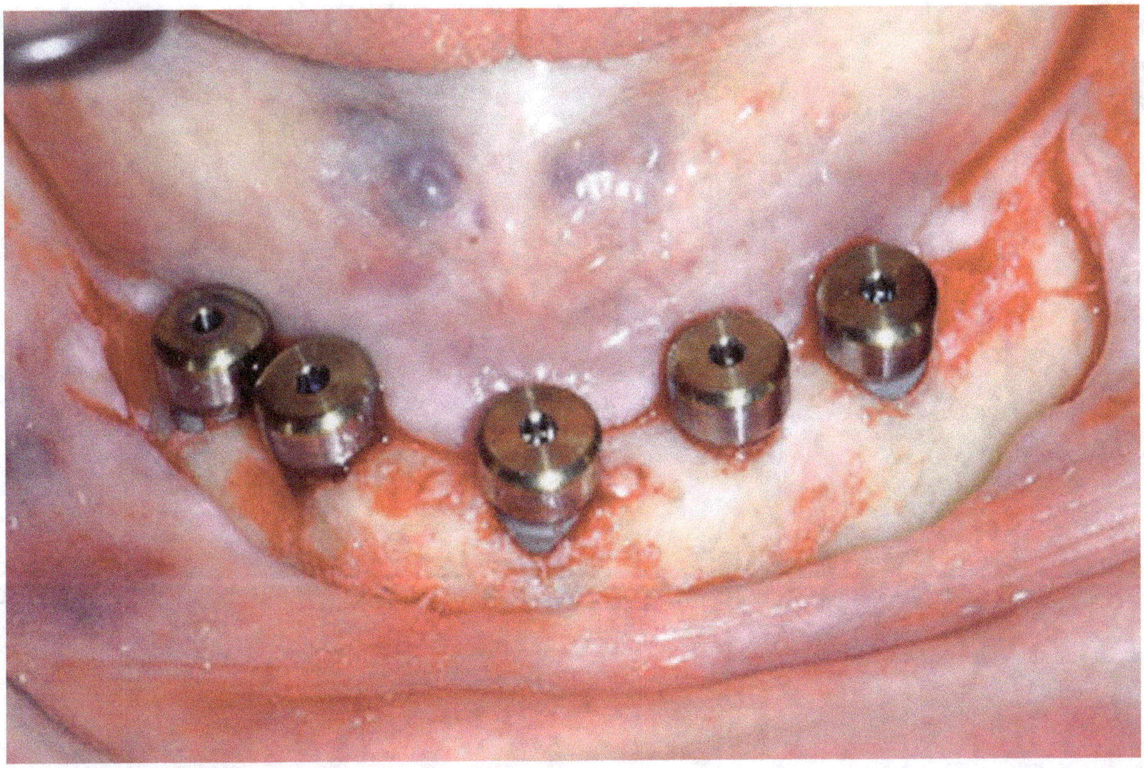

Fig. 26. Clinical view of the five healing abutments on the implants seated immediately after the implant placement.

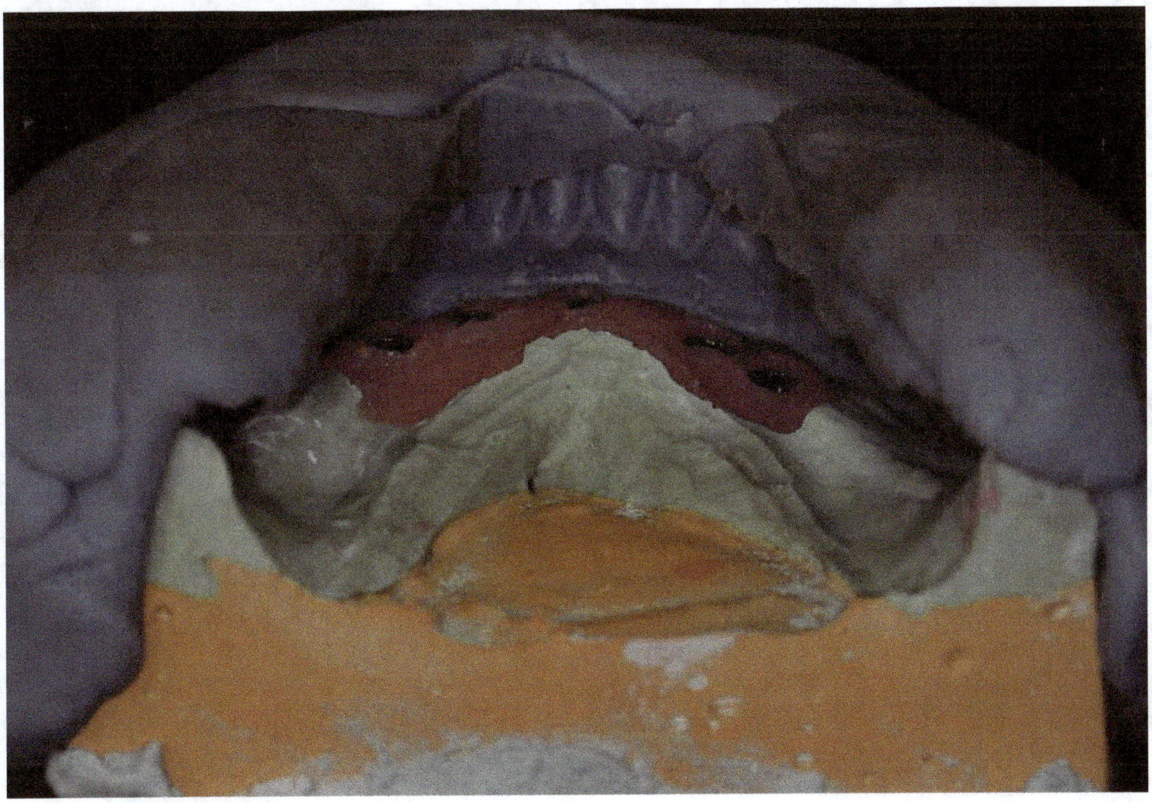

Fig. 27. The lingual view of the mandibular definitive cast with the tooth index, showing the room for the framework.

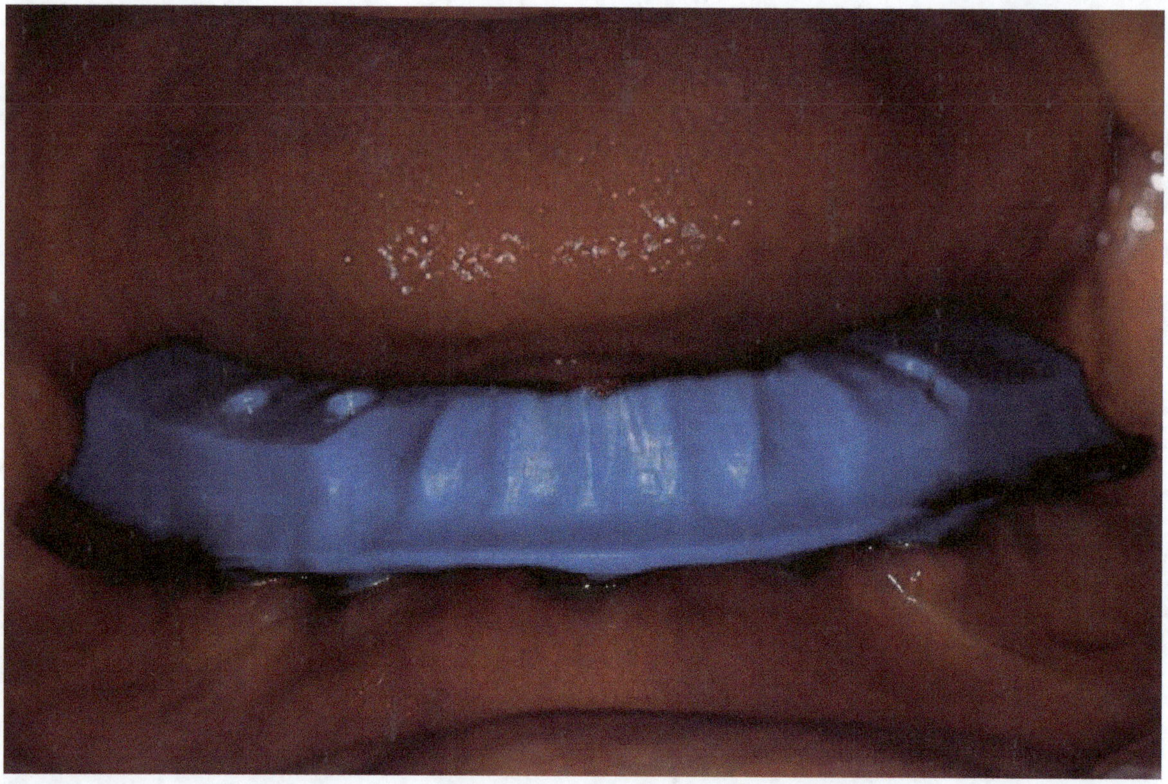

Fig. 28. The fit of the mandibular wax pattern was verified clinically.

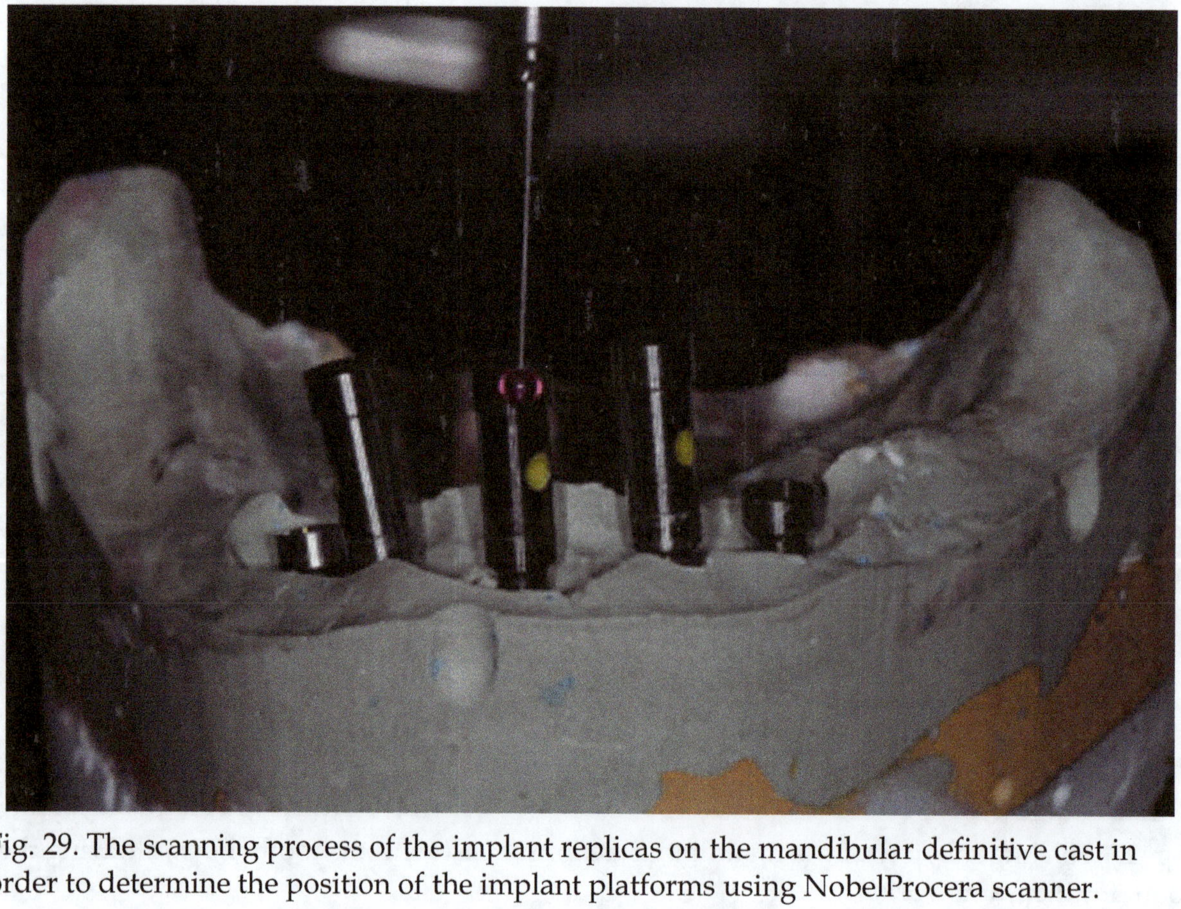

Fig. 29. The scanning process of the implant replicas on the mandibular definitive cast in order to determine the position of the implant platforms using NobelProcera scanner.

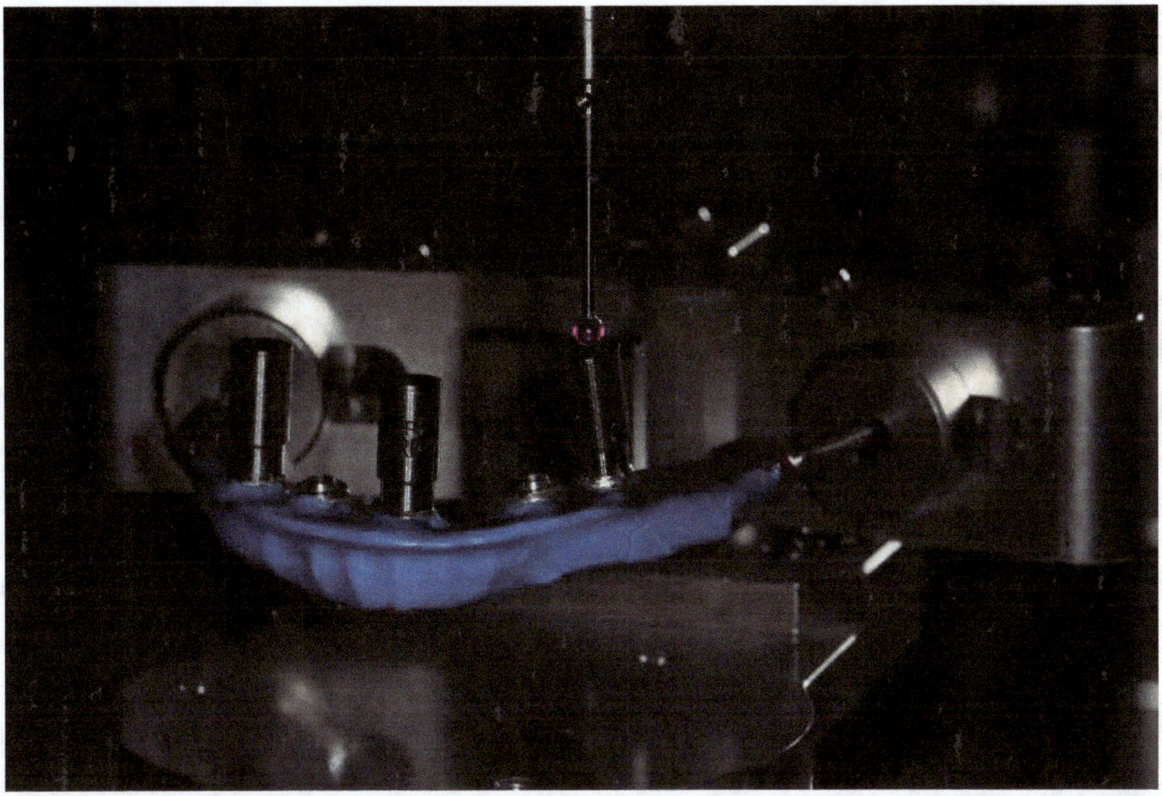

Fig. 30. The scanning process of the implant replicas in the mandibular wax pattern in order to determine the position of the implant platforms using NobelProcera scanner.

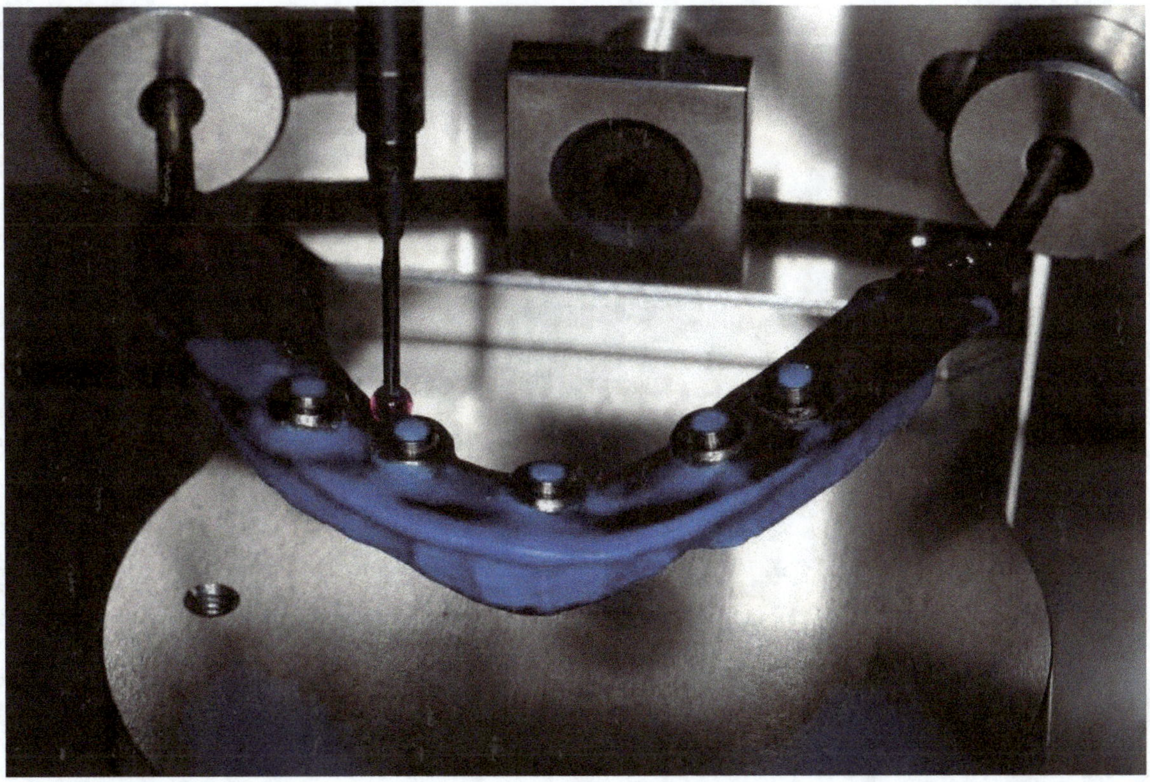

Fig. 31. The scanning process of the gingival surface of the mandibular wax pattern using NobelProcera scanner.

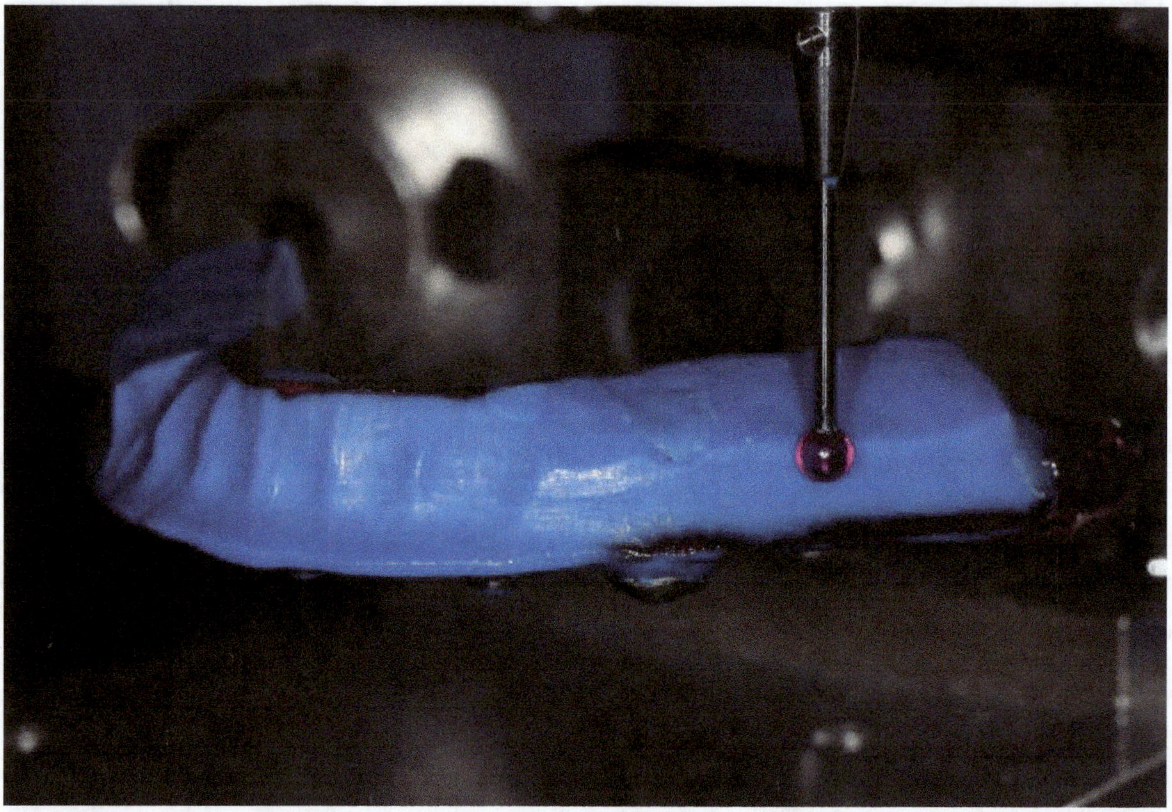

Fig. 32. The scanning process of the occlusal surface of the mandibular wax pattern using NobelProcera scanner.

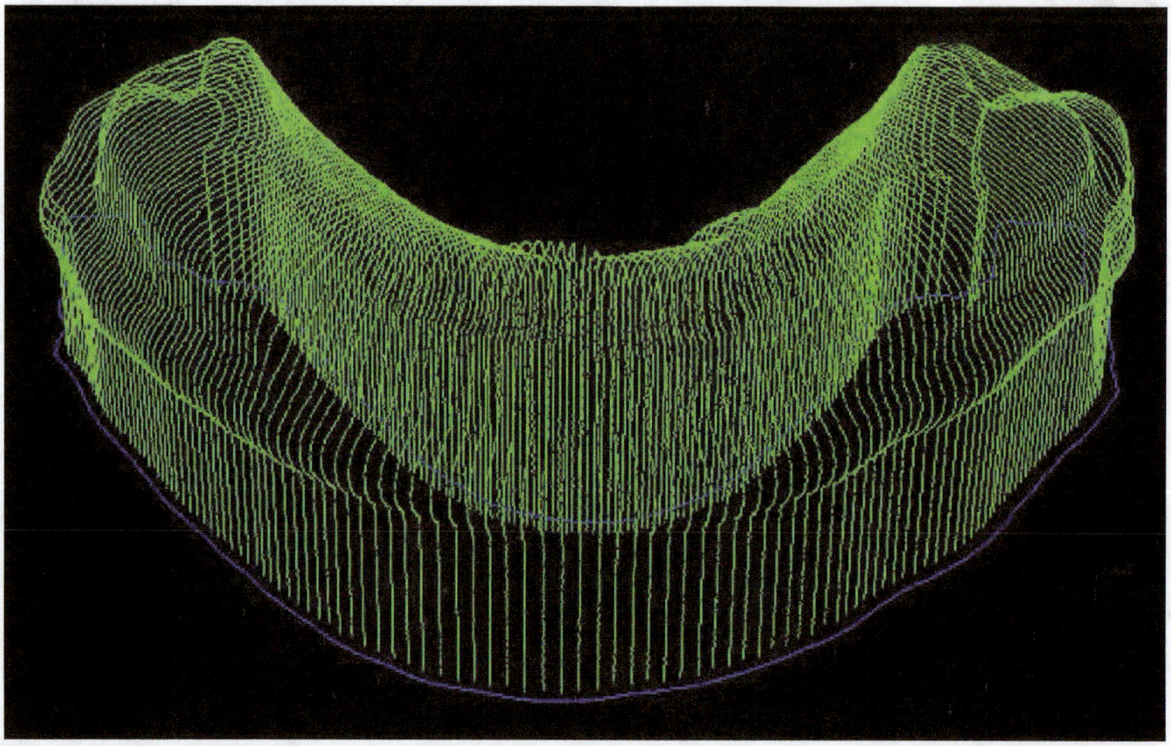

Fig. 33. The design of the occlucal surface of the mandibular framework using NobelProcera scanner.

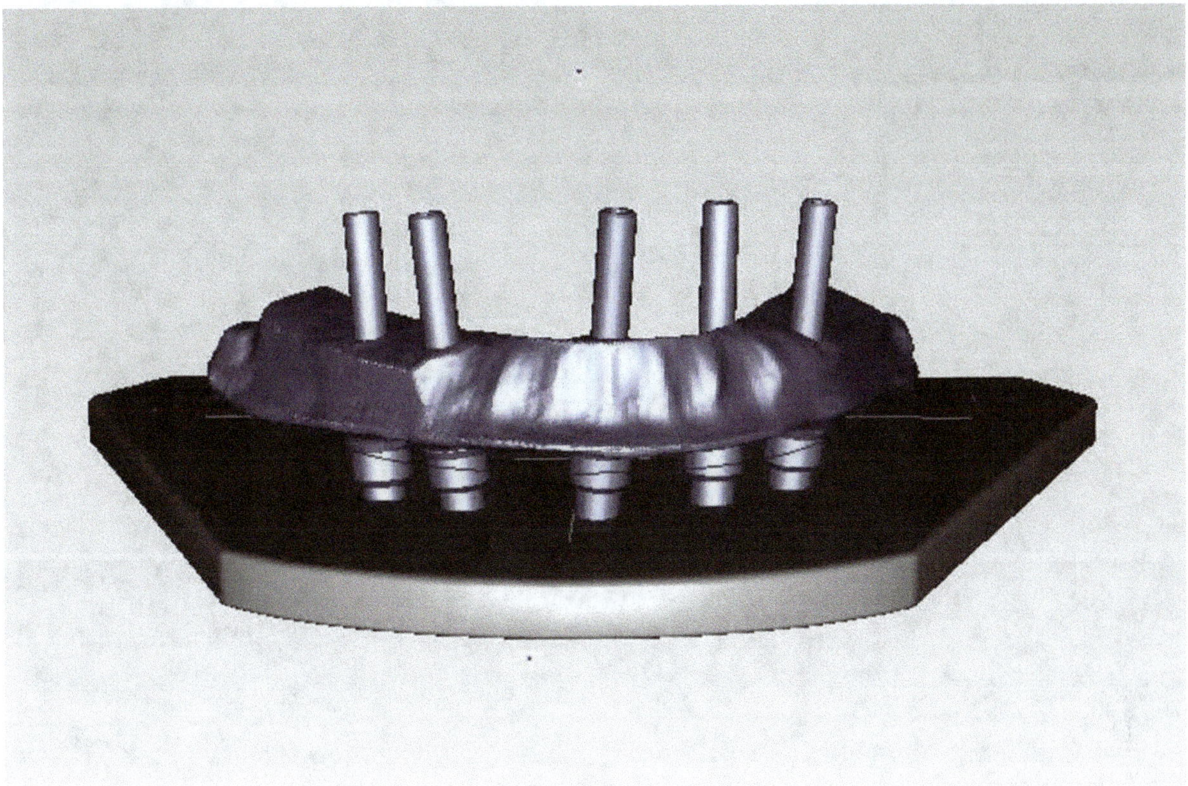

Fig. 34. The final design of the mandibular framework using NobelProcera scanner.

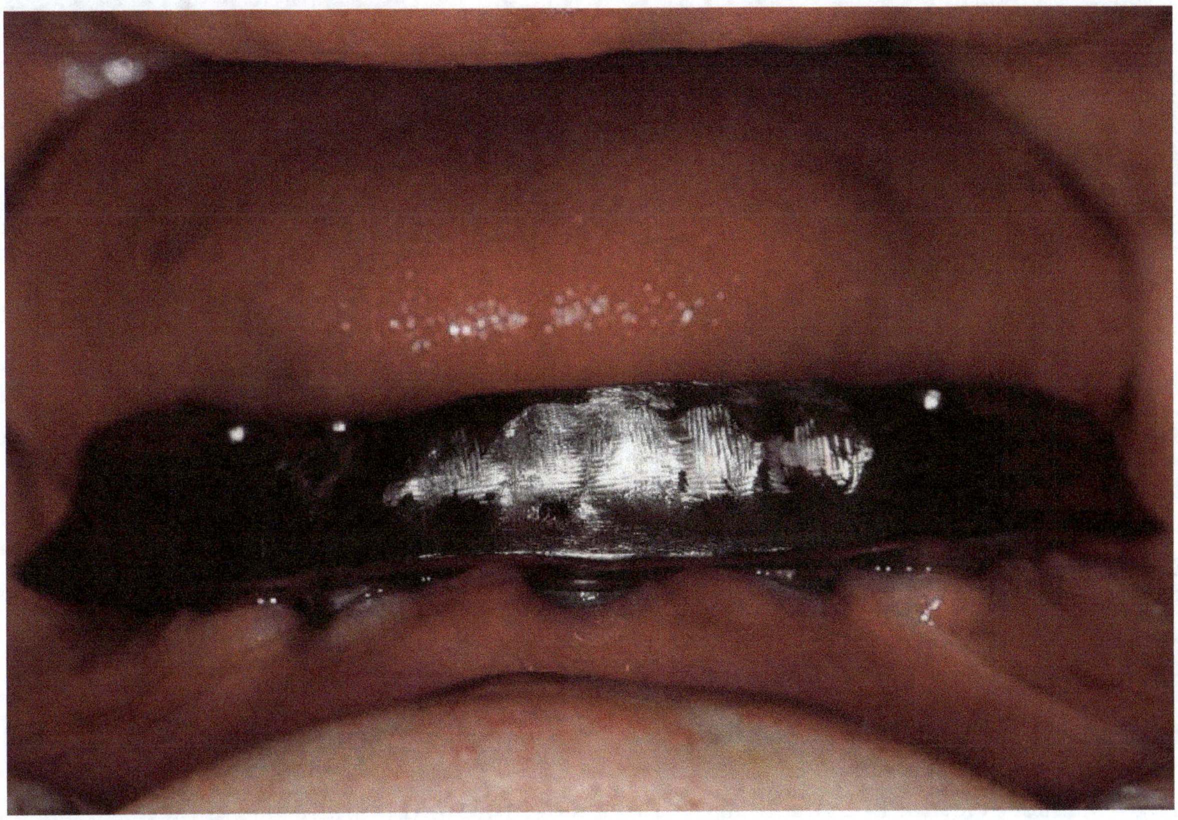

Fig. 35. Clinical fit of the final mandibular framework fabricated was verified.

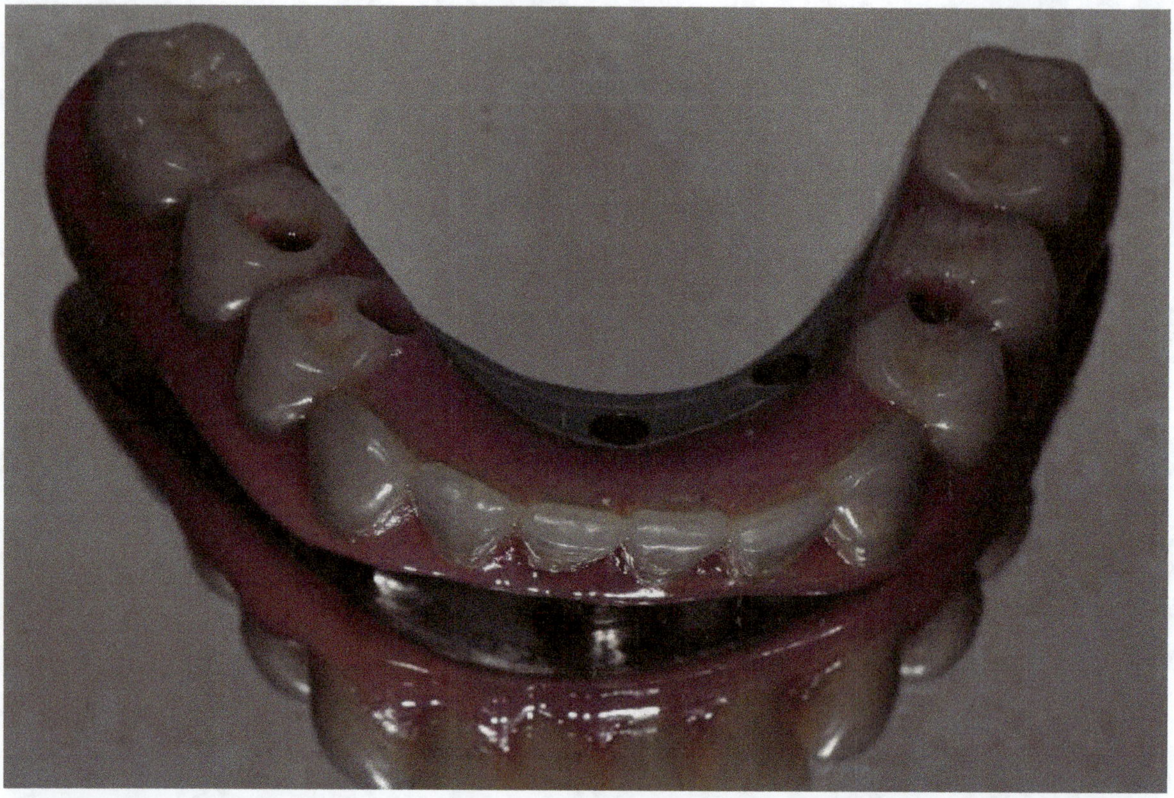

Fig. 36. The implant-supported screw-retained fixed dental prosthesis after processed.

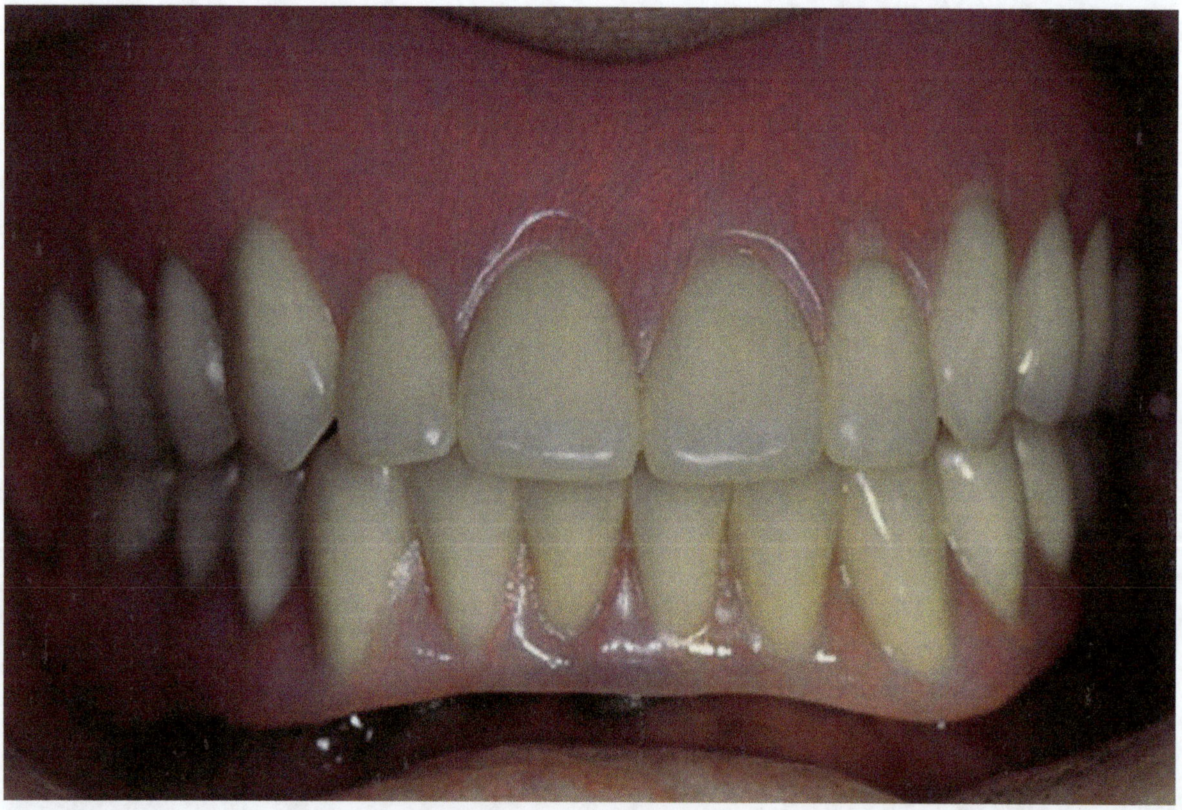

Fig. 37. Clinical view of both maxillary complete denture and mandibular implant-supported screw-retained fixed dental prosthesis.

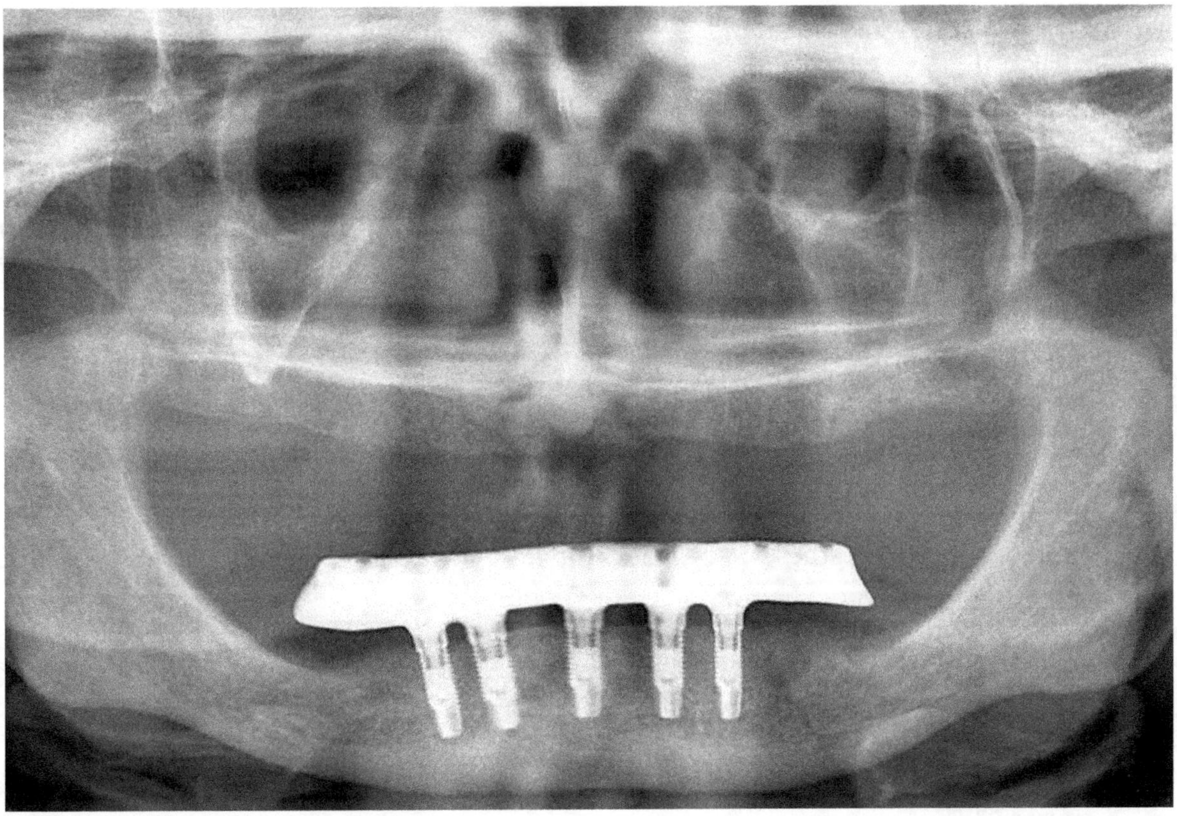

Fig. 38. Panoramic radiograph of the patient a year after the implant placement.

3.5 Comparison of fabrication techniques

An abundance of literature supports the improved accuracy of CAD/CAM over traditional casting, even when corrective procedures are included. A recent publication by Drago et al. (2010), evaluated volumetric misfit of CAM and cast 5-implant frameworks fabricated in three different laboratories. Thirty implant level impressions with verified implant indices were made from one master cast with five intra-foraminal mandibular implants. Fifteen verified master casts were scanned and CAD/CAM frameworks were fabricated. Another fifteen verified master casts served as the base for attachment of UCLA abutments and resin pattern fabrication for casting procedures. A volumetric analysis of fit based on single screw test and "best fit" of individual frameworks to respective master cast revealed that the CAD/CAM frameworks were significantly more accurate than the cast frameworks.

An earlier study by Riedy et al.(1997), showed similar results when comparing one piece cast frameworks to Procera CAD/CAM frameworks. They also found that sectioning and laser welding cast frameworks significantly improved the overall fit. These results are consistent with other studies comparing conventional casting to CAD/CAM techniques (Al-Fadda et al., 2007). Given the significant improvement of fit and decrease in laboratory time, CAD/CAM bars and frameworks, particularly for overdentures and hybrids, will soon be the standard.

4. Conclusion

CAD/CAM technology has revolutionized the field of implant dentistry. CAD/CAM surgical guides have greatly improved the predictability of implant surgery. CAD/CAM bars and framework have proven more accurate, less expensive, and less time-consuming to produce. All of this results in improved experience for the patient, decreased treatment time, and greater accessibility.

The future of dentistry is quickly approaching. Digital impression systems and CAMed models for tooth born restorations are rapidly expanding in the market. Virtual tooth libraries allow CAD/CAM of both provisional and final tooth-born restorations. Numerous implant companies have already designed abutments for compatibility with digital impression systems. Just on the horizon is virtual articulation and virtual tooth arrangement, thus completing the virtual relm of dental technology. It is clear that CAD/CAM technology has transformed all aspects of dentistry, not just implant dentistry.

5. References

Abduo, J., Bennani, V., Waddell, N., Lyons, K., Swain, M. (2010). Assessing the Fit of Implant Fixed Prostheses: A Critical Review. *Int J Oral Maxillofac Implants,* Vol. 25, No.3, pp.506-515.

Albrektsson, T., Zarb, G., Worthington, P., Eriksson. AR. (1986). The long-term efficacy of currently used dental implants: a review and proposed criteria of success. *Int J Oral Maxillofac Implants,* Vol. 1, No. 1, pp:11-25

Al-Fadda, SA., Zarb, GA., Finer, Y. (2007). A comparison of the accuracy of fit of 2 methods for fabricating implant-prosthodontic frameworks. *Int J Prosthodont,* Vol. 20, No.2, pp.125-131.

Allen, PF., McMillan, AS. (2003). A longitudinal study of quality of life outcomes in older adults requesting implant prostheses and complete removable dentures. *Clin Oral Impl Res,* Vol. 14, No. 2 , pp.173-179.

Arisan, V., Karabuda, ZC., Ozdemir, T. (2010). Accuracy of two stereolithographic guide systems for computer-aided implant placement: a computed tomography-based clinical comparative study. *J Periodontol,* Vol. 81, No. 1, pp.43-51.

Awad, MA., Lund, JP., Dufresne, E., Feine, JS. (2003). Comparing the efficacy of mandibular implant-retained overdentures and conventional dentures among middle-aged edentulous patients: satisfaction and functional assessment. *Int J Prosthodont,* Vol.16, No.2, pp.117-122.

Besimo, CE., Rohner, HP. (2005). Three-dimensional treatment planning for prosthetic rehabilitation. *Int J Periodontics Restorative Dent,.* Vol. 25, No. 1, pp.81-87.

Brånemark. PI., Albrektsson, T. (1982). Titanium implants permanently penetrating human skin. *Scand J Plast Reconstr Surg,* Vol. 16, No.1, pp:17-21.

Christensen, GJ. (2005). Dental Laboratory Technology in Crisis: The Challenges Facing the Industry. *J Am Dent Assoc,* Vol. 136, No. 5, pp.653-655.

Drago, C., Saldarriaga, RL., Domagala, D., Almasri, R. (2010). Volumetric determination of the amount of misfit in CAD/CAM and cast implant frameworks: a multicenter laboratory study. *Int J Oral Maxillofac Implants,* Vol. 25, No.5, pp.920-929.

Ersoy, AE., Turkyilmaz, I., Ozan, O., McGlumphy, EA. (2008). Reliability of Implant Placement with Stereolithographic Surgical Guides Generated From Computed Tomography: Clinical Data From 94 Impants. *J Periodontol,* Vol.79, No. 8, pp.1339-1345.

Fortin, T., Bosson, JL., Isidori, M., Blanchet, E. (2006). Effect of flapless surgery on pain experienced in implant placement using an image-guided system. Int J Oral Maxillofac Implants, Vol. 21, No. 2 , pp.298-304.

Friberg, B., Jemt, T. (2010). Clinical experience of TiUnite implants: a 5-year cross-sectional, retrospective follow-up study. *Clin Implant Dent Relat Res,* Vol.12, No. Suppl 1, pp.e95-103.

Heydecke, G., Thomason, JM., Lund, JP. (2005).The impact of conventional and implant supported prostheses on social and sexual activities in edentulous adults: Results from a randomized trial 2 months after treatment. *J Dent,* Vol. 33, No.8, pp. 649-657.

Jacobs, P. (1992) Rapid Prototyping and Manufacturing: Fundamentals of Stereolithography. Vol. 1., Dearborn, MI: Society of Manufacturing Engineers. 434.

Jorneus, L., Jemt, T., Carlsson, L. (1992). Loads and designs of screw joints for single crowns supported by osseointegrated implants. *Int J Oral Maxillofac Implants,* Vol. 7, No.3, pp.353-359.

Kapur, KK., Soman S. (1965) The effect of denture factors on masticatory performance. IV. Influence of occlusal patterns. *J Prosthet Dent,* Vol.15, pp.662-670

Mandelaris, GA., Rosenfeld, AL., King, SD., Nevins, ML. (2010). Computer-guided implant dentistry for precise implant placement: combining specialized stereolithographically generated drilling guides and surgical implant instrumentation. *Int J Periodontics Restorative Dent* Vol. 30, No. 3, pp.275-281.

Misch, CE., Goodacre, CJ., Finley, JM., Misch, CM., Marinbach, M., Dabrowsky, T., English, CE., Kois, JC., Cronin, RJ. (2005). Consensus Conference Panel Report: Crown-Height Space Guidelines for Implant Dentistry--Part I. *Implant Dent,* Vol. 14, No.4, pp.312-318.

Misch, CE., Perel, ML., Wang, HL., Sammartino, G., et. al. (2008). Implant Success, Survival, and Failure: The International Congress of Oral Implantologists (ICOI) Pisa Consensus Conference. *Implant Dent,* Vol.17, No.1, pp.5-15.

Ortorp, A., Jemt, T. (2000). Clinical experiences of CNC-milled titanium frameworks supported by implants in the edentulous jaw: 1-year prospective study. Clin Implant Dent Relat Res. Vol. 2, No.1, pp.2-9.

Ozan, O., Turkyilmaz, I., Ersoy, AE., McGlumphy, EA., Rosenstiel, SF. (2009). Clinical accuracy of 3 different types of computed tomography-derived stereolithographic surgical guides in implant placement. J Oral Maxillofac Surg, Vol. 67, No. 2, pp.394-401.

Pommer, B., Zechner, W., Watzak, G., Ulm, C., Watzek, G., Tepper, G. (2011). Progress and trends in patient's mindset on dental implants. I: level of information, sources of information and need for patient information. *Clin Oral Impl Res,* Vol.22, No.2, pp.223-229.

Riedy, SJ., Lang, BR., Lang, BE. (1997). Fit of Implant Frameworks Fabricated by Different Techniques. *J Prosthet Dent,* Vol. 78, No. 6, pp.596-604.

Sahin, S., Cehreli, M. (2001). The Significance of Passive Framework Fit in Implant Prosthodontics: Current Status. *Implant Dent,* Vol. 10, No.2, pp.85-92.

Sarment, DP., Sukovic, P., Clinthorne, N. (2003). Accuracy of Implant Placement with a Stereolithographic Surgical Guide. *Int J Oral Maxillofac Implants,* Vol;. 18, No. 4, pp.571-577.

Takahashi, T., Gunne, J. (2003). Fit of implant frameworks: an in vitro comparison between two fabrication techniques. *J Prosthet Dent*, Vol. 89, No.3 ,pp.256-260.

Tardieu, P., Vrielinck, I., Escolano, E. (2003). Computer-assisted implant placement. A case report: Treatment of the mandible. *Int J Oral Maxillofac Implants,* Vol. 18, No. 4, pp.599-604.

Turkyilmaz, I., Aksoy, U., McGlumphy, EA. (2008). Two alternative surgical techniques for enhancing primary implant stability in the posterior maxilla: a clinical study including bone density, insertion torque, and resonance frequency analysis data. *Clin Implant Dent Relat Res,* Vol.10, No.4, pp.231-237.

Turkyilmaz, I., Company AM., McGlumphy EA. (2010). Should edentulous patients be constrained to removable complete dentures? The use of dental implants to improve the quality of life for edentulous patients. *Gerodontology,* Vol.27, No.1, pp.3-10.

Valente, F., Schiroli, G., Sbrenna, A. (2009). Accuracy of computer-aided oral implant surgery: a clinical and radiographic study. *Int J Oral Maxillofac Implants,* Vol.24, No.2, pp.234-242.

Van Assche, N., van Steenberghe, D., Quirynen, M., Jacobs, R. (2010). Accuracy assessment of computer-assisted flapless implant placement in partial edentulism. *J Clin Periodontol,* Vol.37, No.4, pp.398-403.

Walter, M., Reppel, PD., Boning, K., Freesmeyer, WB. (1999). Six-year follow-up of titanium and high-gold porcelain fused-to-metal fixed partial dentures. *Journal of Oral Rehabil,* Vol. 26, No.2, pp.91-96.

Weintraub, JA., Burt, BA. (1985). Oral health status in the United States: tooth loss and edentulism. *J Dent Educ,*Vol.49, No.6, pp.368-378.

3

Bisphosphonate-Related Osteonecrosis of the Jaw Around Dental Implants

Tatsuo Shirota[1], Atsushi Nakamura[2], Yoshiro Matsui[3], Masashi Hatori[1], Masanori Nakamura[1] and Satoru Shintani[1]
[1]*Showa University,*
[2]*Yamato Tokushukai Hospital,*
[3]*Kagawa University,*
Japan

1. Introduction

Bisphosphonate is the collective name for compounds in which the backbone of pyrophosphoric acid, a P-O-P structure, is converted to chemically stable P-C-P, and this structure shows the affinity of bisphosphonate for bone hydroxyapatite in the body (Fleisch et al. 2002). Administered bisphosphonate preparations (BPs) transfer to and deposit in bone, exhibiting a bone resorption-inhibitory effect. The chemical structure of the side chain bound to the carbon atom of P-C-P markedly influences bisphosphonate activity, and, particularly, side chains containing nitrogen molecules not only markedly increase the affinity for HA but also bone resorption-inhibitory activity (Migliorati et al. 2005). Because of this potent bone resorption-inhibitory effect, BPs are the first-choice treatment for osteoporosis worldwide (Russell et al. 2007), and their efficacy for malignant tumor-associated hypercalcemia (Body et al.1999), ostealgia complicating bone metastasis of solid tumors (Hortobagyi et al. 1998), and multiple myeloma accompanied by bone destruction (Berenson et al. 1996) has been shown. Adverse effects of BPs were previously considered to be relatively mild, such as digestive symptoms induced by oral preparations and fever induced by injections (Berenson et al. 1996), but the association of BPs with osteonecrosis of the jaw has been frequently described since Marx (2003) initially reported it (Ruggiero et al. 2004; Marx et al. 2005; Khosla et al. 2007)

Bisphosphonate-related osteonecrosis of the jaw (BRONJ) is clinically diagnosed when the following 3 conditions are met: 1) current or previous treatment with BPs, 2) persistent exposure of necrotized bone in the maxillofacial region for 8 weeks or longer, 3) no past medical history of radiotherapy for the jaw bone (AAOMS 2007; Ruggiero et al. 2009). BPs inducing BRONJ mostly contain nitrogen (NBPs). BRONJ frequently develops in patients under NBP treatment upon dental treatment, such as tooth extraction, implant placement, and surgical periodontal treatment accompanied by bone invasion, and inflammatory diseases, such as periodontal disease and abscess (Ruggieri et al. 2009; Vahtsevanos et al. 2009; Yoneda et al. 2010). BRONJ shows poor responses to the standard treatment for common osteomyelitis of the jaw, such as curettage/resection of necrotized tissue and antimicrobial drugs, and its intractability is the most serious problem.

Stack & Epker (1995) initially reported the influence of BPs on dental implant treatment. They introduced a case in which all 5 favorably functioning implants in the lower anterior tooth region were lost after the 5-month administration of a BP containing no nitrogen, etidronatedisodium (Didronel; Procter and Gamble, Cincinnati, OH), for osteoporosis. The details of the bone wound healing process after implant loss or whether BRONJ developed were not described, but the author concluded that Didronel administration is a risk factor for implant treatment. However, several recent studies reported that implant treatment in the presence of NBPs was possible when the NBPs were oral drugs. Fugazzotto et al (2007) evaluated that a retrospective analysis of case records of patients with a history of oral BPs therapy treated as part of routine periodontal and implant treatment. They reported that no osteonecrosis was noted immediately postoperatively or during follow-up period 61 patients, and all implants were functioning successfully 12 to 24 months post-insertion.Grant et al. (2008) evaluated the clinical results of 115 patients who received oral BPs during implant treatment. They showed that there was no significant difference in treatment results between patients with and without oral BPs during implant treatment. It was also reported that no patients developed ONJ after implant treatment. Bell & Bell (2008) reported that bone grafting for implant treatment in 42 patients who received oral BPs for osteoporosis treatment was conducted safely. Therefore, no conclusion has been reached regarding whether oral BPs are contraindicated for implant treatment. On the other hand, it has been clarified that the risk of developing BRONJ upon open dental treatment rises in patients treated with NBP intravenous injection showing a potent bone adsorption-inhibitory action, and implant treatment is considered contraindicated for such cases (Khan et al. 2008; Ruggiero et al. 2009). However, there have been fewer reports on the influence of intravenous BPs on implants which have already acquired osseointegration and are favorably functioning, and the actual state is unclear.

We experienced the case of a patient who developed ONJ around implants in the maxilla, considered to be caused by intravenous BP administration for osteometastasis treatment of breast cancer, and underwent partial maxillectomy to relieve inflammation (Shirota et al. 2009). This chapter introduces clinical findings, the treatment and its outcome, and peri-implant histopathological findings in the patient, and the developmental mechanism of peri-implant BRONJ is discussed with a literature review.

2. Patient and methods

2.1 Outline of the patient

The patient was a 54-year-old female who visited our hospital for chief complaints of peri-implant pain in the upper left molar region and bone exposure. The patient developed breast cancer about 6 years ago and underwent left mastectomy followed by irradiation and chemotherapy. However, multiple cancer metastases occurred about 2 years ago, and the patient underwent cancer chemotherapy and intravenous BPs injection.

The patient underwent implant treatment for the upper left molar region at a dental clinic immediately before the development of breast cancer, in which 2 implants were placed. These implants functioned without a problem for about 6 years, but peri-implant gingival recession, bone exposure, and pain appeared about one month ago, and the patient received antimicrobial drug administration, irrigation, and disinfection at a clinic, but the symptoms did not improve. Thus, the patient visited our department. On the first examination, brown-colored necrotized bone was exposed in the upper left first molar region on the buccal side.

The peri-implant gingiva was painful and swollen with slight flare, but no implant mobility was observed (Fig.1). On panoramic radiography, mild bone resorption was noted in alveolar bone in the implant neck. Computed tomography (CT) revealed sequestration with an irregular trabecular bone structure around the implant (Fig.2). Biopsy was performed in consideration of metastasis of breast cancer to the oral cavity, but only inflammatory cell infiltration was observed without tumor cells.

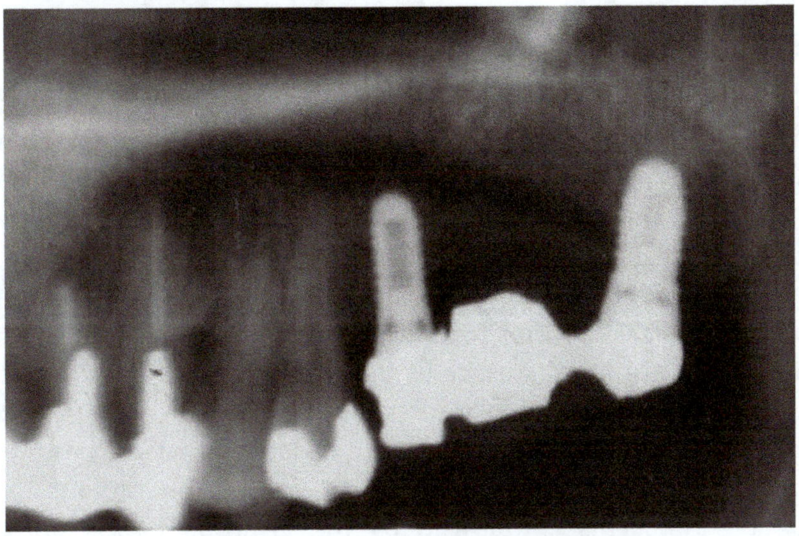

Fig. 1. Radiograph showing slight bone resorption around the implants.

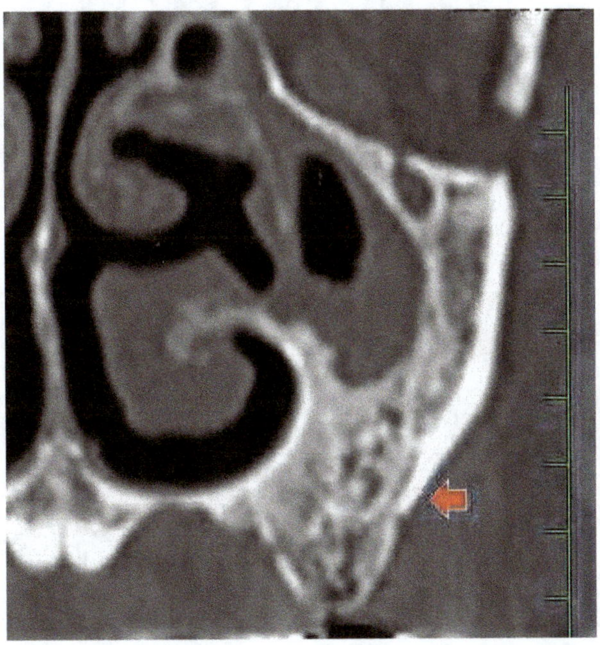

Fig. 2. Computed tomography (CT) image around the implants (arrow).

2.2 Diagnosis and treatment

It is well-known that curative chemotherapy or long-term adrenocortical steroid administration for lymphoblastic leukemia and Hodgkin and non-Hodgkin lymphomas induces osteonecrosis of the femoral head (Kubo et al. 2001; Bojko et al 2003; Karimova et al.

2008). Many anticancer drugs were administered for breast cancer metastasis in this patient, but no osteonecrosis of the jaw caused by these drugs has been reported. In addition, the clinical symptoms of this patient met all diagnostic criteria of BRONJ proposed by AAOMS (AAOMS 2007; Ruggiero et al. 2009). Based on these findings, BP-induced osteonecrosis was diagnosed.

In the treatment, morbid bone tissue including implants was resected in consideration of the following 3 conditions: 1) early chemotherapy for metastatic cancer was necessary, for which removal of the infected lesion was necessary, 2) there was a possibility that continuation of the withdrawal of BPs would aggravate metastatic cancer-associated bone destruction and hypercalcemia, and 3) it was difficult to remit inflammation by employing conservative treatment proposed by the American Association of Oral and Maxillofacial Surgeons (AAOMS 2007; Ruggiero et al. 2009). After considering these points, sequestrectomy of the left maxilla was selected. The gingival margin was incised between the upper left first premolar and implant towards the maxillary tuberosity, and the lesion area was exposed by forming a buccal and palatal mucoperiosteal flap. The bone cortex of the lesion was brownish black, and necrotic bone was confirmed between the distal surface of the second premolar and mesial surface of the implant placed in the second molar area, but particularly around the implant placed in the first molar area (Fig.3a). The area for resection around the living bone in the lesion was determined after the extraction of the second premolar, and the pathological bone tissue including the implant was removed with a Lindeman bar and bone chisel, followed by the grinding of the bone surface of the resection stump until bleeding was confirmed. As a result, the instrument partially perforated the maxillary sinus floor, and the thickened maxillary sinus mucosa was exposed. This sinus mucosa was spared, and the surgical wound was completely closed by suturing the mucoperiosteal flaps (Fig.3b)

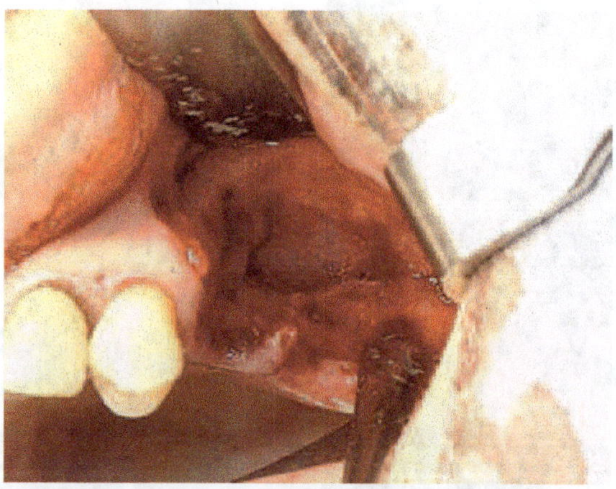

(a) Pathological bone including the implants was removed, and maxillary sinus mucosa was exposed.

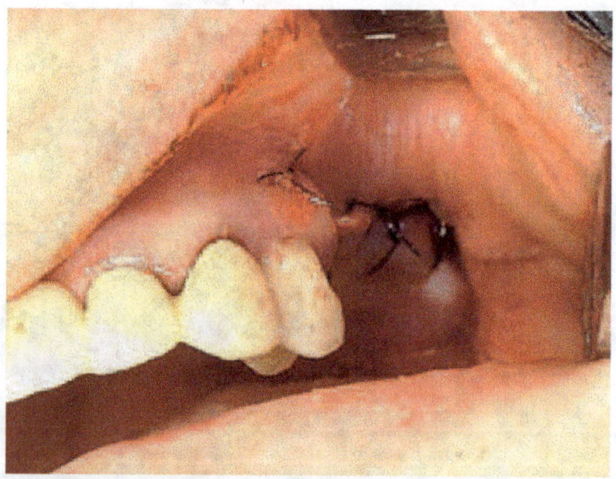

(b) The surgical wound was completely closed by suturing the mucoperiosteal flap.

Fig. 3. Intraoperative view of the sequestomy of the left maxilla.

After surgery, antibiotic was intravenously administered for 3 days and oral antibiotic was administered for 3 days. In addition, hyperbaric oxygen therapy was performed. The efficacy of hyperbaric oxygen therapy for BRONJ is controversial (Ruggiero et al. 2004; Freiberger et al 2009), but, at least, it may be effective to promote mucoepithelial wound healing in the sequestration-resected region. The wound was completely covered with healthy mucosa 2 weeks after surgery (Fig.4.). Since the remission of inflammation could be confirmed, anticancer drug and BP administration was initiated for metastatic cancer and bone metastasis-associated bone destruction. The patient died of multiorgan failure associated with multiple cancer metastasis 8 months after surgery, but BRONJ did not recur before death.

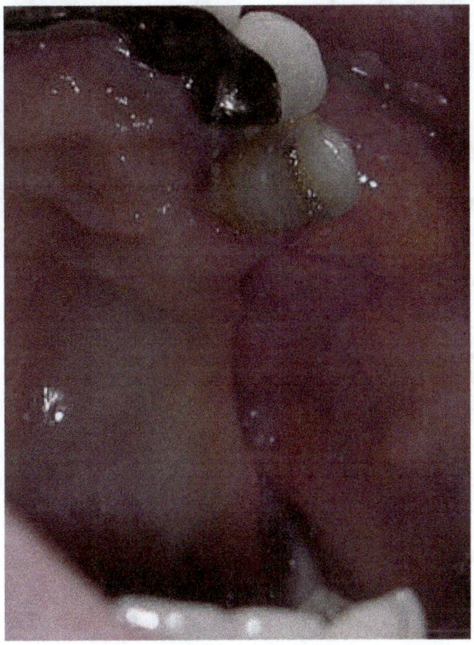

Fig. 4. Intraoral view at 4 weeks after surgery.

2.3 Macroscopic and μCT findings of the resected specimen

Implants were strongly fixed to the bone, and areas of brown sequestration were observed around them (Fig.5.). On μCT, no apparent abnormality, such as trabecular destruction, was observed, and the implant surface was in direct contact with the trabecula at various sites (Fig.6.).

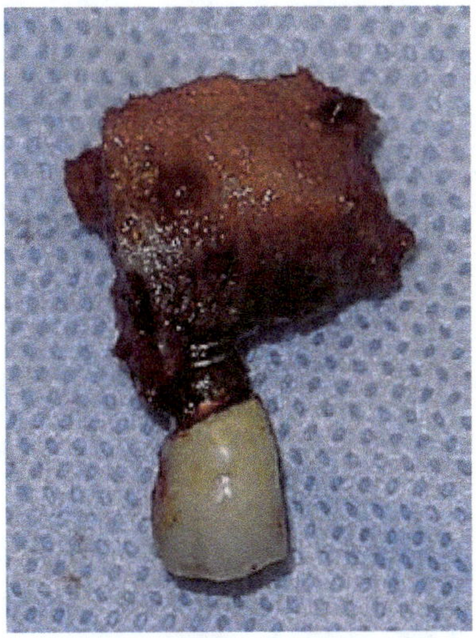

Fig. 5. The resected specimen shows a portion of the left maxilla including two implants.

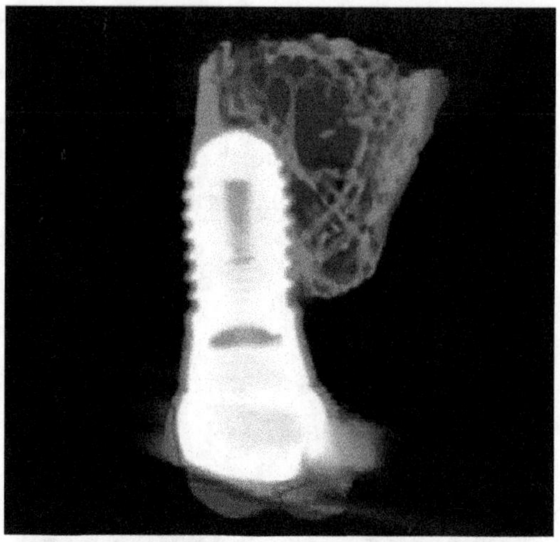

Fig. 6. μCT findings of the resected specimen.

2.4 Histopathological analysis

2.4.1 Histologic preparation

The resected specimen was divided into the lesion including the implants and peri-lesion, i.e., healthy tissue in the resected stump. The bone tissue around the implants was fixed, dehydrated, and embedded in polyester resin (Ligorac®, Wako Pure Chemical Industries, Ltd., Tokyo, Japan). Undecalcified ground sections 15 μm in thickness were cut along the long axis of the implant using the EXAKT Cutting-Grinding System (EXAKT, Norderstedt, Germany) and stained with 1% toluidine blue (pH 7.2), then the bone tissue around the implant was observed under light microscopy. Meanwhile, the bone tissue around the lesion was dehydrated and embedded in paraffin according to the conventional procedure. Some of the sections were stained with hematoxylin-eosin (HE) and AZAAN. Other sections were processed for immunohistochemical analysis by immunostaining with anti-human CD3, CD20, CD45 and CD68 (Daco, Carpinteria, CA).

2.4.2 Peri-implant histopathological findings in undecalcified ground sections

The implant surface was mostly in direct contact with bone tissue, suggesting that osseointegration was maintained until BRONJ development (Fig.7a). No osteocyte was present in the cavity of bone contacting implants or the surrounding trabeculae, nor were there cellular components on the bone surface, and bone tissue mostly showed sequestration (Fig.7b). The marrow cavity was filled with aggregates of actinomycete-like microorganisms, neutrophils, and other necrotized soft tissue (Fig.8a). In addition, adsorption cavities with a worm-eaten appearance were widely present. Normally, bone tissue necrotized in the body is absorbed by osteoclasts, shows sequestration, and is naturally excreted. However, no osteoclasts were present in the resorption cavity, suggesting that active resorption of the bone occurred in the BRONJ developmental process, rather than the resorption of necrotized bone by osteoclasts (Fig.8b).

2.4.3 Histopathological findings around lesions in decalcified sections

Osteocytes were present in the bone cavity (Fig.9a,b). The trabecular surface was smooth, and osteoid formation and osteoblast arrangement were observed. Reactive bone formation was also observed at various trabecular sites. Granulation tissue rich in capillary blood

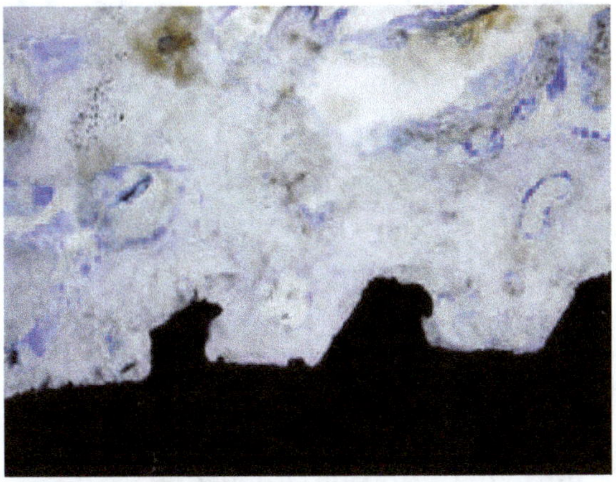

(a) Most of the implant surfaces are in direct contact with the bone (× 40).

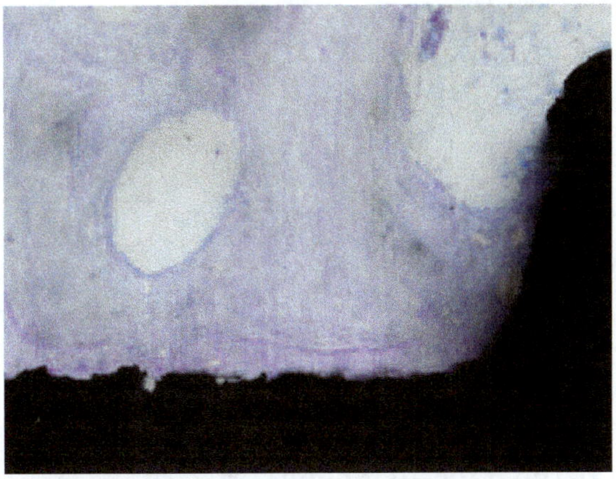

(b) The bone in contact with the implant sureface is necrotic (× 200).

Fig. 7. Histological findings of the tissue from the implants in an undecalcofied sections stained with toluidine blue.

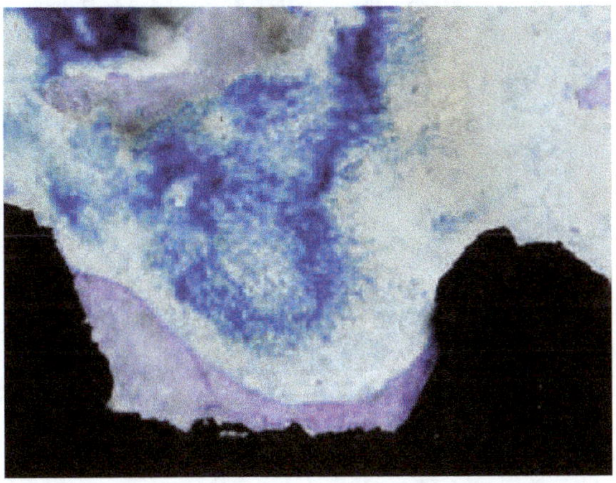

(a) Growth of a bacterial colony into the marrow cavity is observed (× 200).

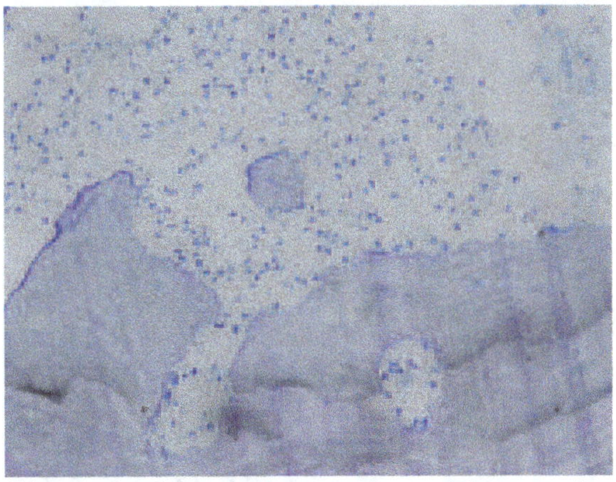

(b) Marked bone destruction with a moth eaten appearance is observed on the necrotic trabecular bone surface (× 200).

Fig. 8. Histological findings of the tissue from the implants in an undecalcofied sections stained with toluidine blue.

vessels invaded the bone marrow region (Fig.10a,b). On immunohistological staining, lymphocytes infiltrating the bone marrow were mostly CD3-positive, showing that the cells were derived from T cells. In contrast, only a few lymphoctyes were positive for CD20 and CD45 (Fig.11a,b), but they were considered not to be significant. Multinucleated giant cells strongly positive for CD68, assumed to be osteoclasts, were present at various sites on the trabecular surface (Fig.12a,b).

3. Discussion on the peri-implant BRONJ developmental mechanism

No viewpoint regarding the pathogenesis of BRONJ has been established. Based on clinical experience, mucosal injuries caused by poorly fitting dentures and oral surgical treatment, such as that for periodontal disease and tooth extraction, have been reported as local risk factors, but this patient received no surgical dental treatment during the BP administration

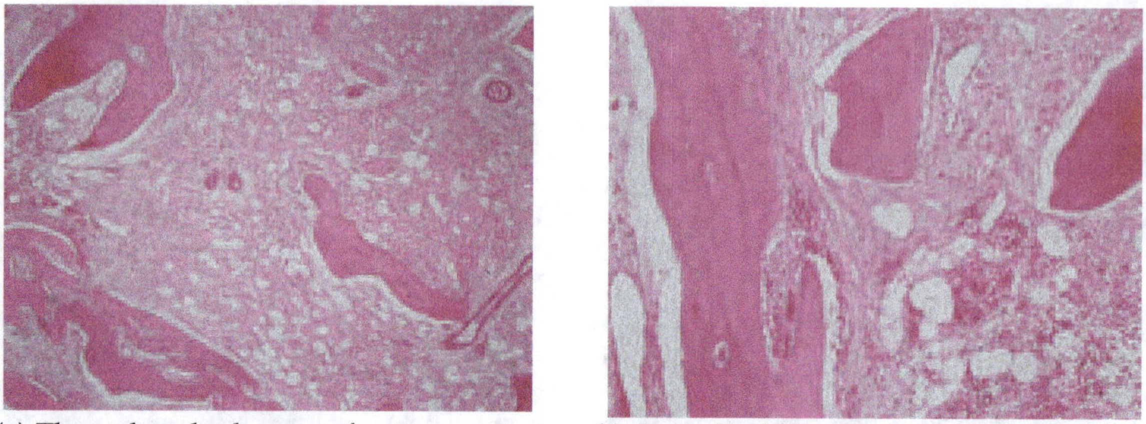

(a) The trabecular bone surface are smooth (HE stain; × 40)

b) Growth of fibrous connective tissue and vascular formation are observed in the marrow(HE stain, × 100).

Fig. 9. Histological findings of the tissue around the lesion in a decalcified thin section.

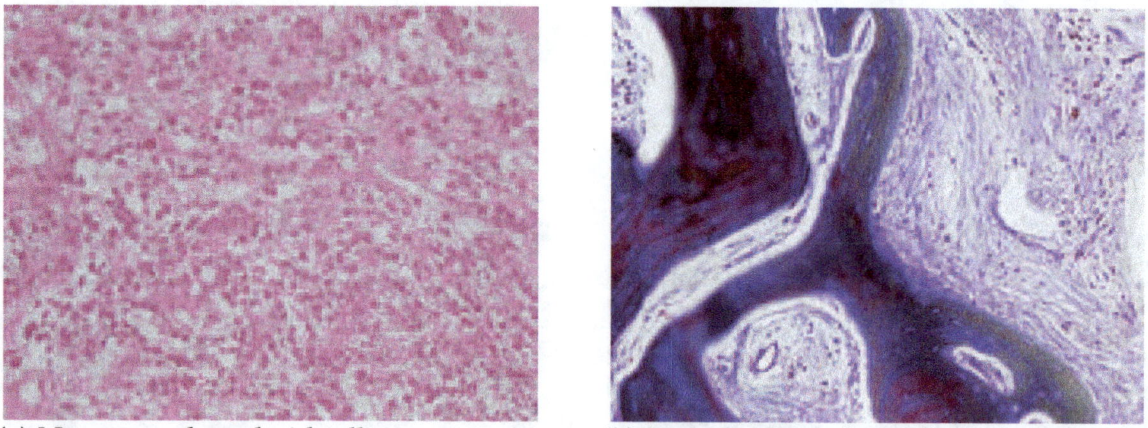

(a) Numerous lymphoid cells are observed in the marrow (HE stain; × 200).

(b) Lining cells and osteoid formation are observed (AZAN; × 100).

Fig. 10. Histological findings of the tissue around the lesion in a decalcified thin section.

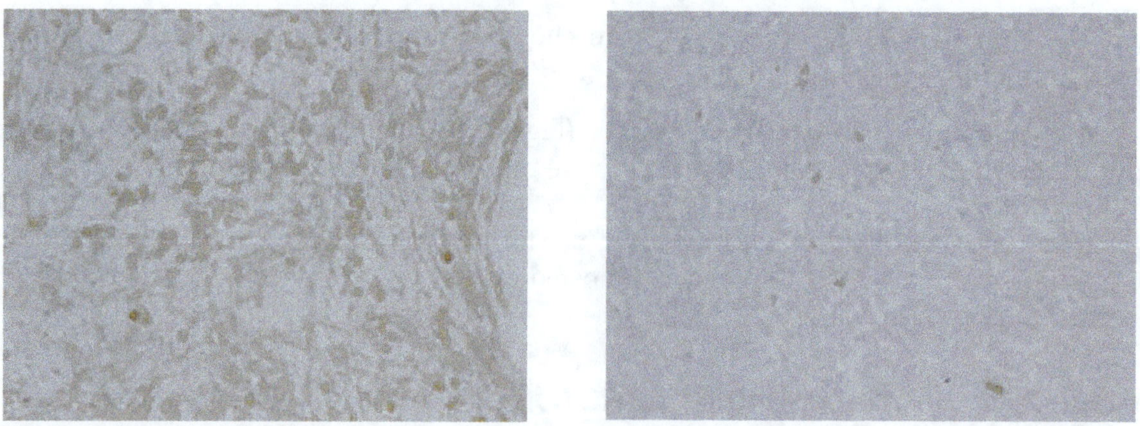

(a) Many lymphoid cells are positive for anti-human CD3 (× 200).

(b) Only a few lymphoctyes are positive for CD20 (× 200).

Fig. 11. Immunohistological staining ot hte tissue around the lesion in a decalcified thin section.

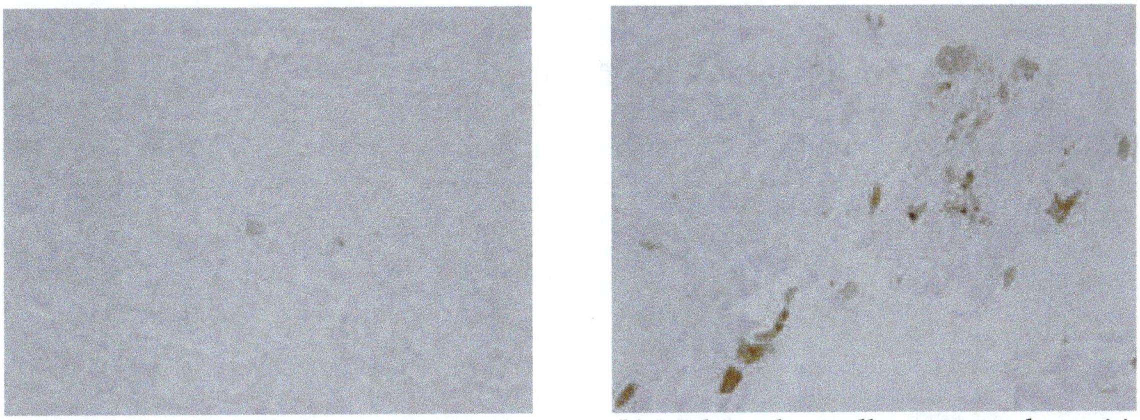

(a) Only a few lymphoctyes are positive for CD45 (× 200).

(b) Multinuclear cells are strongly positive for anti-human CD68 antibody (× 200).

Fig. 12. Immunohistological staining ot hte tissue around the lesion in a decalcified thin section.

period, and no implant mobility was observed in the BRONJ site. Histologically, oseointegration was widely maintained on the implant surface, and no deep overgrowth of gingival epithelium was noted, suggesting that BRONJ in this patient suddenly occurred around favorably functioning implants, and was not induced by peri-implant inflammation. Necrosis of the femoral head (Kerachian et al. 2006) and irradiation-induced osteonecrosis of the jaw (Marx 1983) are widely known as osteonecrotic lesions, and the cause is insufficiency of vascular formation in both diseases. Reportedly, zoledronate exhibits a potent vascularization-inhibitory effect (Giraudo et al. 2004), and the BP-induced obstruction of blood vessels in bone and necrosis of osteocytes around them have been reported (Hansen et al. 2007). Based on these findings, it is hypothesized that insufficiency of the blood supply is also involved in BRONJ, but, histologically, the absence of vascularization inhibition in BRONJ has been reported (Bedogni et al. 2008). Another important hypothesis suggests an influence of reduced bone remodeling due to the BP-induced inhibition of bone resorption by osteoclasts. It has been reported that osteocyte mortality increases when bone remodeling declines, i.e., BPs reduce bone remodeling, increasing osteocyte death, which is involved in BRONJ (Allen et al. 2009). However, many resorption cavities were present on the peri-implant-sequestered bone surface, and the growth of granulation tissue containing abundant capillary blood vessels and reactive bone formation in the resected stump were confirmed in this patient. Thus, it is difficult to explain the cause of BRONJ with insufficient blood supply and the bone remodeling-inhibitory effect of BPs alone.

Pamidronate and zoledronate administered intravenously to this patient are BPs that incorporate nitrogen. BPs containing nitrogen (NBPs) induce an inflammatory reaction by stimulating cells (Hewit et al. 2005; Endo et al. 1993; Nakamura et al. 1996). NBPs also exist on the surface of gram-negative cell walls, and increase inflammatory reactions to lipopolysaccharide (LPS), which has a strong inflammatory effect (Yamaguchi et al. 2000). Therefore, BRONJ may be caused by interactions among several factors differing among cases, not by a single cause. For example, in this patient, the following conditions may have influenced each other and caused BRONJ: 1) the excessive inhibition of bone turnover due to the NBP-related inhibition of bone resorption; 2) the occlusal force loaded on implants was directly transmitted to the bone, which activated local bone metabolism in the surrounding region, releasing BP accumulated in the bone at a high level; 3) free NBP-induced inflammatory reactions, induction of osteoclast apoptosis (Roelofs et al. 2006), and inhibition of epithelial activity (Landesberg et al. 2009); 4) increased risk of bacterial infection due to suppression of the immune system; 5) enhanced inflammatory reactions due to interactions between gram-negative bacterial lipopolysaccharides and NBPs and 6) reduced local blood flow by vascularization inhibition and vascular obstruction (Fig.13).

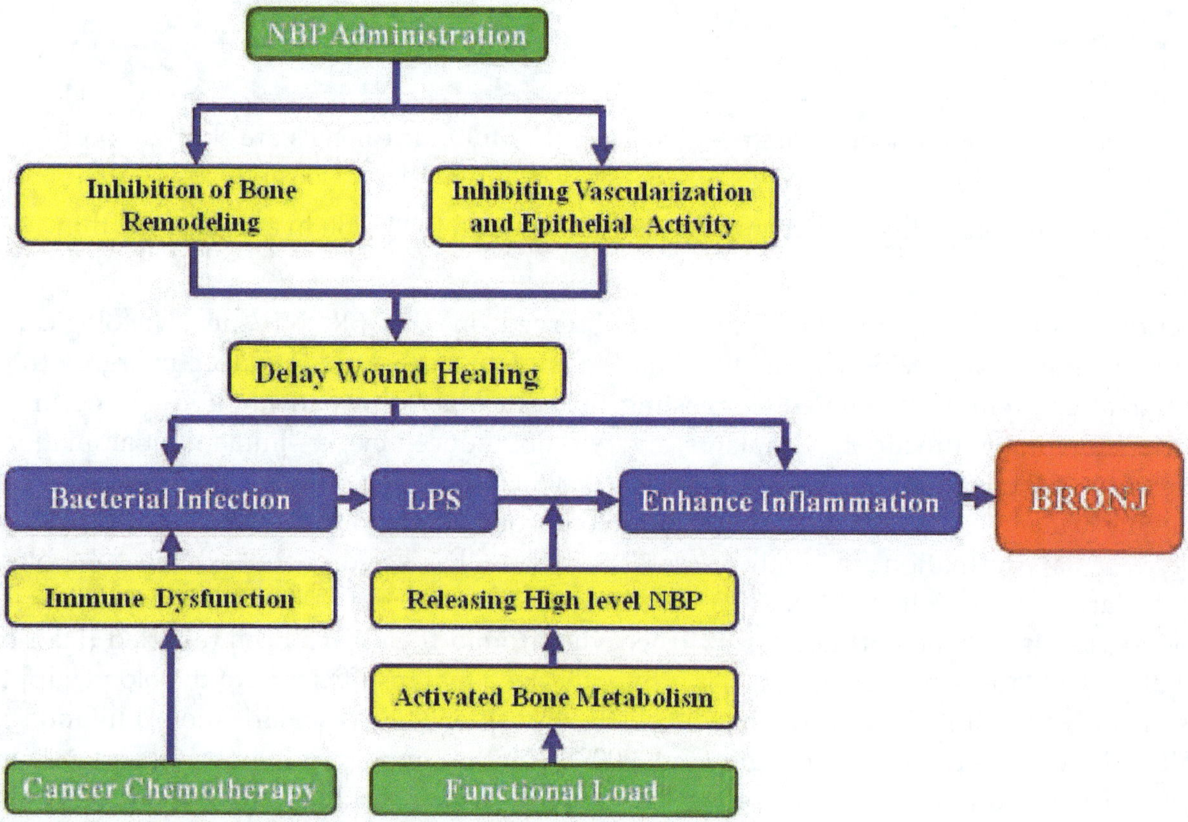

Fig. 13. Hypothetical mechanism of BRONJ aroud the implants.

4. Conclusion

BRONJ is intractable, and no treatment method has been established. Only guidelines mainly concerning prevention and conservative treatment have been proposed. When peri-implant BRONJ occurs, firstly, conservative treatment should be selected following the AAOMS treatment guidelines, placing great importance on the prevention of exacerbation of BRONJ, but when NBPs are administered to control bone metastasis, it should be a priority to re-start BP administration and prevent any delay in cancer chemotherapy. Accordingly, although the appropriateness and timing of sequestration site resection should be carefully investigated, active surgical treatment may be one choice for some patients. Implant treatment is no longer special treatment. It is widely introduced into routine dental practice as a method to recover the occlusal function of defective teeth. Therefore, NBP intravenous injections will be increasingly administered to patients with a past medical history of implant treatment, for which the establishment of a practical clinical policy for the prevention and treatment of BRONJ is strongly desired.

5. References

AAOMS. (2007) American association of oral and maxillofacial surgeons position paper on bisphosphonate-related osteonecrosis of the jaws. *The Journal of Oral and Maxillofacial Surgery*, Vol. 67, No.3, (March 2007), pp. 943-950, ISSN 0278-2391

Allen, M.R. & Burr, D.B. (2009). The pathogenesis of bisphosphonate-related osteonecrosis of the jaw: so many hypotheses, so few data. *The Journal of Oral and Maxillofacial surgaery*, Vol.67 No.5 Supplement 1, (May 2009), pp. 61-70, ISSN 0278-2391

Bedogni, A., Blandamura, S., Lokmic, Z., Palumbo, C., Ragazzo, M., Ferrari, F., Tregnaghi, A., Pietrogrande, F., Procopio, O., Saia, G., Ferretti, M., Bedogni, G., Chiarini, L., Ferronato, G., Ninfo, V., Lo Russo, L., Lo Muzio, L. & Nocini P.F. (2008). Bisphosphonate-associated jawbone osteonecrosis: a correlation between imaging techniques and histopathology. *Oral Surgery, Oral Medicine, Oral Pathology, Oral Radiology and Endodontology*, Vol. 105, No. 3, (March 2009), pp.358-364, ISSN 1079-2104

Bell, B.M., & Bell, R.E. (2008). Oral bisphosphonates and dental implants: a retrospective study. *The Journal of Oral and Maxillofacial Surgaery*, Vol. 66, No.5, (May 2008), pp.1022-1024, ISSN 1079-2104

Berenson, J. R., Lichtenstein, A., Porter, L., Dimopoulos, M.A., Bordoni, R., George, S., Lipton, A., Keller, A., Ballester, O., Kovacs, M. J., Blacklock H.A., Bell, R., Simeone, J., Reitsma, D. J., Hefferman, M., Seaman, J. & Knight, R. D. (1996). Efficacy of pamidronate in reducing skeletal event in patients with advanced multiple myeloma. Myeloma Aredia Study Group. *The New England Journal of Medicine*, Vol. 334, No. 8, (Feburuary 1996), pp.488-493, ISSN 0028-4793

Body, J. J., Lortholary, A., Romieu, G., Vigneron, A. M. & Ford, J. (1999). A dose-finding sudy of zoledronate in hypercalcemic cancer patients. *Journal of Bone and Mineral Research*, Vol.14, No.19, (September 1999), pp.1557-61, ISSN 1523-4681

Bojko, P., Hilger, R.A., Ruehm, S.G., Dirsch, O., Seeber, S. & Scheulen, M.E. (2003). Femoral head necrosis in three patients with relapsed ovarian cancer receiving high-dose chemotherapy followed by autologous peripheral blood stem cell transplantation. *Bone Marrow Teansplantation*, Vol. 31, No.6, (March 2003), pp.487-491, ISSN 0268-3369

Endo, Y., Nakamura, M., Kikuchi, T., Shinoda, H., Takeda. Y., Nitta, Y. & Kumagai, K. (1993) Aminoalkylbisphosphonates, potent inhibitors of bone resorption, induce a prolonged stimulation of histamine synthesis and increase macrophages, granulocytes, and osteoclasts in vivo. *Calcified Tissue International* Vol.52, No.3, (March 1993), pp.248-254, ISSN 0171-967X

Fleisch, H., Reszka, A., Rodan, G. & Rogers, M. (2002). Bisphosphonates: Mechanisms of action, *Principles of Bone Biology*, Bilezikian, J. P., Raisz, L. G. & Rodan, G.A., pp. 13161-1385, Academic Press, ISBN 012-0986-523, San Diego

Freiberger, J.J. (2009). Utility of hyperbaric oxygen in treatment of bisphosphonate-related osteonecrosis of the jaws. *The Journal of Oral Maxillofacial Surgery*. Vol.67, No.5 Supplement 1, (March 2009), pp.96-106, ISSN 1079-2104

Fugazzotto, P.A., Lightfoot, W.S., Jaffin, R. & Kumar, A. (2007). Implant placement with or without simultaneous tooth extraction in patients taking oral bisphosphonates: postoperative healing, early follow-up, and the incidence of complications in two private practices. *Journal of Periodontology*, Vol.78, No.9, (September 2007), pp.1664-1669 ISSN 0022-3492

Giraudo, E., Inoue, M. & Hanahan, D. (2004). An amino-bisphosphonate targets MMP-9-expressing macrophages and angiogenesis to impair cervical carcinogenesis. *The Journal of Clinical Investigation*, Vol.114, No.5, (September 1 2004), pp.623-633, ISSN, 0021-9738

Grant, B.T., Amenedo, C., Freeman, K. & Kraut RA. (2008). Outcomes of placing dental implants in patients taking oral bisphosphonates: a review of 115 cases. *The Journal of Oral and Maxillofacial Surgery*, Vol. 66, No.2, (February 2008), pp.223-230, ISSN 0278-2391

Hansen, T., Kunkel, M., Springer, E., Walter, C., Weber, A., Siegel, E. & Kirkpatrick, C.J. (2007). Actinomycosis of the jaws--histopathological study of 45 patients shows significant involvement in bisphosphonate-associated osteonecrosis and infected osteoradionecrosis *Virchows Archiv* Vol.451, No.6, (December 2007), pp.1009-1017, ISSN 0945-6317

Hewit, R.E., Lissina, A., Green, A.E., Slay, E.S., Price, D.A. & Sewell, D.A. (2005) The bisphosphonate acute phase response: rapid and copious production of proinflammatory cytokines by peripheral blood gd T cells in response to aminobisphosphonates is inhibited by statins. *Clinical Experimental Immunology*, Vol.139, No.1, (January 2005), pp.101-111, ISSN 0009-9104

Hortobagyi, G. N., Theriault, R. L., Lipton, A., Porter, L., Blayney, D., Sinoff, C., Wheeler, H., Simeone, J. F., Seaman, J. J., Knight, R. D., Heffernan, M., Mellars, K. & Reitsma, D. J. (1998). Long-term prevention of skeletal complications of metastatic brest cancer with pamidronate. Protocol 19 Aredia Brest Cancer Study Group. *Journal of Clinical Oncology*, Vol.16, No.6, (June 1998), pp.2038-2044, ISSN 0732-183X

Karimova, E.J., Rai, S.N., Wu, J., Britton, L., Kaste, S.C. & Neel, M.D. (2008). Femoral resurfacing inyoung patients with hematologic cancer and osteonecrosis. *Clinical Orthopaedics Related Research*, Vol. 466, No. 12, (December 2008), pp.3044-3050, ISSN 1528-1132

Kerachian, M.A., Harvey, E. J., Cournoyer, D., Chow, T.Y. & Séguin C. (2006). A vascular necrosis of the femoral head: vascular hypotheses. *Journal of Endothelial Cell Research*, Vol.23, No. 4, (July-August 2006), pp.237-244, ISSN 1062-3329

Khan, A.A., Sándor, G.K., Dore, E., Morrison, A.D., Alsahli, M., Amin, F., Peters, E., Hanley, D.A., Chaudry, S.R., Dempster, D.W., Glorieux, F.H., Neville, A.J., Talwar, R.M., Clokie, C.M., Al Mardini, M., Paul, T., Khosla, S., Josse, R. G., Sutherland, S., Lam, D.K., Carmichael, R.P., Blanas, N., Kendler, D., Petak, S., St-Marie, L.G., Brown, J., Evans, A.W., Rios L. & Compston, J.E.; Canadian Association of Oral and Maxillofacial Surgeons. (2008). Canadian consensus practice guidelines for bisphosphonate associated osteonecrosis of the jaw. *The Journal of Rheumatology*, Vol.35, No.7, (July 2008), pp.1391-1397, ISSN 0315-162X

Khosla, S., Burr, D., Cauley, J., Dempster, D.W., Ebeling, P.R., Felsenberg, D., Gagel, R.F., Gilsanz , V., Guise, T., Koka, S., McCauley, L.K., McGowan, J., McKee, M.D., Mohla, S., Pendrys, D.G., Raisz, L.G., Ruggiero, S.L., Shafer, D.M., Shum, L., Silverman, S.L., Van Poznak, C.H., Watts, N., Woo, S.B. & Shane, E.; American Society for Bone and Mineral Research. (2007). Bisphosphonate-associated osteonecrosis of the jaw: Report of a task force of the American Society for Bone and Mineral Research. *Journal of Bone and Mineral Research*, Vol.22, No. 10, (October 2007), pp.1479-1491, ISSN 1523-4681

Kubo, T., Kojima, A., Yamazoe, S., Ueshima, K., Yamamoto, T. & Hirasawa, Y. (2001). Osteonecrosis of the femoral head that developed after long-term topical application. *Journal of Orthopaedic Science*, Vol.6, No.1, (January 2001), pp.92-94, ISSN 0949-2658

Landesberg, R., Eisig, S., Fennoy, I. & Siris, E. (2009). Alternative indications for bisphosphonate therapy. *The Journal of Oral and Maxillofacial Surgery*, Vol.67, No.5 Supplement 1, (May 2009), pp.27-34, ISSN 1079-2104

Marx, R. E. (1983). Osteonecrosis: a new concept of its pathophysiology. J *The Journal of Oral and Maxillofacial Surgery*, Vol.41, No.5, (May 1983), pp. 283-288, ISSN 1079-2104

Marx, R. E. (2003). Pamidronate (Aredia) and Zoledronate (Zometa) Induced Avascular Necrosis of the Jaws: A growing epidemic. *Journal of Oral and Maxillofacial Surgery*, Vol.61, No.9, (September 2003), pp.1115-1117, ISSN 1079-2104

Marx, R. E., Sawatari, Y., Fortin, M. & Broumand, N. (2005). Bisphosphonate-induced exposed bone (osteonecrosis/osteopetrosis) of the jaws. Journal of Oral and Maxillofacial Surgery, Vol.63, No.11, (November 2005), pp.1567-1575, ISSN 1079-2104

Migliorati, C.A., Casiglia, J., Epstein, J., Jacobsen, P.L., Siegel, M.A. & Woo, S.B. (2005). Managing the care of patients with bisphosphonate-associated osteonecrosis: an American Academy of Oral Medicine position paper. *Journal of the American Dental Association*, Vol.136, No.12, (December 2005), pp.1658-68, ISSN 0002-8177

Nakamura, M., Ando, T., Abe, M., Kumagai, K & Endo, Y. (1996) Contrast between effects of aminobisphosphonates and non-aminobisphosphonates on collagen-induced arthritis in mice. *British Journal of Pharmacology*, Vol.119, No.2, (September 1996), pp.205-212, ISSN 1476-5381

Roelofs, A.J., Thompson, K., Gordon, S. & Rogers, M.J. (2006). Molecular mechanisms of action of bisphosphonates: current status. *Clinical Cancer Research*, Vol.12, No.20 Pt 2, (October 2006), pp.6222s-6230s, ISSN1557-3265

Ruggiero, S. L., Mehrotra, B., Rosenberg, T.J. & Engroff, S. L. (2004). Osteonecrosis of the Jaws associated with the use of bisphosphonates: a review of 63 cases. *The Journal of Oral and Maxillofacial Surgery*, Vol.62, No.5, pp.527-534, ISSN 1079-2104

Ruggiero, S.L., Dodson, T.B., Assael, L.A., Landesberg, R., Marx, R.E. & Mehrotra, B.; American Association of oral and Maxillofacial Surgeons. (2009). American Association of Oral and Maxillofacial Surgeons Position Paper on Bisphosphonate-Related Osteonecrosis of the Jaws – 2009 update. *The Journal of Oral and Maxillofacial Surgery*, Vol.67, No.5 Supplement, pp.2-12, ISSN 1079-2104

Russell, R.G., Xia, Z., Dunford, J.E., Oppermann, U., Kwaasi, A., Hulley, P.A., Kavanagh, K.L., Triffitt, J.T., Lundy, M.W., Phipps, R.J., Barnet, B.L., Coxon, F.P., Rogers, M.J., Wattss, N.B. & Ebetino, F.H. (2007). Bisphosphonates an update on mechanisms of action and how these relate to clinical efficacy. *Annals of the New York Academy of Sciences* Vol.1117, (November 2007), pp.209-257, ISSN 1749-6632

Shirota, T., Nakamura, A., Matsui, Y., Hatori, M., Nakamura, M. & Shintani, S. (2009) Bisphosphonate-related osteonecrosis of the jaw around dental implants in the maxilla: report of a case. *Clinical Oral Implants Ressearch*, Vol.20, No.12, (December 2009), pp. 1402-1408, ISSN 0905-7161

Starck, W.J. & Epker, B.N. (1995). Failure of osseointegrated dental implants after diphosphonate therapy for osteoporosis: a case report. *The International Journal of Oral & Maxillofacacial Implants*, Vol. 10, No.1, (January-February 1995), pp.74-78, 0882-2786

Vahtsevanos, K., Kyrgidis, A., Verrou, E., Katodritou, E., Triaridis, S., Andreadis, C.G., Boukovinas, I., Koloutsos, G.E., Teleioudis, Z., Kitikidou, K., Paraskevopoulos, P., Zervas, K. & Antoniades, K. (2009). Longitudinal cohort study of risk factors in cancer patients of bisphosphonate-related osteonecrosis of the jaw. Journal of *Clinical Oncology*, Vol.27, No.32, (November 2009), pp.5356-5362, ISSN 0732-183X

Yamaguchi, K., Motegi, K., Iwakura, Y. & Endo, Y. (2000). Involvement of interleukin-1 in the inflammatory actions of aminobisphosphonates in mice. *British Journal of Pharmacology*, Vol.130, No.7, (August 2000), pp.1646-1654, ISSN 1476-5381

Yoneda, T., Hagino, H., Sugimoto, T., Ohta, H, Takahashi, S., Soen, S., Taguchi, A., Toyosawa, S., Nagata, T. & Urade, M. (2010). Bisphosphonate-related osteonecrosis of the jaw: position paper from the Allied Task Force Committee of Japanese Society for Bone and Mineral Research, Japan Osteoporosis Society, Japanese Society of Periodontology, Japanese Society for Oral and Maxillofacial Radiology, and Japanese Society of Oral and Maxillofacial Surgeons. *Journal of Bone and Mineral Metabolism*, Vol.28, No.4, pp.365-383, ISSN 1435-5604

4

Computer-Guided Implantology

Rogério Margonar[1], Cássia Bellotto Corrêa[2], Ana Lúcia Roselino Ribeiro[2], Erika Oliveira de Almeida[3,4], Elcio Marcantonio[2] and Luís Geraldo Vaz[2]
[1]*Araraquara University Center - UNIARA, Araraquara, SP,*
[2]*São Paulo State University - UNESP, College of Dentistry, Araraquara, SP,*
[3]*São Paulo State University - UNESP, College of Dentistry, Araçatuba, SP,*
[4]*New York University - NYU, College of Dentistry, New York, NY,*
[1,2,3]*Brazil,*
[4]*USA*

1. Introduction

Anatomically planned and functionally optimal implant placement has long been a major goal of implant dentistry (Drago, 1994.; Garber & Belser, 1995). Many surgical procedures are necessary to the optimal placement of the implant. Thus, it would be of great clinical advantage for patients to have dental implants placed flapless and immediately loaded with prosthesis, delivered just after surgery. Post-operative morbidity and treatment times could be reduced significantly (Cannizzaro et al., 2008; Meloni et al., 2010). Thereby the growing interest for flapless surgery in conjunction with immediate loading of the edentulous patients has led to the development of software programs that allow treatment planning, fabrication of a surgical template, as well as the production of a prosthesis that can be secure to the patient immediately after the placement of the implants (Fuster-Torres et al., 2009).

However, the accurate diagnostic is the main factor for the treatment success. The edentulous patients generally have resorption when they loose their teeth.

The resorption can be related to bone loss and bone loss associated with the soft tissue. The type of resorption is decisive to determine the kind of fixed implant supported prosthesis. Patients who lost soft tissue and underlying supporting bone in addition to teeth may be considered to have a composite defect. To evaluate the relative amount of soft tissue deficiency, it is suggested to utilize a denture or denture set-up in wax that has been confirmed for proper tooth position, border extension, and relationship between the arcs (Bedrossian et al., 2008). So, an appropriate selection of the type of prosthesis is fundamental in the beginning of the treatment planing using implants.

There are two main objectives of computer-aided design (CAD), computer-aided machining (CAM): guided dental implant placement and restoration. The first allow the precise planning of implant positions on computed tomography scans, and the second is to generate an accurate surgical guide that permits the surgeon to place implants precisely into planned positions allowing the immediate prosthesis placement (Fuster-Torres et al., 2003).

Thus the objective of this chapter is to discuss the indications, contraindications, protocol preparation, maintenance problems and postoperative-guided in implantology.

2. Guided surgery

The use of software associated with digital images, acquired from computerized tomography, it is a new trend in dentistry. The CAD/CAM technologies associated with stereolithography provide to the professional tools to improve the planning and the rehabilitation with more security.

The use of software combined with three-dimensional images obtained by computerized tomography enables the professional to evaluate the optical density, to measure the bone thickness and, therefore, to choose the implant size and its appropriate positioning in the arch (Spin-Neto et al. 2011).

The guided surgery is a highly accurate in implantology. By this technique, the extensive amount of information obtained in a virtual planning is transferred for the surgical field by means of surgical guides manufactured in stereolithography (Parel & Triplett, 2004). Later, the advantages and limitation of the surgical guide will be discuss.

2.1 Indications

The guided surgery is indicated both for total edentulous patients (Casap et al., 2005 ;Van Steenberghe et al., 2004) as for partially edentulous patients (Fortin et al. 2003; Kupeyan et al., 2006; Marchack, 2007; Serry et al., 2007).

The guided surgery is counter-indicated for patients with reduced mouth opening that jeopardizes positioning of surgical instruments on the guide (Almeida et al., 2010).

This technique has several advantages compared to the conventional open flap surgery. These are the preservation of the vital anatomical structures, minimal invasive surgery, faster and simpler technique and leads to less discomfort to the patient after the surgery (Kupeyan et al., 2006; Van Steenberghe et al., 2004; Becker et al., 2005; Widmann et al., 2010) as well as lower risk of infection. However, due to the use of a range of sophisticated technology and specialized instrumentals, the guided surgery technique has a higher cost compared to the conventional surgery. In addition, some authors reports that the surgical guide can be unstable for completely edentulous patient mainly when only remaining soft tissue is present. (Bedrossian, 2007; Holst et al., 2004).

2.2 Technique

Before the tomography, some steps are necessary to assist the planning, as a specific clinical exam. In this session, it is important to evaluate the existing prosthesis of the patient, relationship between the arches, the dental oclusal pattern and the inter maxillary distance. An initial clinical exam is accomplished to evaluate the relationship among the arches, the oclusal pattern and the inter maxillary distance.

For the total edentulous patients, it is fabricated the total prosthesis with appropriate vertical dimension of occlusion (Figure 1). After that, the prosthesis should be duplicated to facilitate the tomography guide construction. To associate the edentulous arches to the tomographic guide at the software the radiopaque marks of barium sulfate are made in the guide near the canine or molar region (Figure 2). The relationship of the maxillary and mandibular arches is registered using condensation silicone.

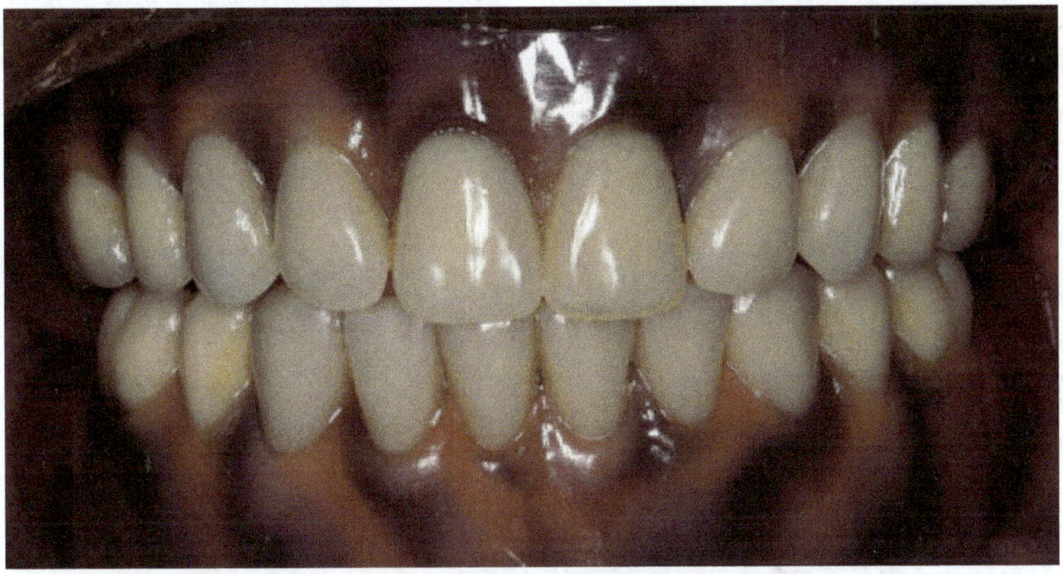

Fig. 1. Total prosthesis with appropriate vertical dimension of occlusion.

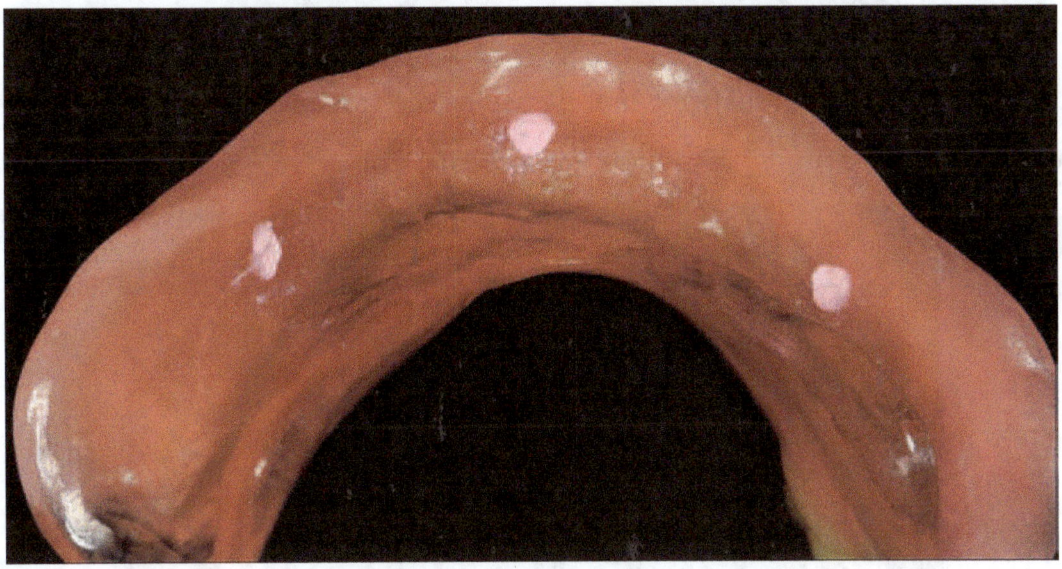

Fig. 2. Tomographic guide with radiopaque marks.

Virtual planning:

The virtual planning has two steps in the computed tomography (CT): the double scanning technique of the patient (Widmann et al., 2007) with both tomographic guide in position and the CT of the guide alone to superimpose the images later in the software. During the CT the complete denture should have adequate positioning in relation to the antagonist arch and the anatomy of the soft tissues. The patient can be asked to use an adhesive to improve stabilization of the denture during the scanning (Almeida et al., 2010). Afterwards, the CT is transformed in 3D images with DICOM extension. It is necessary conversion to a planning guide software, as DentalSlice® (Bioparts, prototipagem biomédica, São Paulo, Brazil).

At this moment, the virtual planning can be made into the software by the prosthodontics and surgery professionals. They can choose the best three-dimensional position of each implant based in the quantity and quality of bone and at emergence profile of the artificial teeth represented by the image of the guide. Wherever possible, it is recommended to plan the posterior implant more distant to the anterior in order to reduce the cantilever. (Figure 3).

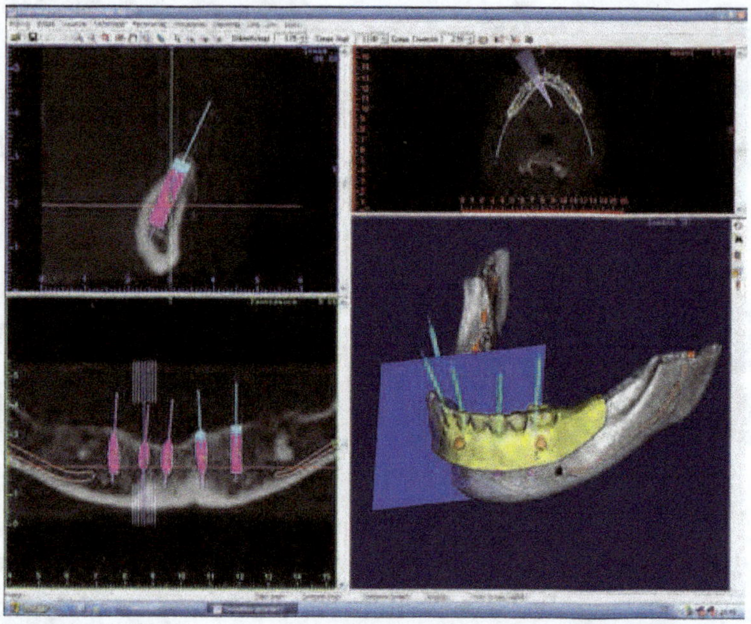

Fig. 3. Virtual planning of the surgery in the DentalSlice Software (Bioparts, Brazil).

Technique description:

After the prototyping and the guide confection, the guide is tested to verify the adequate position to the edentulous area and the dental position. The guide should touch the edentulous area being passive and avoiding ischemic areas (Figure 4).

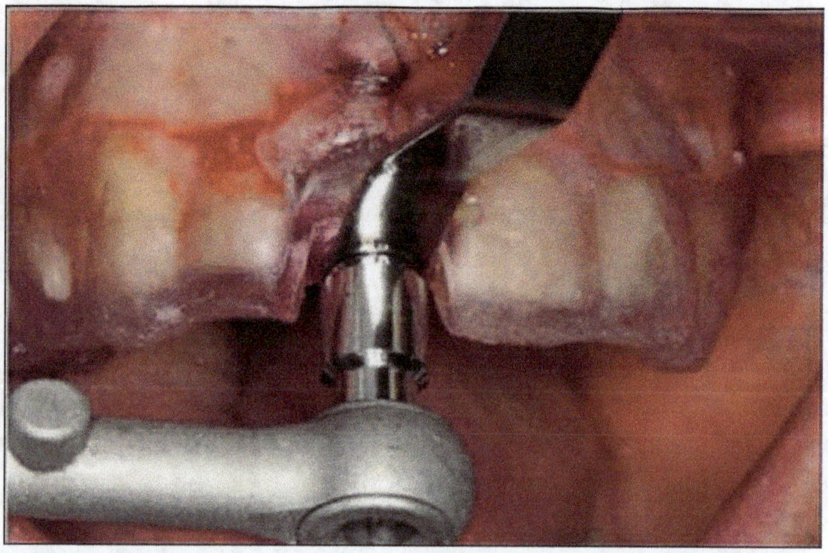

Fig. 4. Surgical guide for partially edentulous patient.

The drill guide inside the guide is important to assist the direction of the surgical drill during perforation to avoid lateral deviations (Valente et al., 2009) (Figure 5).
The guides should be sterilized according to the manufacturer indications.

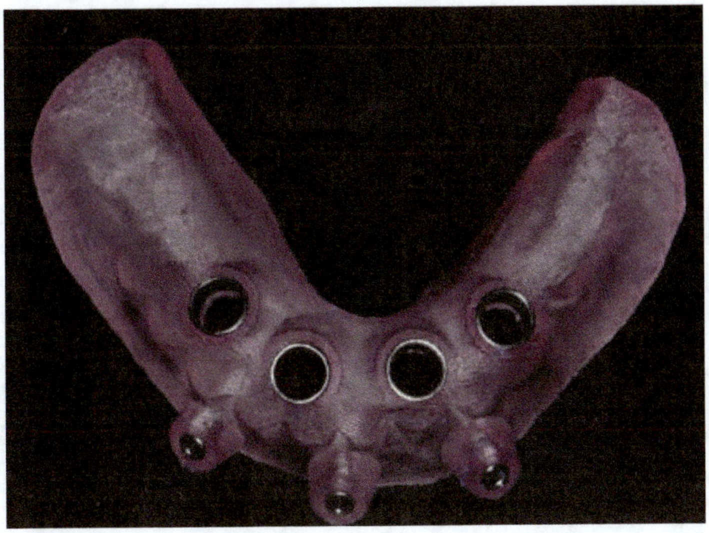

Fig. 5. Mandible surgical guide.

At the moment of the surgery, the first step is the distant local anesthesia because the region can develop edema areas and prevent the guide adaptation.
Later, the guide is stabilized at the planned dental occlusion using the silicone and the retaining pins are screwed at the buccal region to stabilize the guide in the correct position (Figure 6).

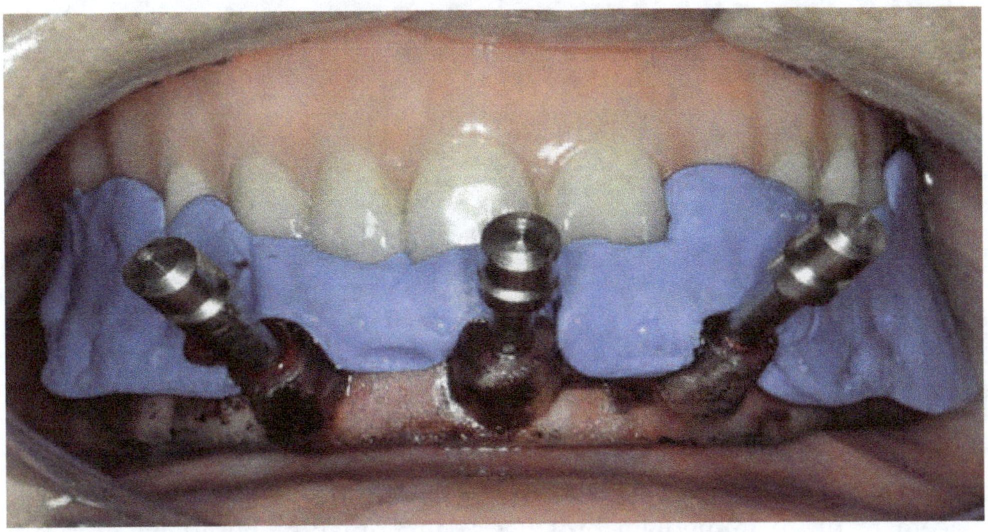

Fig. 6. Surgical guide stabilization at the planned dental occlusion.

Afterwards, the mucous membrane can be removed bellow the drill guide by punch (Figure 7). The perforations should respect the progressive sequence of drills with their guides corresponding to the diameter of the drill to be used (Slice-guide, Conexão Sistema de Prótese Ltda, Arujá, SP).
The sequence of drill was used with its respective guide with intermittent movement and abundant irrigation to avoid heating of the bone tissue. The speed of the drill can vary from 400 to 800 rpm, depending on the bone quality. The long length of the drill is a limitation of this technique for reduced mouth opening.
After the drill perforations, it is recommended to start the installation of the implants by the intermediary positions ones to avoid the guide displacement (Figure 8).

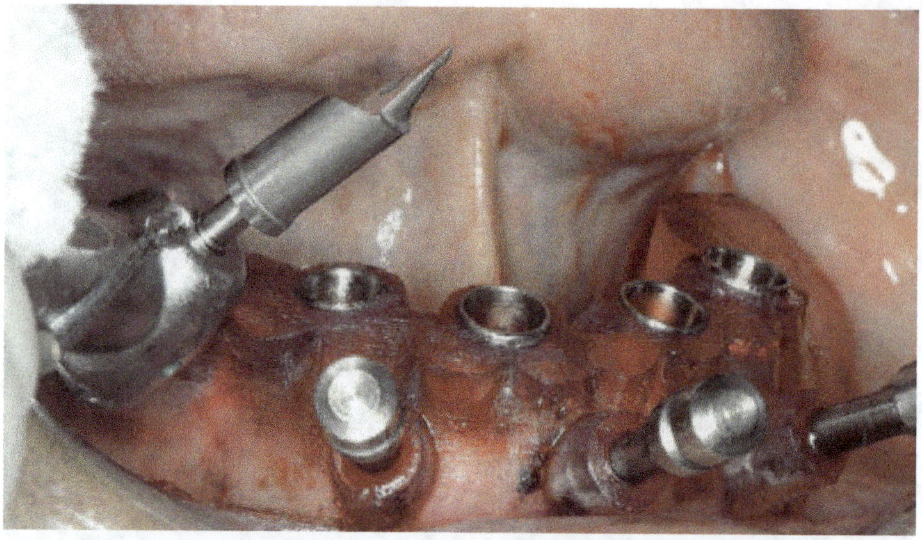

Fig. 7. Punch used to remove the mucous membrane bellow the drill guide.

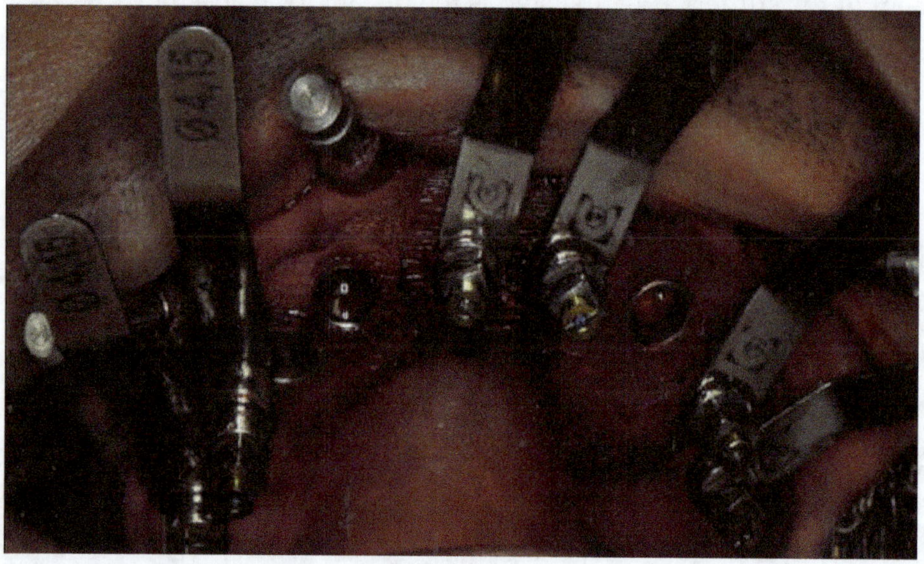

Fig. 8. Placement of implants.

When the last implant is installed, all screws and the palate fixation are removed together with the guide (Figure 9).

For the placement of an immediate prosthesis, all implants should have an appropriate primary stability, in other words, an initial torque around 40N.cm.

There are two options for prosthesis confection: prosthesis fabricated before the implants installation surgery or prosthesis fabricated after the surgery.

2.3 Manufacturing of the prosthesis

Prosthesis fabricated after the guided surgery:

Firstly, the impression cooping are attached to the implant and the surgical guide is positioned (Figure 10). Thereafter, the impression cooping are conected with auto polimerized resin (Pattern Resin LS; GC America, Alsip, Ill) to record the implant position (Figure 11).

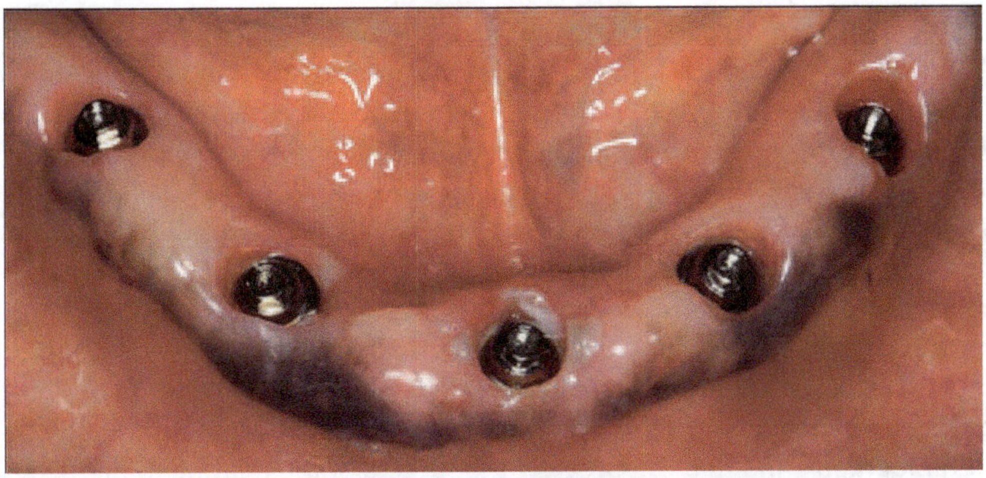

Fig. 9. Final aspect of the soft tissue after the surgical guide been removed.

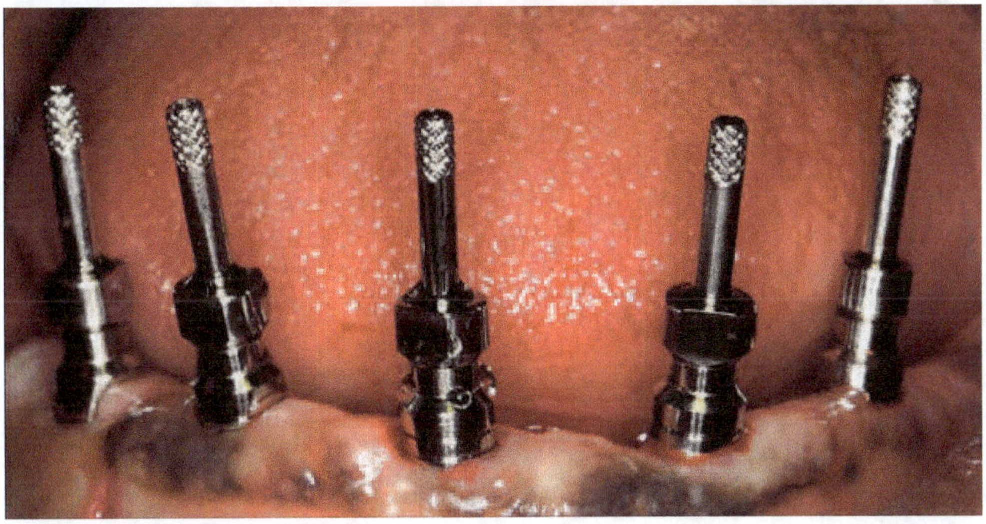

Fig. 10. Impression cooping attached at the implants.

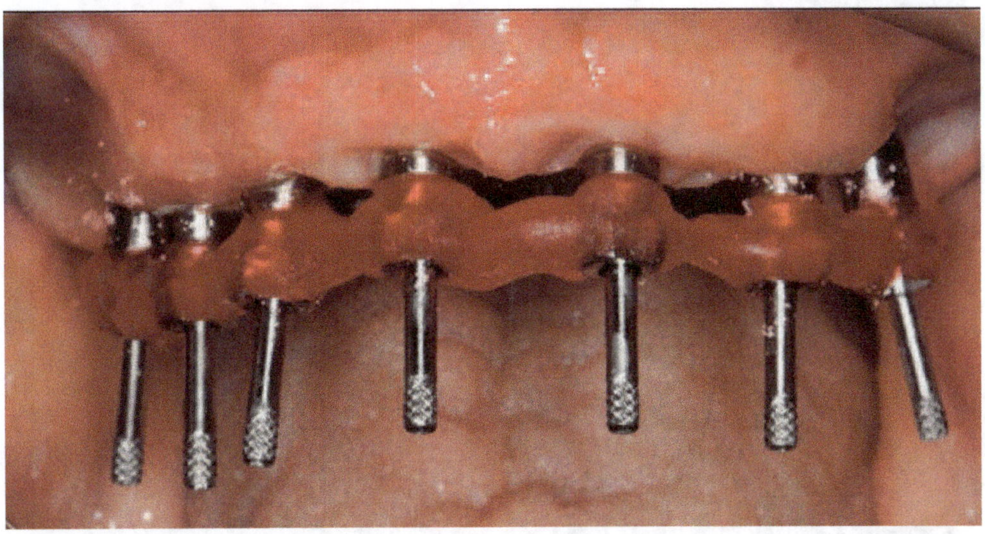

Fig. 11. Impression cooping connected with autopolymerized acrylic resin (Patter Resin LS) to record the implant position

Impression cooping are carried out in both arches using the same surgical guide and condensation silicone (Zetaplus/Oranwash; Zhermack, Rovigo, Italy) (Figure 12). Then, the analogs are attached to the transfer copings before dental stone pouring. In laboratorial phase, the implant superstructure and the teeth in wax are positioned on a base of light-polymerized resin on the working cast (Margonar et al., 2010a). The implant superstructure is attached to the implant to verify the passive fit (Figure 13). Later, the teeth in wax on the base of light-polymerized resin are tested on the superstructure (Sterngold ImplaMed, São Paulo, Brazil) during the same clinical session (Margonar et al., 2010a) (Figure 14).
On the second day, the immediate implant-supported fixed dentures are inserted and the occlusion is evaluated in order to favor the force distribution (Figure 15). The appropriate three-dimensional positioning of the implants was verified by panoramic radiography and computed tomography and that can preview the success of the treatment (Figure 16 and 17).

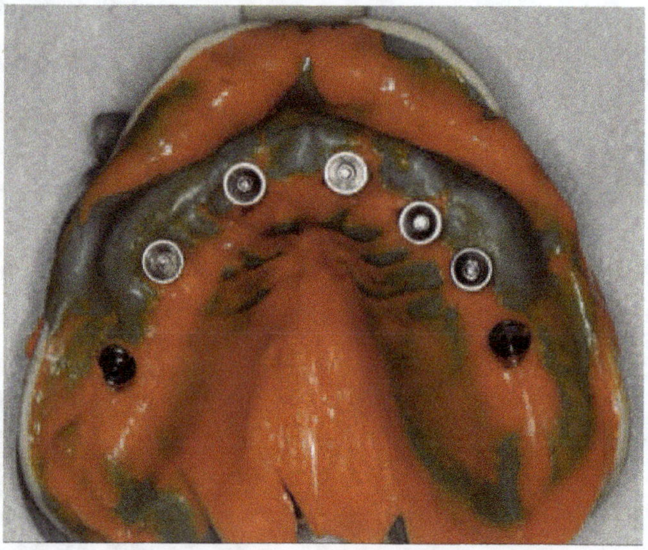

Fig. 12. Mold obtained.

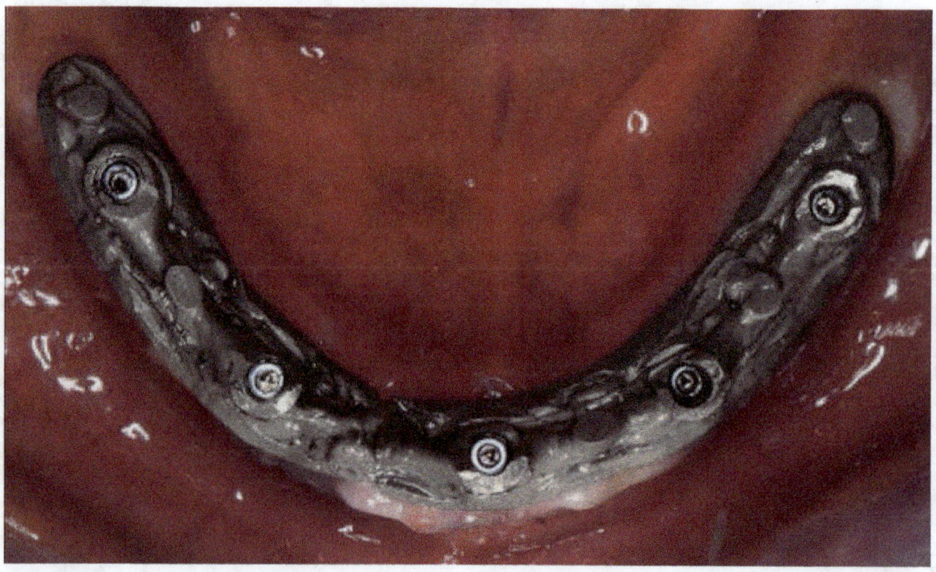

Fig. 13. The implant superstructure attached to the implant to verify the passive fit.

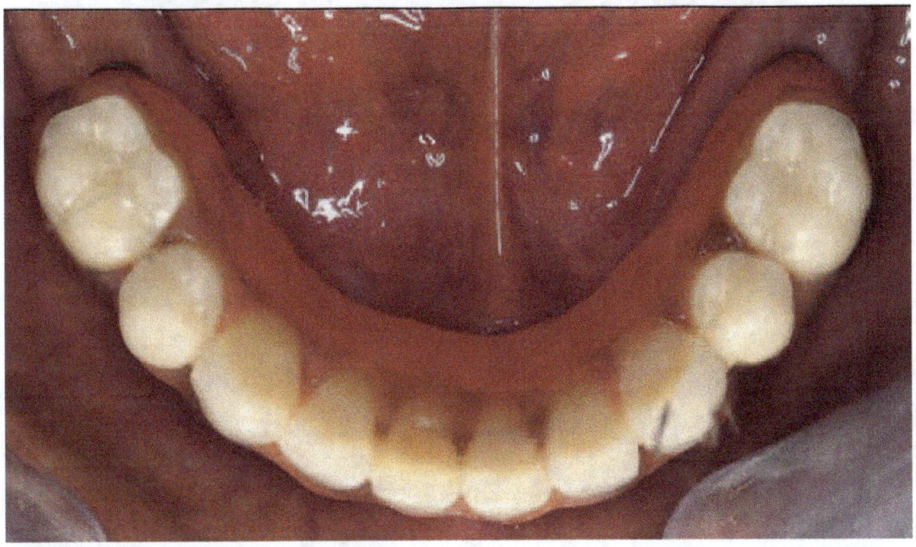

Fig. 14. Teeth in wax on the light-polymerized resin plate.

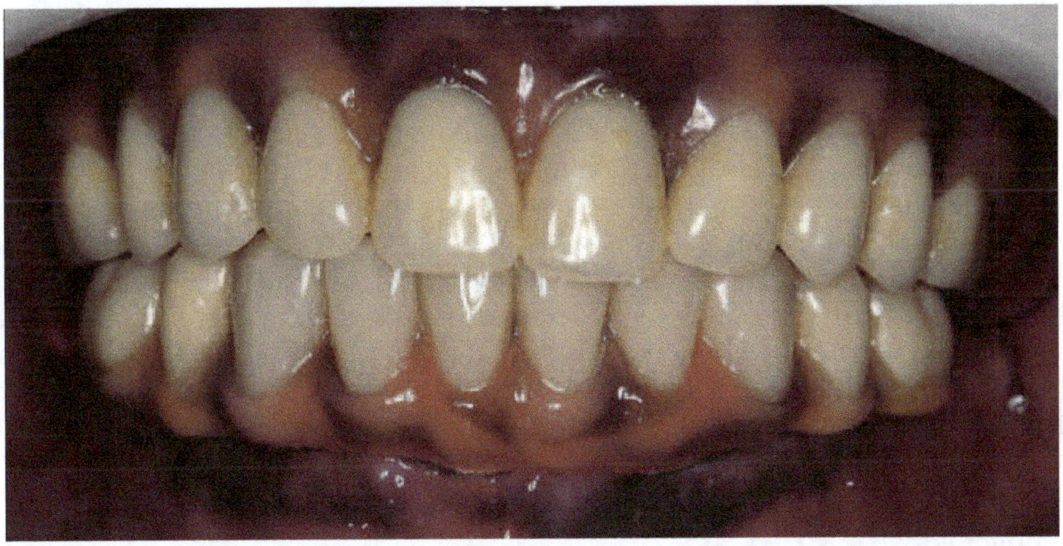

Fig. 15. Final view of the immediate implant-supported fixed denture installed.

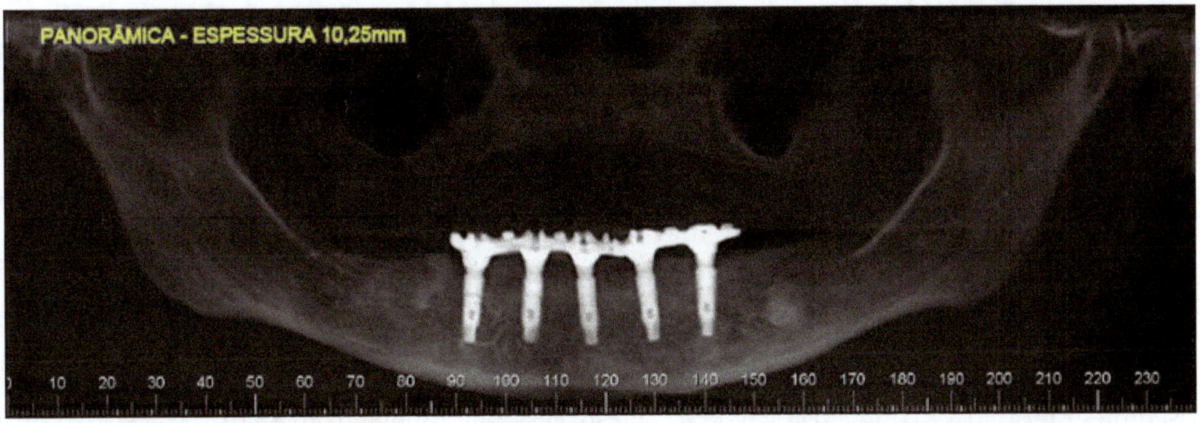

Fig. 16. Panoramic radiography showing the appropriate positioning of the implants.

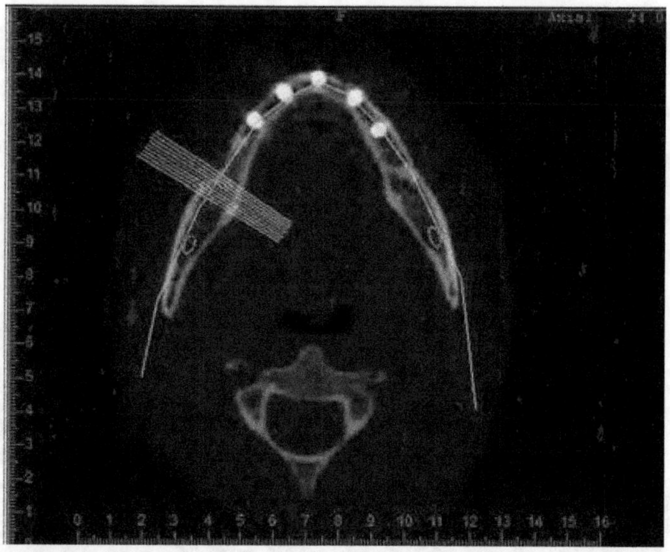

Fig. 17. Computed tomography showing the appropriate three-dimensional positioning of the implants.

Prosthesis fabricated before the guided surgery:

Some techniques have been cited in the literature for the fabrication of prosthesis before the guided surgery. These techniques use the passive cementation. One of them uses the Nobel Biocare system. In this technique the surgical guide is used to make a master model, the abutments are selected, and then the titanium cylinders are placed onto the abutments for the bridge manufacture, that is immediately secured to the implants, installed by the guided surgery (Bedrossian et al., 2008).

Another technique is the technique of the cemented cylinder (Siirilä et al. 1988; López, 1995). In this technique the components installation in the mouth is done after the guided surgery. They are selected previously with torque from 20 to 32N.cm. It is accomplished the molding of the components for the fabrication of an index. And it is made the cementation of the cylinders inside the prosthesis in agreement with the index. Then, it is made the cementation of the prosthesis in the mouth (Siirilä et al. 1988; López, 1995).

2.3 Complications

The complications in guided surgery can be divided in early complications and late complications:

Early complications: lack of primary stability (Yong & Moy, 2008), loosening of prosthesis screw (Young & Moy, 2008), slight genial tumefaction (Gillot et al., 2010), difficulty in speech and bilateral cheek occlusion (Young & Moy, 2008), jugal hematoma (Gillot et al., 2010) and heating of tissues (Figure 18).

Margonar et al., 2010b, evaluated bone tissue heating and the wear drills after repeated osteotomies for implants, simulating the guided surgery technique and comparing it with the classical technique. According to that study, the heating of the bone tissue due to the guide surgery technique was higher when compared with the conventional open flap surgery during the preparation of the surgical site, but both techniques have not reached the threshold temperature that causes immediate necrosis.

Late complications: persistent pain (Gillot et al., 2010), gingival recession (Yong & Mo, 2008), osseointegration loss (Yong & Moy, 2008). The success rate ranges from 83 to 100% (Canizzaro et al., 2008; Komiyama et al., 2008; Schneider et al., 2009; Van Steenberghe et al., 2005).

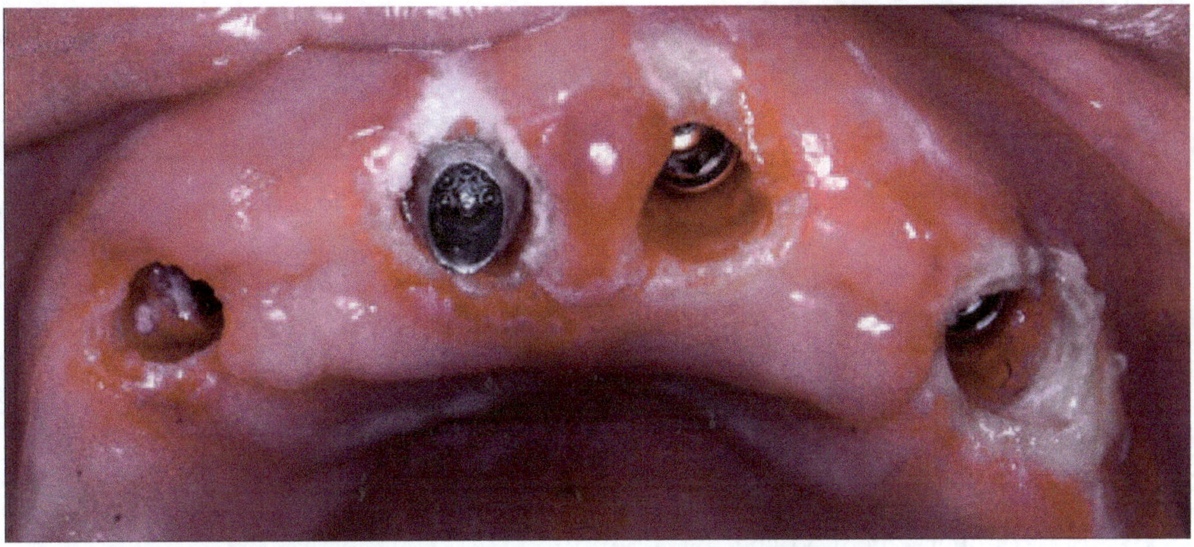

Fig. 18. Soft tissue with necrotic aspect due to heating in the region.

2.4 Mistakes in guided surgery

The computer-guided surgery has a sequence from the diagnostic stage to the prosthetic, and mistakes may occur in different stages. The most common mistakes found in the literature are as follows:

1. Mistake on acquisition of tomographic image or incorrect processing (mean of error <0.5 mm) (Reddy et al., 1994; Valent et al., 2009).
2. Deviation of 0.1 a 0.2 mm on fabrication of the surgical guide (Valent et al., 2009; Van Steenberghe et al., 2002.)
3. Inaccurate fixation of the guide resulting in displacement during perforation (Valent et al., 2009).
4. Mechanical errors caused by angulation of the drills during perforation that may cause lateral deviations (Valent et al., 2009).
5. Changed positioning of surgical instruments due to reduced mouth opening (Valent et al., 2009).
6. Human mistakes as not using the whole length of the drill during perforation (Valent et al., 2009).

3. Conclusion

The guided surgery is an excellent option of treatment for patients with satisfactory bone quantity for implant insertion. The guided surgery can be indicated for complete and partially edentulous arches in the maxilla and/or mandible.

When properly prescribed and monitoring, the virtual planning and the guide surgery are excellent tools used in implantology to perform surgical procedures with more safety, confort and predictability to the patient.

4. Acknowledgment

The authors gratefully acknowledge "Conexão Sistemas de Próteses Ltda" for supplying the implants, "DVI: Diagnóstico Volumétrico por Imagem" for providing the tomographies and "BIOPARTS: prototipagem biomédica" for supplying prototyping used in this study.

5. References

Almeida, E.O.; Pellizzer, E.P.; Goiatto, M.C; Margonar, R.; Rocha, E.P.; Freitas-Jr, A.C. & Anchieta, R.B. (2010). Computer-Guided Surgery in Implantology: Review of Basic Concepts. *The Journal of Craniofacial Surgery.* Vol.21, No. 6, pp,1917-1921, ISSN 1049-2275.

Azari, A. & Nikzard, S. Computer-ssisted implantology: historical background and potential outcomes - a review (2008). *The International Journal of Medical Robotics and Computer Assisted Surgery.* Vol.4, No.2, pp.95-104, ISSN 1478-596X.

Becker, W.; Goldstein, M.; Becker, B.E. & Sennerby, L. (2005). Minimally invasive flapless surgery: a prospective multicenter study. *Clinical Implant Dentistry and Related Research.* Vol.7 (Supp1), pp.21-27, ISSN1523-0899.

Bedrossian E. (2007). Laboratory and prosthetic considerations in computer-guided surgery and Immediate Loading. *International Journal of Oral & Maxillofacial Surgery,* Vol.66, No.1 (January 2008), Vol.65 , No.7 Suppl 1, pp.47-52, ISSN 0901-5027.

Bedrossian, E.; Sullivan, R.M.; Fortin, Y.; Malo, P. & Intedresano, T. (2008). Fixed-prosthetic implant restoration of the edentulous maxilla: a systematic pretreatment evaluation method. *International Journal of Oral & Maxillofacial Surgery,* Vol.66, No.1 (January 2008), pp.112-122, ISSN 0901-5027.

Cannizzaro, G.; Leone, M.; Consolo, U.; Ferri, V. & Esposito, M (2008). Immediate functional loading of implants placed with flapless surgery versus conventional implants in partially edentulous patients. A 3-year randomized controlled clinical trial. *The International Journal of Oral & Maxillofacial Implants,* Vol.23, No.5, pp. 867-875, ISSN 0882-2786.

Casap, N.; Terazi, E.; Wexler, A.; Sonnenfeld, U. & Lustmann, J (2005). Intraoperative computerized navigation for flapless implant surgery and immediate loading in the edentulous mandible. *The International Journal of Oral & Maxillofacial Implants,* Vol.20, No.1, pp.92-98, ISSN 0882-2786.

Drago, C. J. (1994). Prosthodontic complications related to compromised implant placement. *Journal of Oral Maxillofacial Surgery,* Vol.52, No.1, (January 1994), pp. 15–22, ISSN 0278-2391.

Fortin, T.; Bosson, J.L.; Coudert, J,L.& Isidori, M. (2003). Reliability of preoperative planning of an image-guided system for oral implant placement based on 3-dimensional images: an in vitro study. *The International Journal of Oral & Maxillofacial Implants,* Vol.18, No.6, pp.886-893, ISSN 0882-2786.

Fuster-Torres, M.A.; Albalat-Estrela, S.; Alcañiz-Raya, M. & Peñarrocha-Diao, M.; (2009). CAD / CAM dental systems in implant dentistry: update. *Medicina Oral , Patología Oral y Cirugía Bucal.* Vol.14, No.3 (March 2009), pp.141-145 , ISSN 1698-4447.

Garber, D. A. & Belser, U. C. (1995). Restoration-driven implant placement with restoration-generated site development. *Compendium of Continuing Education in Dentistry,* Vol.16, No.8, (August 1995), pp. 796,798–802,804, ISSN 1548-8578.

Gillot, L.; Noharet, R. & Cannas, B. (2010). Guided Surgery and Presurgical Prosthesis: Preliminary Results of 33 Fully Edentulous Maxillae Treated in Accordance with the NobelGuide® Protocol. *Clinical Implant Dentistry and Related Research.* Vol.12, Suppl 1, ISSN 1523-0899.

Holst, S.; Blatz, M.B.; Wichmann, M. & Eitner, S. (2004). Clinical application of surgical fixation screws in implant prosthodontics – Part I: positioning of radiographic and surgical templates. *Journal of Prosthetic Dentistry*. Vol.92, No4, pp395-398, ISSN 0022-3913.

Komiyama, A.; Klinge, B. & Hultin, M. (2008). Treatment outcome of immediately loaded implants installed in edentulous jaws following computer-assisted virtual treatment planning and flapless surgery. *Clinical Oral Implants Research*. Vol.19, No.7, pp.677–685.

Kupeyan, H.K.; Shaffner, M. and Armstrong, J. (2006). Definitive CAD/CAM-guided prothesis for immediate loading of bone-grafted maxilla: a case report. *Clinical Implant Dentistry and Related Research*. Vol.8, No.3, pp.161-167, ISSN1523-0899.

Lal, K.; White, G.S.; Morea, D.N. & Wright, R.F. (2006). Use of stereolithographic templates for surgical and prosthodontics implant planning and placement. Part I. The concept. *Journal Prosthodontics*. Vol.15, No.1 (January-February 2006), pp.51-58, ISSN:1059-941X.

López, V.J. (1995). Prótese sobre implantes: oclusão, casos clínicos e laboratório. São Paulo - Brazil. Ed. Quintessence.

Marchack, C.B. (2007). CAD/CAM-guided implant surgery and fabrication of an immediately loaded prosthesis for a partially edentulous patient. The Journal of Prosthetic Dentistry. Vol.97, No.6, pp.389-394, ISSN 0022-3913.

Margonar, R.; Almeida, E.O.; Queiroz, T.P.; Marcantonio, E. (2010a). Wax Teeth and Metallic Superstructure Trials at the Same Session: Simplified Technique for Implant-Supported Prosthesis. *The Journal of Craniofacial Surgery*. Vol.21, No.6, (November 2010), ISSN 1049-2275.

Margonar, R.; Queiroz, T.P; Santos, P.L.; Carvalho, E.R.; & Luvizuto, E.R.; Souza, F.A.; Okamoto, R.; Magro-Filho, O.; Hochuli-Vieira, E. & Garcia-Júnior, I.R. (2010b) Bone heating after implant osteotomies using the guided surgery. *Journal of Dental Research*, Vol. 89, Special Issue B, Retrieved from
<URL>
http://iadr.confex.com/iadr/2010barce/webprogramcd/Paper137398.html

Meloni, S.M.; De Riu, G.; Pisano, M.; Cattina, G. & Tullio, A. (2010). Implant treatment software planning and guided flapless surgery with immediate provisional prosthesis delivery in the fully edentulous maxilla. A retrospective analysis of 15 consecutively treated patients. *European Journal of Oral Implantology*, Vol.3, No.3, pp. 245-251, ISSN 1756-2406.

Parel, S.M. & Triplett, R.G. (2004). Interacive imaging for implant planning, placement, and prosthesis construction. *International Journal of Oral & Maxillofacial Surgery*, Vol.62, No.9 (Suppl 2), pp.41-47, ISSN 0901-5027.

Reddy, M.S.; Mayfiel-Donahoo, T.; Vanderven, F.J. & Jeffcoat M.K. (1994). A comparison of the diagnostic advantages of the panoramic radiography and computed tomography scanning for placement of root-form dental implants. *Clinical Oral Implants Research*. Vol.5, No.4, pp.229-238.

Schneider, D.; Marquardt, P.; Zwahlen, M. & Jung, R.E. (2009). A systematic review on the accuracy and the clinical outcome of computerguided template-based implant dentistry. *Clinical Oral Implants Research*. Vol.20, Suppl. 4, pp.73–86, ISSN 0905-7161.

Serry, J.S.; Sims, L.O. & Balshi, S.F. (2007). A simple technique for immediate placement of definitive engaging custom abutments using computerized tomography and flapless guided surgery. *Quintessence International.* Vol.38, No. 9, pp.755–76, ISSN 0033-6572.

Siirilä, H.S.; Nordberg, L.; Oikarinen, V.J. (1988). Technique for converting an existing complete denture to a tissue-integrated prosthesis. *The journal of Prosthetic Dentistry.* Vol 59, No.4, pp463-467, ISSN 0022-3913.

Spin-Neto, R,; Marcantonio-Jr, E., Gotfredsen, E. & Wenzel, A. (2011). Exploring CBCT-Based DICOM Files. A Systematic Review on the Properties of Images Used to Evaluate Maxillofacial Bone Grafts. *Journal of Digital Imaging.* Retrieved from <URL>
http://www.ncbi.nlm.nih.gov/pubmed/21448762.

Valente, F.; Schiroli, G. & Sbrenna, A. (2009). Accuracy of computer-aided oral implant surgery: a clinical and radiographic study. *The International Journal of Oral & Maxillofacial Implants,* Vol.24, No.2, pp.234-242, ISSN 0882-2786.

Van Steenberghe, D.; Naert, I.; Andersson, M.; Brajnovic, I.; Van Cleynenbreugel, J. & Suetens P. (2002). A custom template and definitive prosthesis allowing immediate implant loading in the maxilla: a clinical report. *The International Journal of Oral & Maxillofacial Implants,* Vol.17, No.5, pp.663-670, ISSN 0882-2786.

Van Steenberghe, D.; Glauser, R.; Blomback, U.; Andersson, M.; Schutyser, F.; Pettersson A. & Wenelhag I. (2005). A computed tomographic scan-derived customized surgical template and fixed prothesis for flapless surgery and immediate loading of implants in fully edentulous maxillae : a prospective multicenter study. *Clinical Implant Dentistry and Related Research.*Vol.8, No.3, pp.111-120, ISSN1523-0899.

Widmann, G.; Stoffner, R.; Schullian, P.; Widmann, R.; Keiler, M.; Zangerl, A.; Puelacher, W. & Bale, R.J. (2010). Comparison of the Accuracy of Invasive and Noninvasive Registration Methods for Image-Guided Oral Implant Surgery. *International Journal of Oral & Maxillofacial Surgery,* Vol.25, No.3, pp.491-498, ISSN 0901-5027.

Widmann, G.; Widmann, R.; Widmann, E.; Jaschke, W. & Bale, R. (2007). Use of a surgical navigation system for CT-guided template production. *The International Journal of Oral & Maxillofacial Implants,* Vol.22, No.1, pp.72-78, ISSN 0882-2786.

Yong, L.T. & Moy, L.T. (2008). Complications of Computer-Aided-Design/Computer-Aided-Machining-Guided (NobelGuide™) Surgical Implant Placement: An Evaluation of Early Clinical Results. *Clinical Implant Dentistry and Related Research.* Vol.10, No.3, (September 2008), pp.123-127, ISSN 1523-0899.

5

Intuitive Surgical Navigation System for Dental Implantology by Using Retinal Imaging Display

Satoshi Yamaguchi[1], Takafumi Ohtani[2], Shinji Ono[1], Yasufumi Yamanishi[1], Taiji Sohmura[3] and Hirofumi Yatani[1]
[1]*Graduate School of Dentistry, Osaka University*
[2]*Graduate Prosthodontics, University of Washington*
[3]*Bionic Inc.*
[1,3]*Japan*
[2]*USA*

1. Introduction

As dental implants have become an established treatment, their application to aggressive cases with insufficient quantity and quality of bone has increased. To perform safe and precise surgery, overcoming these difficulties, computer-assisted systems have been developed (Jabero et al., 2006). There are two major classes of these systems, that is, a computer-guided (static) system (Schneider et al., 2009) and a computer-navigated (dynamic) system (Jung et al., 2009). The computer-guided system such as SimPlant software and SurgiGuide (Materialize Dental Inc., USA), NobelGuide (Nobel Biocare Management AG, Sweden), and 10DR (10DR JAPAN Co., Ltd., Japan) are a surgical template based system which can simulate an optimal implant location, angle, direction, depth and size pre-operatively. Our system, BoneNavi (Bionic Inc., Japan), has also been developed to simulate implant placement and the surgical template fabrication for dental implant surgery (Ohtani et al., 2009) and applied in more than 200 clinical cases in Japan (Sohmura et al., 2009). On the other hand, the computer-navigated system such as IGI system (Image Navigation Ltd., USA) offers freehand implant navigation empowered by highly accurate motion tracking technology that tracks the positions of the dental drill and patient throughout the surgery (Casap et al., 2004). It has also already been applied in clinical cases (Casap et al., 2005 & 2008). Advantages and disadvantages of the computer-guided system and the computer-navigated system are shown in Table 1.

Unlike an open chest surgery and an open abdominal surgery, looking away from the oral cavity (narrow space (Fig.1)) intra-operatively involve a risk of operation errors in case of a dental implant surgery. However, with conventional systems, surgeons have to manipulate instruments in the patient's oral cavity while watching a surgical monitor as shown in Fig.2(a) and they feel anxious during operations.

To overcome this problem, we have been developed a novel surgical navigation system by combining the retinal imaging display (RID) and the augmented reality (AR) techniques

	Advantages	Disadvantages
Computer-guided system	General familiarity High degree of precision	Difficulties in cases of poor edentulous ridge form or loose teeth
Computer-navigated system	Modifiable surgical plan intra-operatively	Complications and difficulties for mounting markers on patiens or hand-piece

Table 1. Comparison between advantages and disadvantages of the computer-guided system and the computer-navigated system

(Azuma, 1997) that can directly overlay pre-operative simulation images onto the real view of the surgeon (Yamaguchi et al., 2009) as shown in Fig. 2 (b). In the last few decades, AR techniques have been applied in wide areas such as medical treatment (Peters et al., 2006) and education (Dede, 2009; Thomas, 2010). Moreover, various possibilities are still expected (Buxton et al., 2008). However, only few attempts have so far been made at an application in dentistry (Birkfellner et al., 1999) because of challenging field by means of image registration accuracy. It is because I believe that our system lead to progress in future dentistry that I have written this chapter.

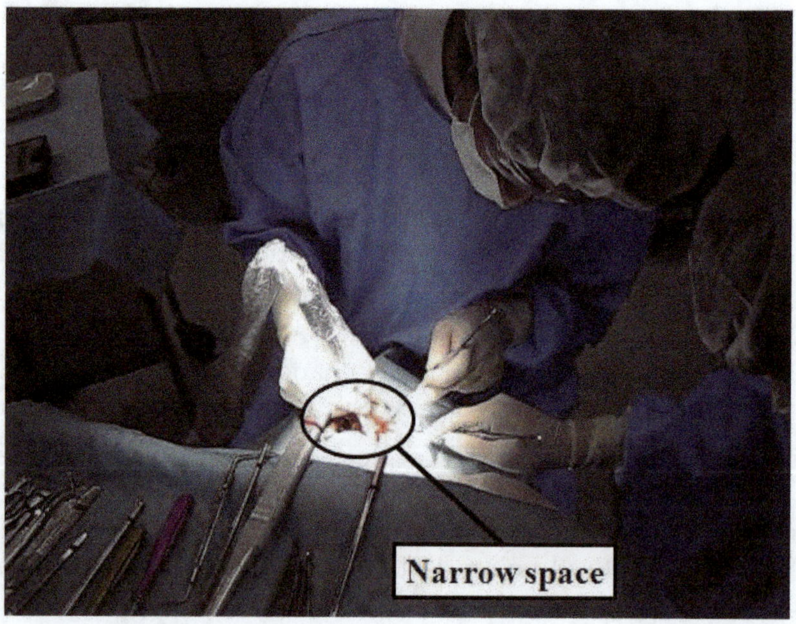

Fig. 1. Scene of dental implant surgical operation in narrow space of patient's oral cavity

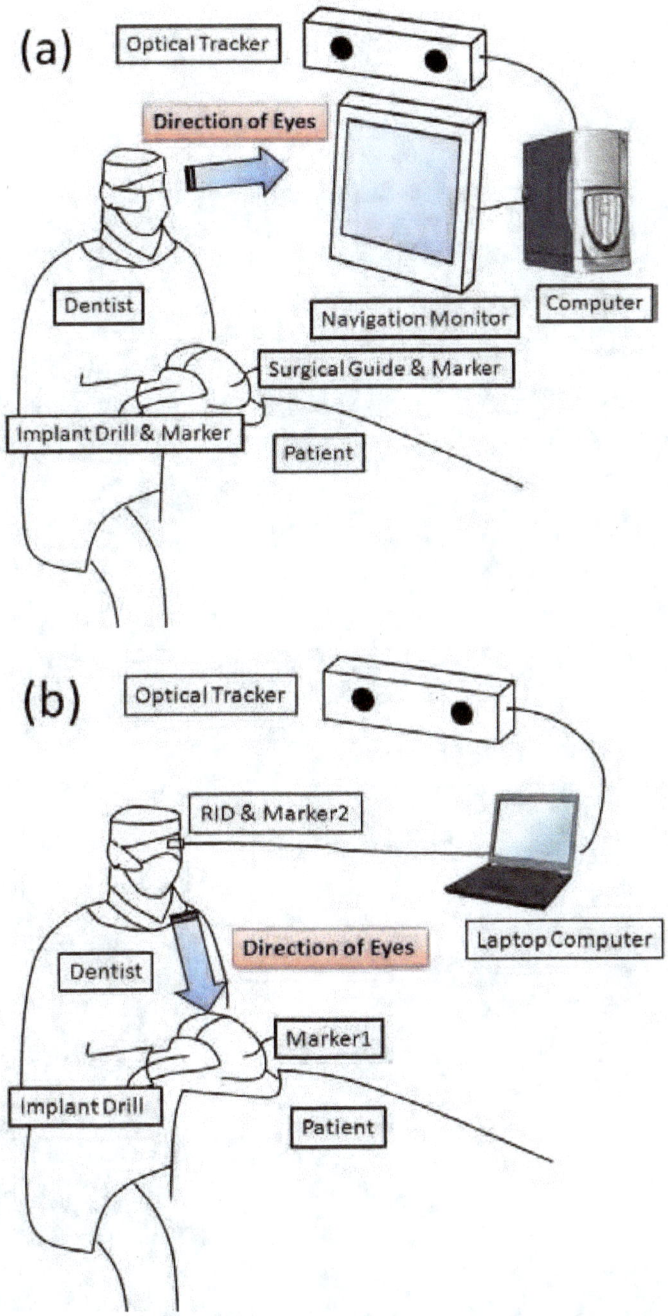

Fig. 2. Schematic illustrations of a surgical navigation system for dental implantology. (a) Conventional approach: A direction of eyes of a dentist is directed to a navigation monitor. (b) Our approach: The direction of eyes of the dentist is directed to an oral cavity of a patient.

2. Materials and methods

2.1 System configurations

As shown in Fig. 3 system configurations, our system consists of a retinal imaging display (Prototype of RID (RID), Brother Industries, Ltd., Japan), an optical tracker (Micron Tracker 2 Sx60 (MT2), Claron Technology Inc., USA), and a laptop computer (Thinkpad X32, IBM, Japan). The RID have an image projection technology that focuses light, of an intensity

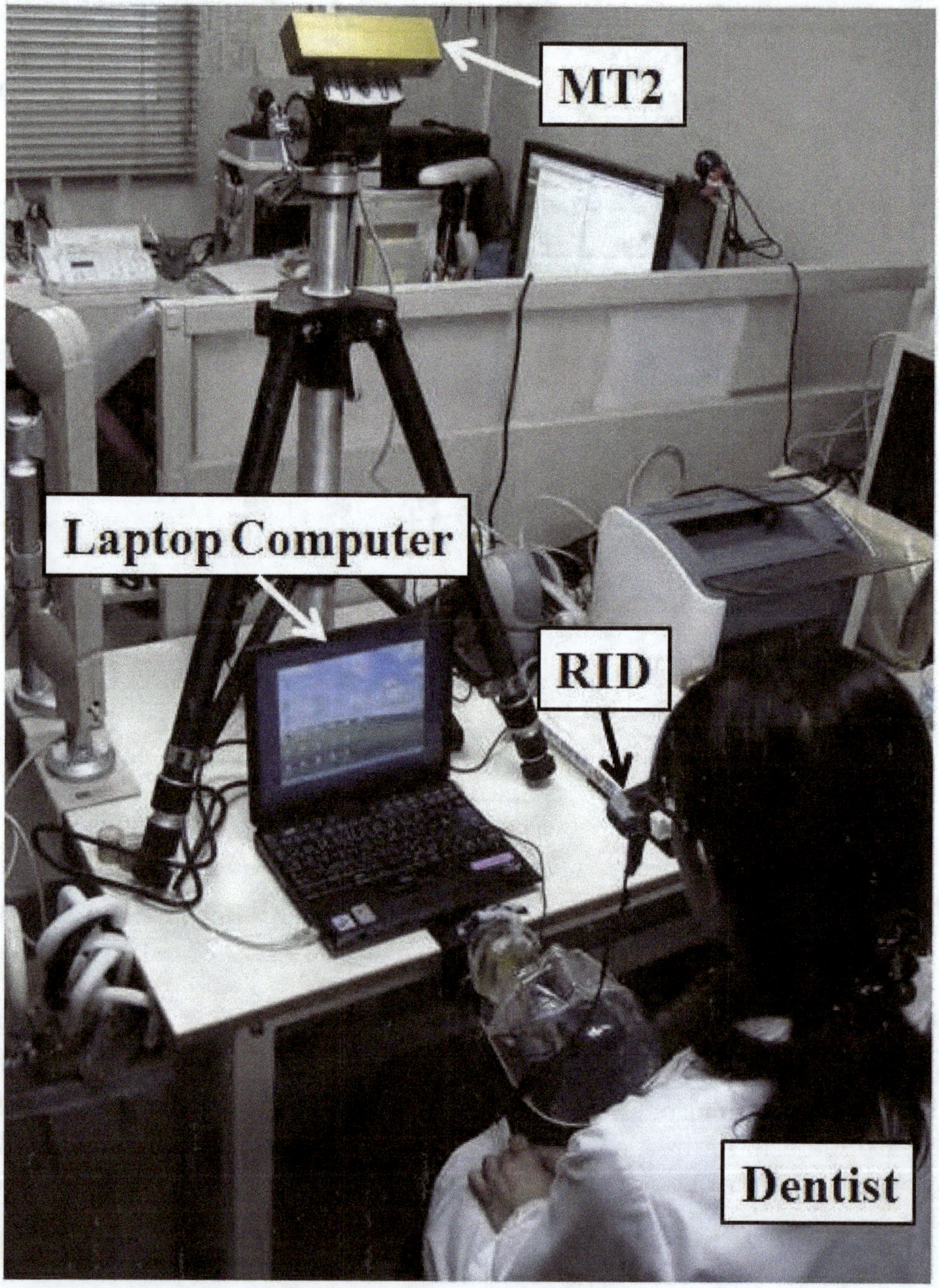

Fig. 3. System configurations

harmless to the eyes, onto the retina and then moves the light at high speed to create after images. This technology differs from an optical see-through head mounted display and a half mirror in respect of projection principle for eyes and has many advantages for dentists. Dentists can intuitively confirm an ideal implant placement without an uncomfortable feeling. And, dentist's view is not interrupt by lenses such as glasses. Moreover, dentist can view private images and personal data of patients away from being viewed by others intra-operatively. To track a position and a pose of marked patient's oral cavity, computer vision technologies are implemented on MT2 instead of conventional optical tracker by using infrared light emission. Thus, MT2 is a cost-effective and high accurate (jitter for moving target is less than 70 micron) optical tracker. A laptop PC receive signals from RID and MT2 and calculate a translate matrix for real-time image overlay.

2.2 Pre-operative procedures

1. To measure the position and orientation of a marker 1, the marker 1 is placed onto a partially edentulous model.
2. A placement position of dental implants for the scanned images is simulated by CAD software (FreeFormModeling, SensAble Technologies, Inc., USA) and the three-dimensional simulation image is generated as a computer graphics (CG). At this time, a translation matrix ${}^{implant}_{marker1}\mathbf{D}$ from the marker 1 to implants is recorded.
3. A translation matrix ${}^{eye}_{marker2}\mathbf{A}$ to dentist's eye from the RID with a marker 2 attached thereto is calculated. By using the marker 1 for calibration, the ${}^{eye}_{marker2}\mathbf{A}$ is calculated from three-dimensional positions on the RID coordinate system and its corresponding two-dimensional positions on the dentist's eye coordinate system (Kato et al., 1999).

2.3 Intra-operative procedures

1. Translation matrixes ${}^{marker1}_{tracker}\mathbf{D}$ and ${}^{marker2}_{tracker}\mathbf{D}$ are measured by the MT2 in real-time intra-operatively.
2. A translation matrix ${}^{eye}_{implant}\mathbf{P}$ is calculated from simulated dental implant CG image to the dentist's eye as per a following equation (1). Finally, the CG image is projected onto the dentist's view,

$$ {}^{eye}_{implant}\mathbf{P} = {}^{marker1}_{implant}\mathbf{D}\,{}^{tracker}_{marker1}\mathbf{D}\,{}^{marker2}_{tracker}\mathbf{D}\,{}^{eye}_{marker2}\mathbf{A} \tag{1} $$

where, ${}^{marker1}_{implant}\mathbf{D} = {}^{implant}_{marker1}\mathbf{D}^{-1}$ and ${}^{tracker}_{marker1}\mathbf{D} = {}^{marker1}_{tracker}\mathbf{D}^{-1}$.

2.4 Design of markers and partially edentulous model

CAD models of the marker 1 and the marker 2 were designed by the CAD software (Fig. 4). A partially edentulous model was scanned by three-dimensional measurement system (Rexcan scanner, Solutionix Corp., Korea). The marker 1, the marker 2, and the partially edentulous model were fabricated by rapid-prototyping machines (Connex500 (two-color process) and EDEN260 (one-color process), Objet Geometries Ltd., Israel). In clinical case, the marker 1 will be placed inside oral cavity of the patient. As shown in Fig.4 and Fig.5, the markers consist of three faces. Sizes of all faces were set to 26 × 21 mm. Both two faces were tilted to a center marker. Its tilt angle was 30 degree. Unlike a white and a black color, a grey and a black color were adopted to improve a contrast ratio for MT2. Both the marker 1 and the marker 2 have different patterns. Fig. 6 shows a pre-operative simulation result including five implant models and simplified models of a mandibular canal which was extracted from a CT data by using a volume rendering software (VG Studio Max 2.0, Volume Graphics GmbH, Germany).

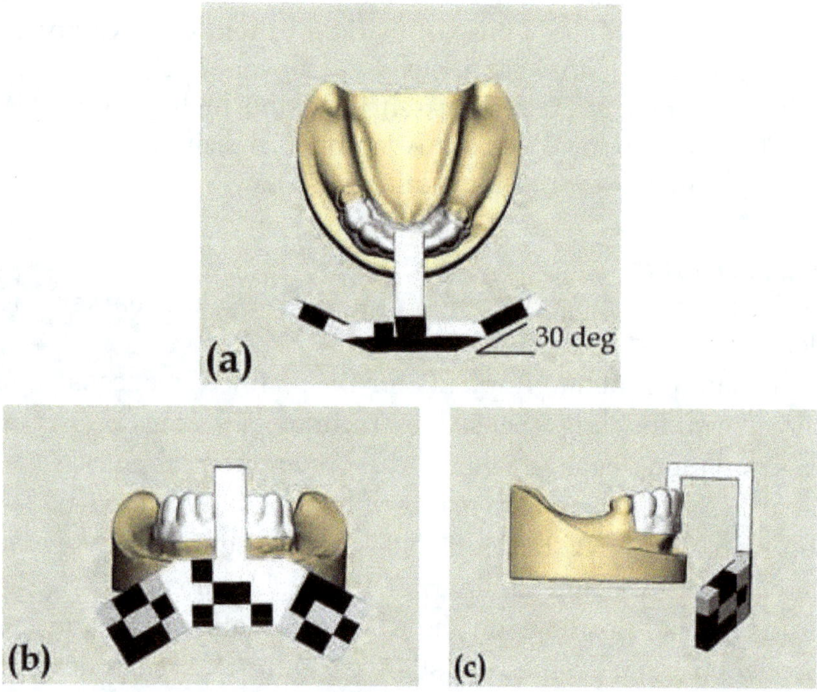

Fig. 4. The CAD model of the marker 1 and the scanned model of the partially edentulous model: (a) top view, (b) front view, (c) lateral view

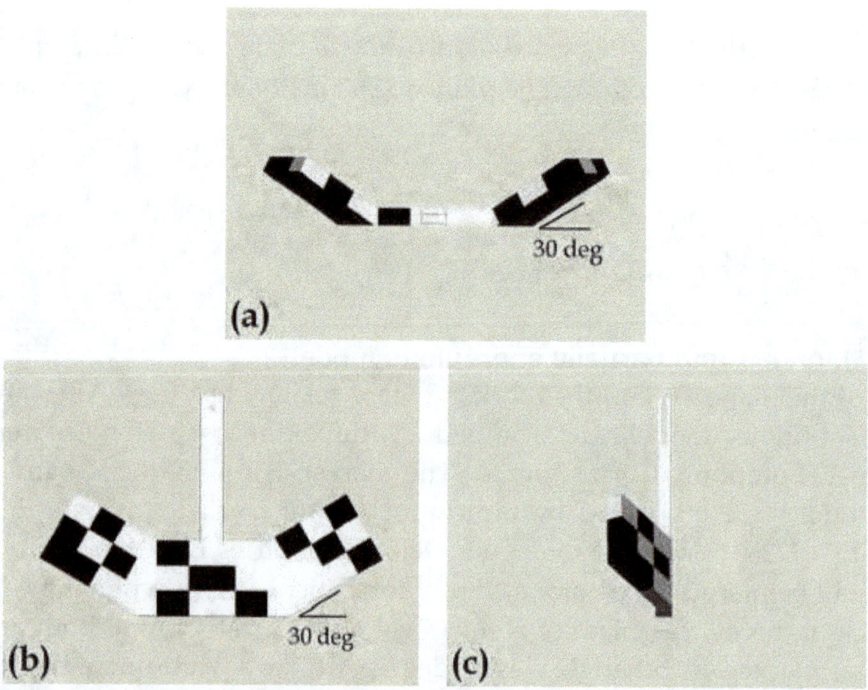

Fig. 5. The CAD model of marker 2: (a) top view, (b) front view, (c) lateral view

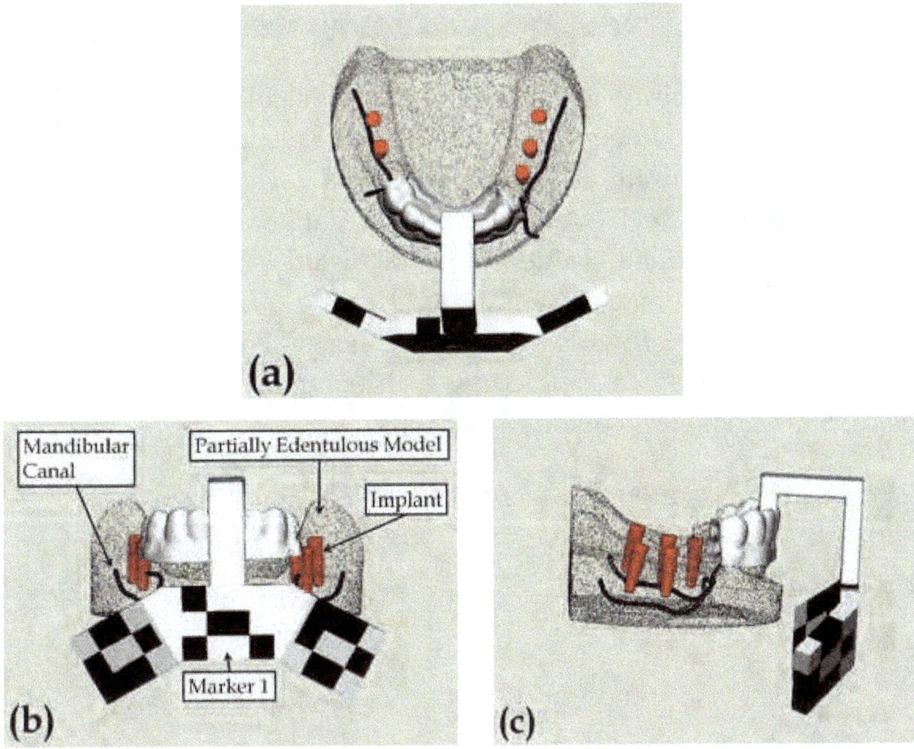

Fig. 6. Pre-operative simulation result: (a) top view, (b) front view, (c) lateral view

2.5 Calculations of ${}^{eye}_{implant}\mathbf{P}$

2.5.1 DLT (Direct Linear Transformation)

Direct linear transformation is a gold standard calibration method (Hartley, R. & Zisserman, A., 2003). By using the marker 1 for calibration, A translation matrix ${}^{eye}_{marker2}\mathbf{A}$ was calculated from three-dimensional positions on the RID coordinate system $\mathbf{p}(x,y,z)$ and its corresponding two-dimensional positions on the dentist's eye coordinate system $\mathbf{P}(X_C,Y_C)$. A transform relationship between a RID coordinate value $\mathbf{p}$ and a dentist's eye coordinate value $\mathbf{P}$ was represented as per a following equation (2).

$$[H_C X_C, H_C Y_C, H_C] = [x,y,z,1]\begin{bmatrix} C_{11} & C_{21} & C_{31} \\ C_{12} & C_{22} & C_{32} \\ C_{13} & C_{23} & C_{33} \\ C_{14} & C_{24} & C_{34} \end{bmatrix} \quad (2)$$

These twelve parameters represent constant values such as a relative position, an orientation, and a focal length. A translation matrix C calls camera parmeters. The camera parameters were calculated by collecting some three-dimensional positions on the RID coordinate system $\mathbf{p}_i(x_i,y_i,z_i)$ and its corresponding two-dimensional positions on the dentist's eye coordinate system $\mathbf{P}_i(X_{Ci},Y_{Ci})$. Once a coordinate value x_1,y_1,z_1 of a three-dimensional position $\mathbf{p}_1$ on the RID coordinate system and its corresponding coordinate value X_{C1},Y_{C1} of a two-dimensional position $\mathbf{P}_1$ on the dentist's eye coordinate system was determined, an equation (3) was derived from the equation (2).

$$\begin{aligned} C_{11}x_1 + C_{12}y_1 + C_{13}z_1 + C_{14} - C_{31}x_1X_{C1} - C_{32}y_1X_{C1} - C_{33}z_1X_{C1} = C_{34}X_{C1} \\ C_{21}x_1 + C_{22}y_1 + C_{23}z_1 + C_{24} - C_{31}x_1Y_{C1} - C_{32}y_1Y_{C1} - C_{32}z_1Y_{C1} = C_{34}Y_{C1} \end{aligned} \tag{3}$$

Six noncoplaner fiducial points were required for calculation of twelve parameters $C_{11} \cdots C_{34}$ because we have two equations once a fiducial point. Actually, a least square method was applied for accurate calculations by using over six fiducial points. In this chapter, we collected fifteen fiducial points for the calculation. Here, we just have to collect a relative (not absolute) coordinate value of $\mathbf{p}_i$ (a distance between each point and an orientation) on the RID coordinate system. If a set of n > 6 fiducial points were given, an equation (4) was derived. There is no problem either C_{34} or H_C are set to a value of constant because a scaling was determined by both parameter. Therefore, we assume that the C_{34} in the camera parameters equal to 1.

$$\mathbf{AC} = \mathbf{R} \tag{4}$$

where

$$\mathbf{A} = \begin{bmatrix} x_1 & y_1 & z_1 & 1 & 0 & 0 & 0 & 0 & -x_1X_{C1} & -y_1X_{C1} & -z_1X_{C1} \\ 0 & 0 & 0 & 0 & x_1 & y_1 & z_1 & 1 & -x_1Y_{C1} & -y_1Y_{C1} & -z_1Y_{C1} \\ \vdots & \vdots & \vdots & \vdots & \vdots & \vdots & \vdots & \vdots & \vdots & \vdots & \vdots \\ x_n & y_n & z_n & 1 & 0 & 0 & 0 & 0 & -x_nX_{Cn} & -y_nX_{Cn} & -z_nX_{Cn} \\ 0 & 0 & 0 & 0 & x_n & y_n & z_n & 1 & -x_nY_{Cn} & -y_nY_{Cn} & -z_nY_{Cn} \end{bmatrix}, \tag{5}$$

$$\mathbf{C} = \begin{bmatrix} C_{11} \\ C_{12} \\ C_{13} \\ \vdots \\ C_{32} \\ C_{33} \end{bmatrix}, \mathbf{R} = \begin{bmatrix} X_{C1} \\ Y_{C1} \\ \vdots \\ X_{Cn} \\ Y_{Cn} \end{bmatrix}. \tag{6}$$

If n fiducial points were given, translation matrixies $\mathbf{A}$, $\mathbf{C}$ and $\mathbf{R}$ are represent as $2n \times 11$, 11×1 and $2n \times 1$ respectively. In cases where n > 6 fiducial points including measurement errors were given, each value of $\mathbf{C}$ could not be calculate because of mathematically impossible problem. Consequently, a task is to find the matrix $\mathbf{C}$ that minimizes a norm $\|\mathbf{AC} - \mathbf{R}\|$. In the case of a determination of the camera parameters, eleven unknown parameters $\mathbf{C}_{11} \cdots \mathbf{C}_{33}$ were given and a number of equations is $2n$ (a number of fiducial points $= n$), that is, the impossible problem $\mathbf{AC} = \mathbf{R}$ was solved by means of a least square solution. Its solution $\langle \mathbf{C} \rangle$ was derived as an equation (7).

$$\mathbf{A}^\mathrm{T}\mathbf{A}\langle \mathbf{C} \rangle = \mathbf{A}^\mathrm{T}\mathbf{R} \tag{7}$$

2.5.2 LMedS (Least Median Square)

Our system was operated not only by researchers in engineering and engineers but also dentists without technical knowledge. Therefore, our system was expected that anyone could perform an image overlay easily in not only laboratories but also operating rooms. In conventional system, we adopted a least square method which is best used in statistical methods to calculate a projection matrix. The least square method which determine parameters by minimizing a sum of square of fitting errors is used as a general calibration method. However, an unchanged application of the least square method is not enough. In case of including exception values, the projection matrix which is estimated by the least square method could not be trusted. If the exception values could be automatically eliminated by fitting a model to a major part in data set, parameters in the major part will be able to estimated accurately. To solve this problem, we introduce a least median square (LMedS) method as a typical robust statistics. A method and an algorithm are as follows. A least square criterion is

$$LMS = \min \sum_{i} \varepsilon_i^2 . \tag{8}$$

A LMedS criterion is

$$LMedS = \min med \varepsilon_i^2 \tag{9}$$

where med means median. In case that the least square criterion, a solution is affected by one big exception value. However, even if a half of all data set were exception values, the solution of the LMedS criterion is not affected. Thus, the LMedS criterion is suitable for this situation.

Step 1. n click of a mouse for an origin position of the marker 1 on the view through the RID, varing location of the marker 1. By this task, n set of three-dimensional points on the marker 1 coordinate system and its corresponding two-dimensional points on the dentist eye's coordinate system are collected. By selection F points from n set of corresponding points, candidates of the projection matrix are calculated by the calibration using the least square method.

Step 2. Calculate error values of the candidate of solution as following equation.

$$err^2 = med\left(\left(X_{Ci} - \bar{X}_{Ci}\right)^2 + \left(Y_{Ci} - \bar{Y}_{Ci}\right)^2\right) \tag{10}$$

where (X_{Ci}, Y_{Ci}) is two-dimensional coordinate value correspoinding to ith origin of the marker 1 on the dentist eye's coordinate system and $(\bar{X}_{Ci}, \bar{Y}_{Ci})$ is reprojected two-dimensional coordinate value which is calculated by the candidate of solution. $med(f(i))$ represent a median of $f(i)$ in all i.

Step 3. Repeat Step 1 and Step 2 q times. F correspoinding points that minimizing err^2 in equation (10) are calculated as following equation (11). Then, camera parameters which is calculated by F corresponding points are selected. A required repitation time in this algorithm can be determined considering a probability that exception values are not included in at least one sample in q random samplings. Let ε be a ratio of exception value in all data. This probability is represented as following equation (11).

$$P = 1 - \left\{1 - (1 - \varepsilon)^F\right\}^q \tag{11}$$

For instance, the number of random samplings in $\varepsilon = 0.3, F = 3$ is $q = 11$. In other words, this means the number of random samplings is over eleven. In our system, $F = 10, n = 15, \varepsilon = 0.3, P = 0.99$ are adopted emprically.

Next, we shall focus on a measurement range. Let A be a measurable range of both the marker 1 and the marker 2 on the MT2 coordinate system. Let B be a measurable range of the marker 2 on the RID corrdinate system. A measurable range of our system represent $A \cap B$. Within this measurable range, the calibration is available.

3. Results and discussions

Fig. 7 (a) shows fabricated models of the marker 1 and the partially edentulous model. Fig. 7 (b) shows the marker 2 attached to the RID. Few systematic errors are expected because both markers were fabricated together. Moreover, a stable intra-operative navigation is achieved even if any one of a pattern of the makers which consists of multiple patterns is hide out in surgical instruments.

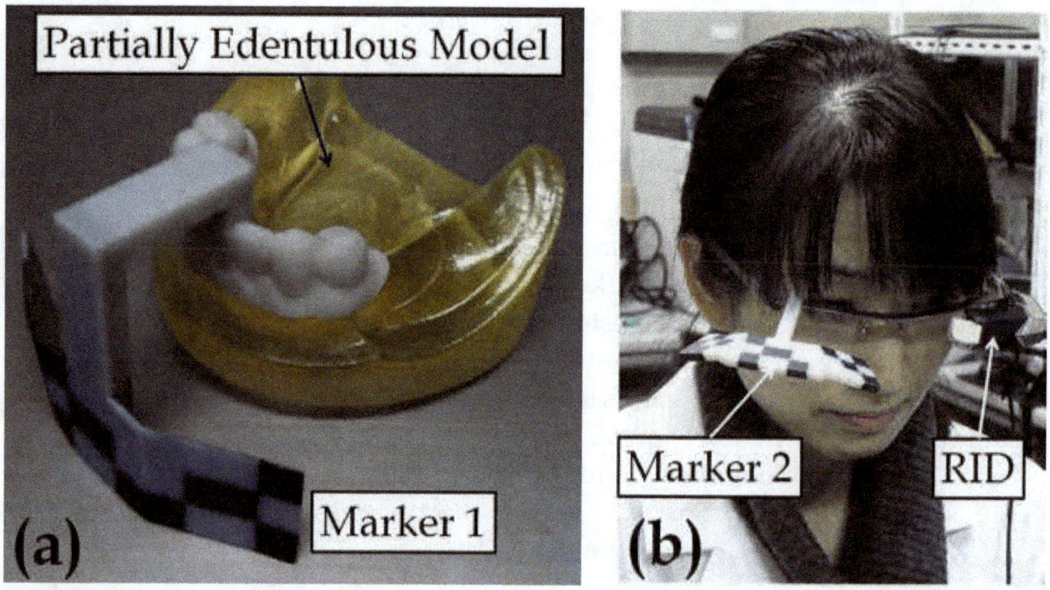

Fig. 7. Fabricated models: (a) The marker 1 and the partially edentulous model, (b) The marker 2 attached to the RID

We adjusted a contrast ratio of colours using the markers on the grounds that the contrast ratio of a grey and black (GB) colour is 20 times higher than that of a white and black (WB) colour. Fig. 8 shows an adjustment result of the contrast ratio. Fig. 8 (a) shows a condition of no spot light in case of a combination with the white and the black colour. Fig. 8 (b) shows the condition of a spotlight in case of a combination with WB. Fig. 8 (c) shows the condition of the spotlight in case of the combination with the grey and the black colour. In the condition of Fig. 8 (b), the WB marker was not measurable because of halation cause the spotlight. However, as shown in Fig. 8 (c), the GB marker was measurable under the condition of the spotlight. Accordingly, we adopt the GB marker around the marker 1 attached to patient's oral cavity with the spotlight and the WB marker 2 around the RID with an environmental light.

As shown in Fig. 9, a measurable range of a new marker was about 2.6 times higher than that of a conventional marker. A tilt angle was set to opposite direction between the marker

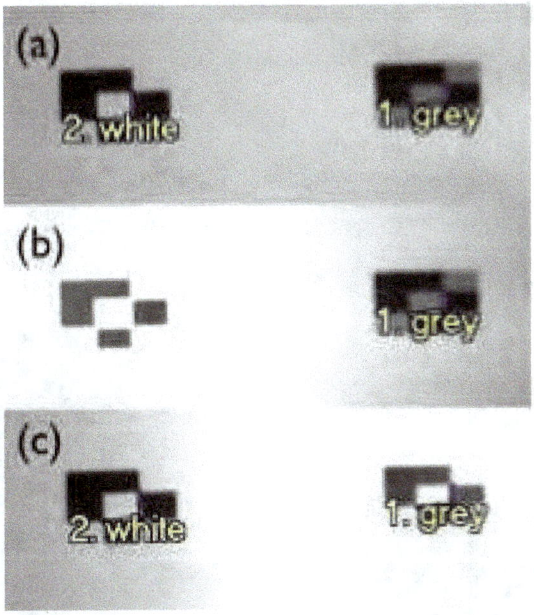

Fig. 8. Adjustment result of contrast ratio. Left marker is combined with a white and black colour (WB). Right marker is combined with a grey and black colour (GB). (a) No spot light, (b) WB marker with spot light, (c) GB marker with spot light

1 and the marker 2 to prevent a false recognition. Fig. 10 shows reprojection errors between the DLT and the LMedS method. An average and a standard deviation of the reprojection errors in the LMedS method indicated decreasing trend in comparison with the DLT method. One of the reasons for the reprojection errors in the LMedS method is dentist's hand movement while sampling. As we have mentioned before, the sampling is performed manually by clicking a mouse in our system. Therefore, some errors may be observed cause dentist's hand movement. So, there is room for further investigatioin about the sampling. And, it must be notice that calibration will be required again in case that a movement of dentist's own misalign relationship between the RID and the dentists.

Fig. 11 and Fig. 12 show real-time image overlay results on the conventional head mounted display and the RID respectively. As shown in Fig. 12 (a) and (b), an image overlay result through the RID was crucially clear view in comparison with that of a conventional head-mounted display (Fig. 11 (a) and (b)). To take Fig. 11 and Fig. 12, we used an off-the-shelf USB camera in place of dentist's eye. Therefore, actual view was better because of direct overlay onto dentist's retina in case of the RID.

4. Conclusion

We proposed the dental implant surgical navigation system by combining the AR technology and the RID and its image overlay procedure, and our procedure proved to be performed as a real-time image overlay. By implementation of the LMedS method, more robust calibration was achieved. Further development of the markers will be planned to decrease the reprojection errors by using the other markers including known sampling points fixed on patient's oral cavity. To achieve clinical applications of this system, evaluation of a fiducial registration error (FRE) and a target registration error (TRE) (Fitzpatrick et al., 1998) and the procedure by real CT data is in progress.

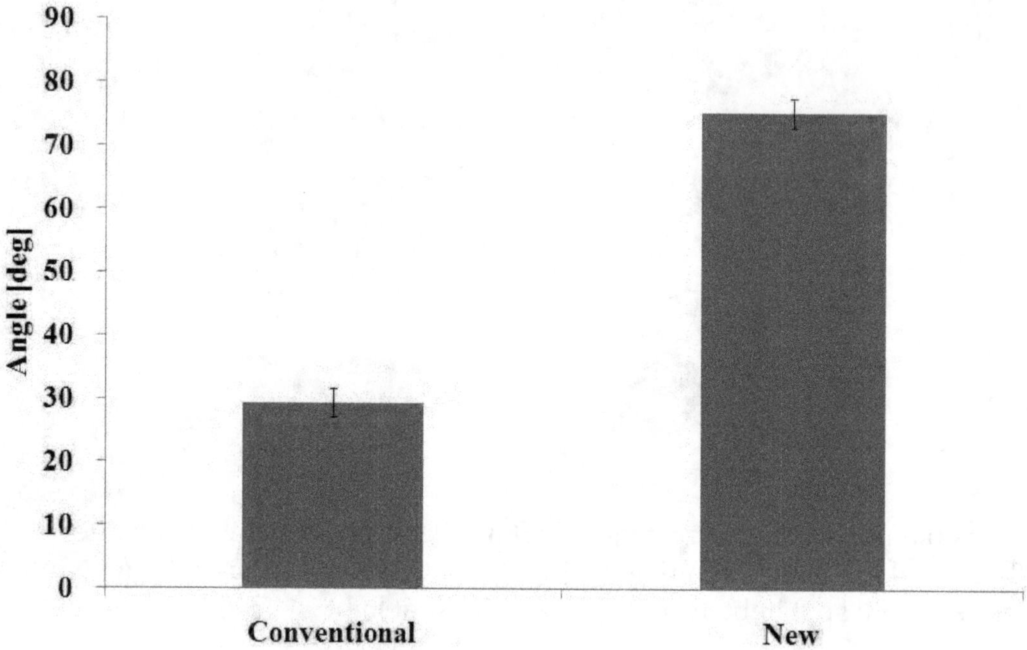

Fig. 9. Comparison with conventional and new measurable range

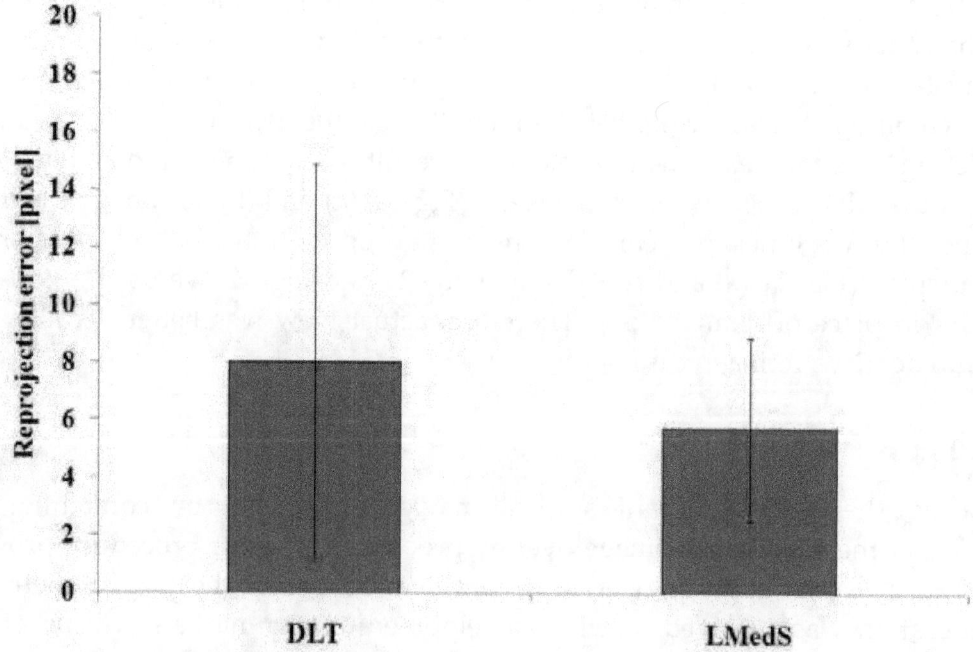

Fig. 10. Comparison with reprojection errors of the DLT method (Yamaguchi et al., 2009) and the LMedS method

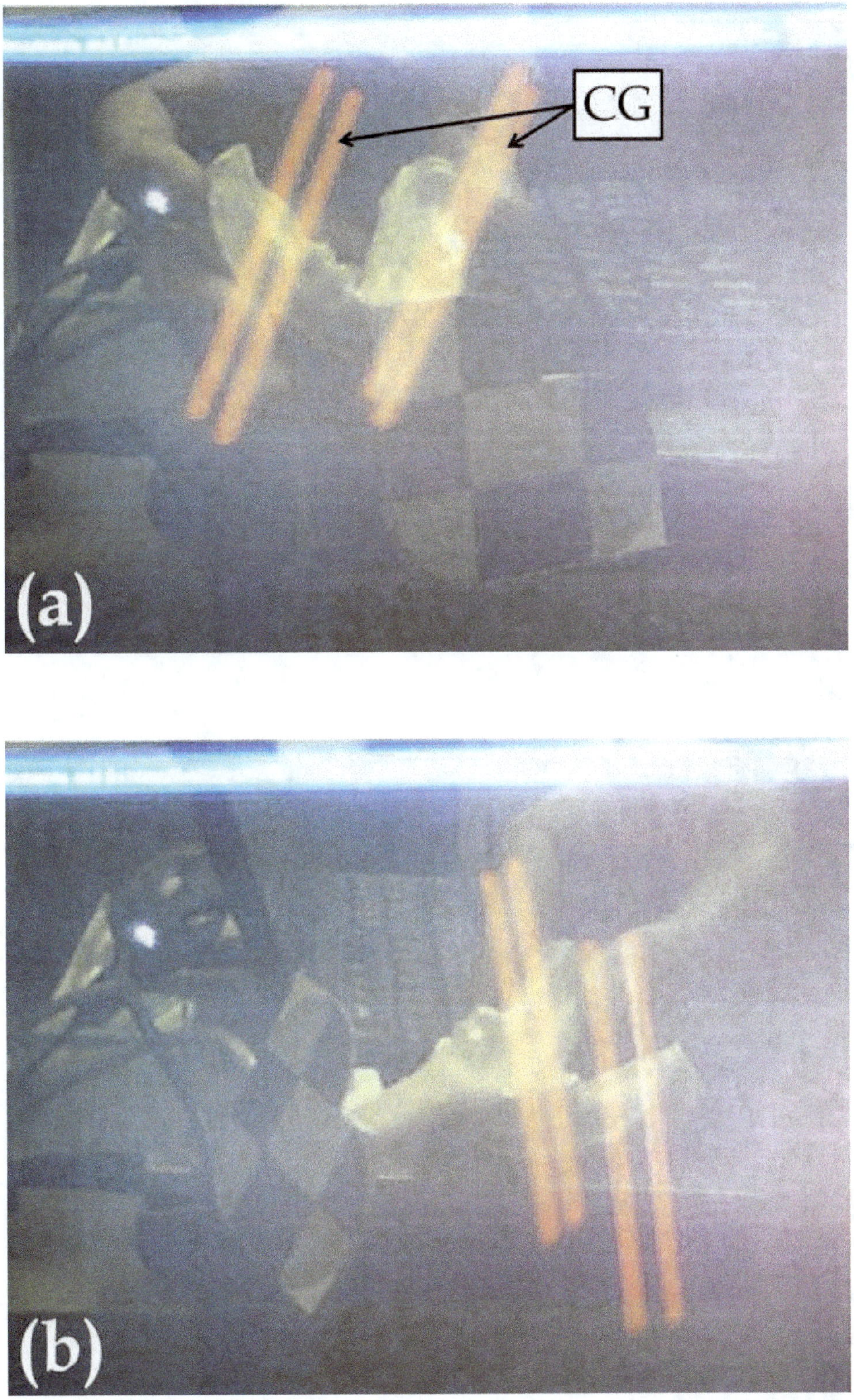

Fig. 11. Real-time image overlay result on the conventional head mounted display: (a) scene 1, (b) scene 2

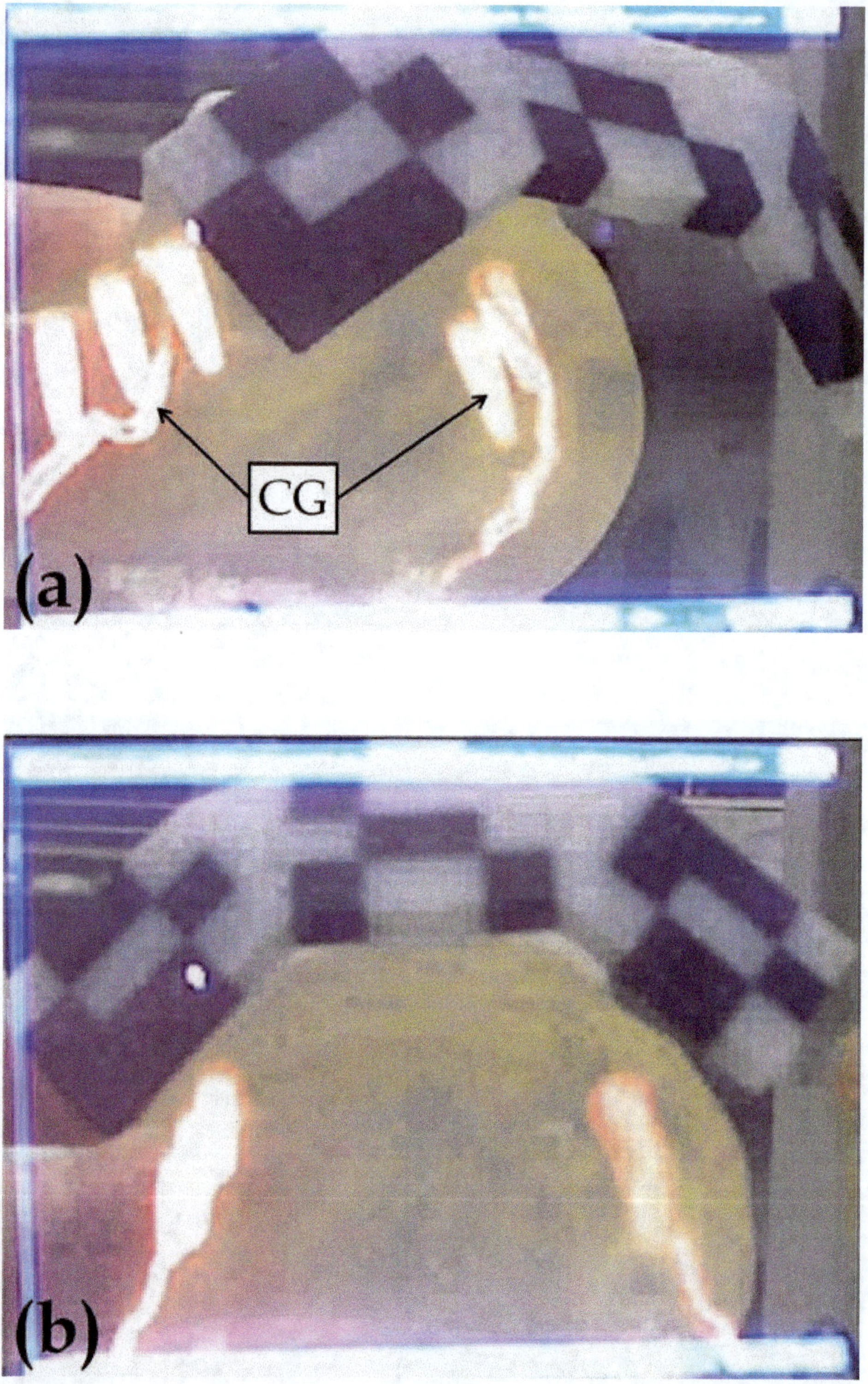

Fig. 12. Real-time image overlay result on the RID: (a) scene 1, (b) scene 2

5. Acknowledgment

This study was supported by Grants-in-Aid for Scientific Research No. 21791937 from the JSPS. For the taking pictures, grateful thanks are due to Noriko Negi at School of Dentistry Osaka University. For the use of RID, grateful thanks are due to Hirokuni Kato and Hideki Tani at Brother Industries, Ltd in Japan. For the advice of calibration techniques, grateful thanks are due to Prof. Hirokazu Kato at Nara Institute of Science and Technology in Japan.

6. References

Azuma, R. T. (1997). A Survey of Augmented Reality, *In Presence : Teleoperators and Virtual Environments*, Vol.6, No.4, pp.355-385.

Birkfellner, W.; Solar, P.; Gahleitner, A.; Huber, K.; Kainberger, F.; Kettenbach, J.; Homolka, P.; Diemling, M.; Watzek, G. & Bergmann, H. (1999). Computer-Aided Implant Dentistry - An Early Report -, *Lecture Notes in Computer Science : MICCAI'99*, Vol.1679, pp.883-891.

Buxton, B.; Hayward, V.; Pearson, I.; Kärkkäinen, L.; Greiner, H.; Dyson, E.; Ito, J.; Chung, A.; Kelly, K. & Schillace, S. (2008). Big data: The next Google, *Nature*, Vol.455, pp.8-9.

Casap, N., et al. (2004). Navigation Surgery for Dental Implants : Assessment of Accuracy of the Image Guided Implantrology System, *Journal of Oral Maxillofacial Surgery*, Vol.62, pp.116-119.

Casap, N., et al. (2005). Application of a surgical navigation system for implant surgery in a deficient alveolar ridge postexcision of an odontogenic myxoma. *Journal of Oral Maxillofacial Surgery*. Vol.63, No.7, pp.982-988.

Casap, N. ; Wexler, A. & Eliashar, R. (2008). Computerized Navigation for Surgery of the Lower Jaw : Comparison of 2 Navigation Systems, *Journal of Oral Maxillofacial Surgery*,

Dede, C., (2009). Immersive Interfaces for Engagement and Learning, *Science*, Vol.323, pp.66-69.

Fitzpatrick, J. M.; West, J. B.; Maurer, C. R., Jr. (1998). Predicting Error in Rigid-Body Point-Based Registration, Transaction on Medical Imaging, Vol.17, No.5, pp.694-702.

Hartley, R. & Zisserman, A. (2003). *Multiple View Geometry in computer vision* (Second edition), Cambridge University Press, ISBN 0-521-54051-8, Cambridge, UK.

Jabero, M. & Sarment D.P. (2006). Advanced Surgical Guidance Technology : A Review, *Journal of Implant Dentistry*, Vol.15, No.2, pp.135-142.

Jung, R. E. ; Schneider, D. ; Wismeijer, D. ; Zwahlen, M. ; Hammerle, C. H. F ; Tahmaseb, A. (2009). Computer Technology Appolications in Surgical Implant Dentistry : A Systematic Review : *Journal of Oral & Maxillofacial Implants*, Vol.24, Suppl. pp.92-109.

Kato, H. & Billinghurst, M. (1999). An Augmented Reality System and its Calibration based on Marker Tracking, *Transaction on Virtual Reality Society of Japan*, Vol.4, No.4, pp.607-616.

Ohtani, T. ; Kusumoto, N. ; Wakabayashi, K. ; Yamada, S. ; Nakamura, T. ; Kumazawa, Y. ; Yatani, H. & Sohmura, T. (2009). Application of Haptic Device to Implant Dentistry - Accuracy Verification of Drilling into a Pig Bone, *Dental Material Journal*, Vol.28, No.1, pp.75-81.

Peters, T. M., (2006). Image-guidance for surgical procedures, *Physics in Medicine and Biology*, Vol. 51, R505 - R540.

Schneider, D. ; Marquardt, P. ; Zwahlen, M. ; Jung, R. E. (2009). A systematic review on the accuracy and the clinical outcome of computer-guided templete-based implant dentistry : *Clinical Oral Implant Research*, Vol.20, Suppl.4, pp.73-86.

Sohmura, T. ; Kusumoto, N.; Otani, T.; Yamada, S.; Wakabayashi, K. & Yatani, H. (2009). CAD/CAM fabrication and clinical application of surgical template and bone model in oral implant surgery, *Journal of Clinical Oral Implant Research*. Vol.20, pp.87–93.

Thomas, R. G.; John, N. W. & Delieu, J. M., (2010). Augmented Reality for Anatomical Education, *Journal of Visual Communication in Medicine*, Vol.33, No.1, pp. 6-15.

Yamaguchi, S.; Ohtani, T.; Yatani, H. & Sohmura, T. (2009). Augmented Reality System for Dental Implant Surgery, *Lecture Notes in Computer Science : Virtual and Mixed Reality*, Vol.5622, pp.633-638.

6

Digital Engineering of Bio-Adaptable Dental Implants

Chahine Gilbert[1], Smith Pauline[2], Kovacevic Radovan[1],
Ajlouni Raed[3] and Ajlouni Khaldoun[3]
[1]*Southern Methodist University, Dallas, Texas,*
[2]*Army Research Lab, Aberdeen, Maryland,*
[3]*Baylor College of Dentistry, Dallas, Texas,*
USA

1. Introduction

Dental implants are the most integral part of modern dentistry (Brånemark, et al., 1969); they provide a permanent and effective solution for a wide range of dental complications and diseases (Tatum, 1988). The prominence of dental implantology is demonstrated by the increase of the number of dental implants used in the U.S. by ten folds from 1983 to 2002, leading to an increase in production capital from $19 million (1983) to $150 million (2002), with a projected yearly growth of 9.4% over the following few years (NIH, 1988; MRG, 2003) According to a report submitted by Merrill Lynch in 2007, the world dental industry is estimated around $2.2 billion (Jüngling, et al., 2006).

From a technological and clinical advancement stand-point, the field of dental implantology has rapidly expanded since its introduction in the late 60s' by Branemark (Spiekermann, et al., 1995). With the introduction of more complex and capable technologies in design, manufacturing, and testing, the dental implant converged to its dominant design of the three-piece assembly (rootform, abutment, and abutment screw) due to incremental changes driven by clinical research and feedback from patient monitoring and the attached trends of success and failure. The prominent design was also crystallized with an attached implant insertion protocol and corresponding pre- and post- implantation routines. The protocol includes biological, functional, and biomechanical assessments, which results into the formulation of different implantation factors such as implant position, amount of available alveolar bone, soft tissue biotype and morphology, implant design and material, abutment, and permanent crown (Sadan, et al., 2004; Poggio, et al., 2002; Touati, et al., 1999). An implantation requirement of great importance is the one devised by Brånemark and Breine et al. (1969), which suggests the countersinking of the implant below the level of crestal bone, while maintaining a soft tissue enclosure for 3-6 months, enforcing a non-loading period before a second-stage surgery would be required in order to uncover the implant and place the abutment and the permanent dental prosthesis. This loading prevention period was discussed in several subsequent studies, where it was concluded that the amount of motion provoked at the implant/alveolar bone interface in early stages of implantation strongly affects the implantations success. Pilliar et al. (1986) states that successful bone integration is only possible in the case of micromotion, not macromotion, suggesting a threshold of 100 μm of micromotion would induce fibrous repair instead of osseointegration (Pilliar, 1991). A finding that was also discussed by Brunski et al. (1993) who considered that displacements of 150 μm to 500 μm are excessive micromotion that would disrupt the process of osteogenesis jeopardizing the implantation's success. Such thresholds prove to be dependent on surface and design characteristics; e.g. porosity (Szmuckler-Moncler, et al., 1998).

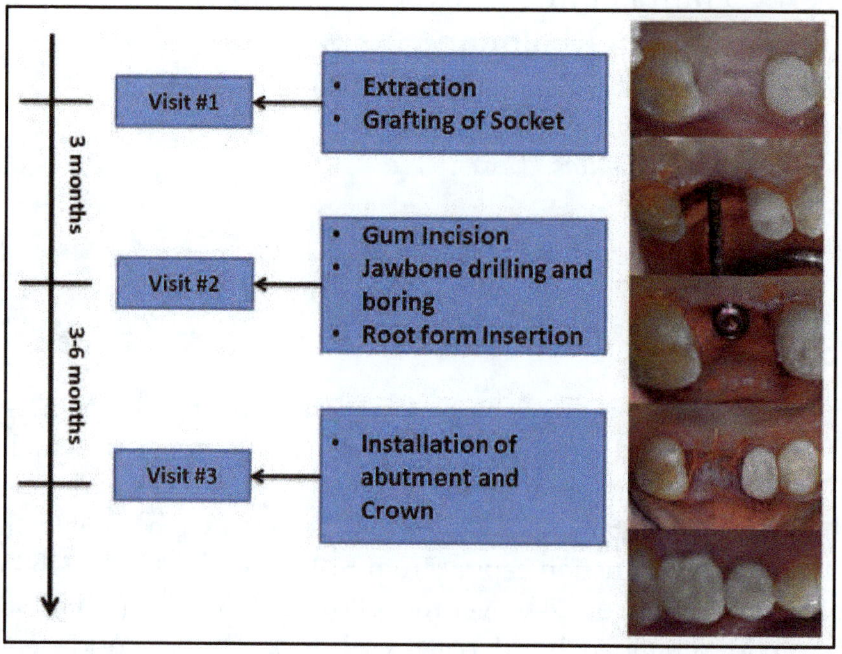

Fig. 1. Traditional post-extraction implantation protocol of a first molar

One area of traditional implantology that is of interest in the current Chapter is the replacement of a decaying unrepairable multi-root posterior dentition. While the survival rates of current implants can reach 95% (Buser, et al., 2002), this is only restricted to anterior single root dentitions. Fig. 1 exhibits a timeline of a traditional replacement of a first molar; it starts with an initial visit to the dentist, where the decaying dentition is extracted and the socket produced is packed with grafting material and enclosed for a healing period reaching 3 months. The second visit includes the surgical insertion of the implant, which is preceded by soft tissue incision, drilling, and boring of the jawbone in preparation of the insertion of the rootform. After insertion, the gum incision is enclosed in order to enforce the aforementioned non-loading period of 3-6 months. The third visit includes the discovery of the rootform and a subsequent installation of the abutment and the permanent dental prosthetic. In summary, the process spans over a period of 6-9 months costing three dentist visits, and a considerable period of incomplete esthetics or function.

In addition to the clinical complications that are imposed by the replacement of a decaying multi-root tooth, when comparing the dental implant to the organ in consideration (natural dentition), several discrepancies are eminent from the functional and physical perspective. In contrast to other load-bearing endosseous implants where a function is being replaced; e.g. hip joint replacement, or knee joint replacement a dental implant is replacing a complete organ which constitutes of a plurality of functions which drastically affect the well-being of a patient. One general discrepancy is the difference in micromotion provided by a dental implant, when compared to natural teeth. A summary is portrayed in Table 1, extracted from (Misch, 2008), where a difference in functionality between natural dentition and dental implants is prominent due to a lack of initial movement (micromotion) in the latter.

Type of Movement	*Natural Tooth*	*Dental Implant*
Vertical Clinical Mobility	0 μm (Misch, 2008)	0 μm (Misch, 2008)
Initial Vertical Movement	28 μm (Parfitt, 1960)	2-3 μm (Sekine, et al., 1986)
Horizontal tooth mobility	56-108 μm (Rudd, et al., 1964)	<73 μm (Sekine, et al., 1986)

Table 1. Comparison of micromotion found in a natural tooth and a dental implant

Another important incongruity between a dentition and the device replacing it is the mismatch in elasticity between the biomaterial (Ti6Al4V 110 GPa (Collin, 1984)) and the surrounding alveolar bone (3-20 GPa (Abe et al., 1996)). A common complication in endosseous implants, the elasticity mismatch causes "stress shielding" which results in disuse bone atrophy manifesting in crestal bone loss in the case of dental implants and a higher risk of implant loosening (Vaillancourt, et al., 1996). In addition to a mismatch in mechanical properties, a mismatch in geometrical aspects is more pronounced in the case of posterior dentition. In a manual published by Zimmer Inc. (Zimmer Dental, n.d.), the average surface area of natural dentition was shown to vary from 154 mm^2 in the case of a mandibular central dentition, to 433 mm^2 in the case of a mandibular first molar. In contrast to a traditional implant that can reach a textured surface of only 310 mm^2.

The multi-component aspect of the traditional design of a dental implant provokes certain impediments that relate to three modes of deterioration which were investigated by Williams (1977): Stress Corrosion Cracking, Galvanic Corrosion, and fretting Corrosion. The latter is mostly pronounced at the abutment/rootform interface and it causes fatigue loading failure.

All the mentioned deviations in physical aspects and functionalities when comparing the modern dental implant to the organ that it replaces lead to a series of shortcomings which seems to be more pronounced in the case of posterior teeth; with the complex implantation surgery and the divergent functionality of the traditional medical device. Accordingly, a series of innovations were suggested over the past few years in order to overcome the mentioned shortcomings, while employing emerging technologies in design, data acquisition and manufacturing. Discussed in the next section, the prior art of new concepts of dental implants, which lead to the crystallization of the concept of bio-adaptable implant that is discussed in the current Chapter.

2. Prior art

Due to the different complications that aroused from traditional dental implantology, several alternative rationales were addressed along the years, which deal with shortcomings found in the function of dental implants, and the prescribed insertion protocol. Hodosh et al. (1969) introduced the concept of root-analogous implants, which enables insertion right after extraction. Some in-vivo testing proved root-analogous dental implant to provide some initial success, however portrayed poor success results (48%) 9 months after implantation (Kohal, et al., 1997), rendering the concept as unattractive. More recent work done by Pirker et al. (2008), employs CAD/CAM techniques to produce root-analogous zirconia implants with macro-retention on the surface. A main improvement is the reduction of the implant size where it comes in contact with the brittle crestal bone, which was one main factors affecting the poor success rates of older versions of the concept.

Fig. 2 displays a few patents that provide alternative concepts of dental implants. Uckleman et al. (2004), introduced the use of laser-based additive manufacturing for the production of a customized abutment, which when coated produces the dental prosthesis. Hayashi et al. (2009), provided a similar concept of using additive manufacturing, where an abutment is produced on top of an abutment screw; hence, reducing the assembly of the implant to two components (in contrast to the traditional three-piece assembly). Rubbert et al. (2005) proposed the use of intraoral scanning for diagnostics and treatment pre-planning purposes, in addition to producing patient-specific dental devices. Mount et al. (2008), patented the concept of a root-mimicking dental implant that exhibits macro-retentions on the surface.

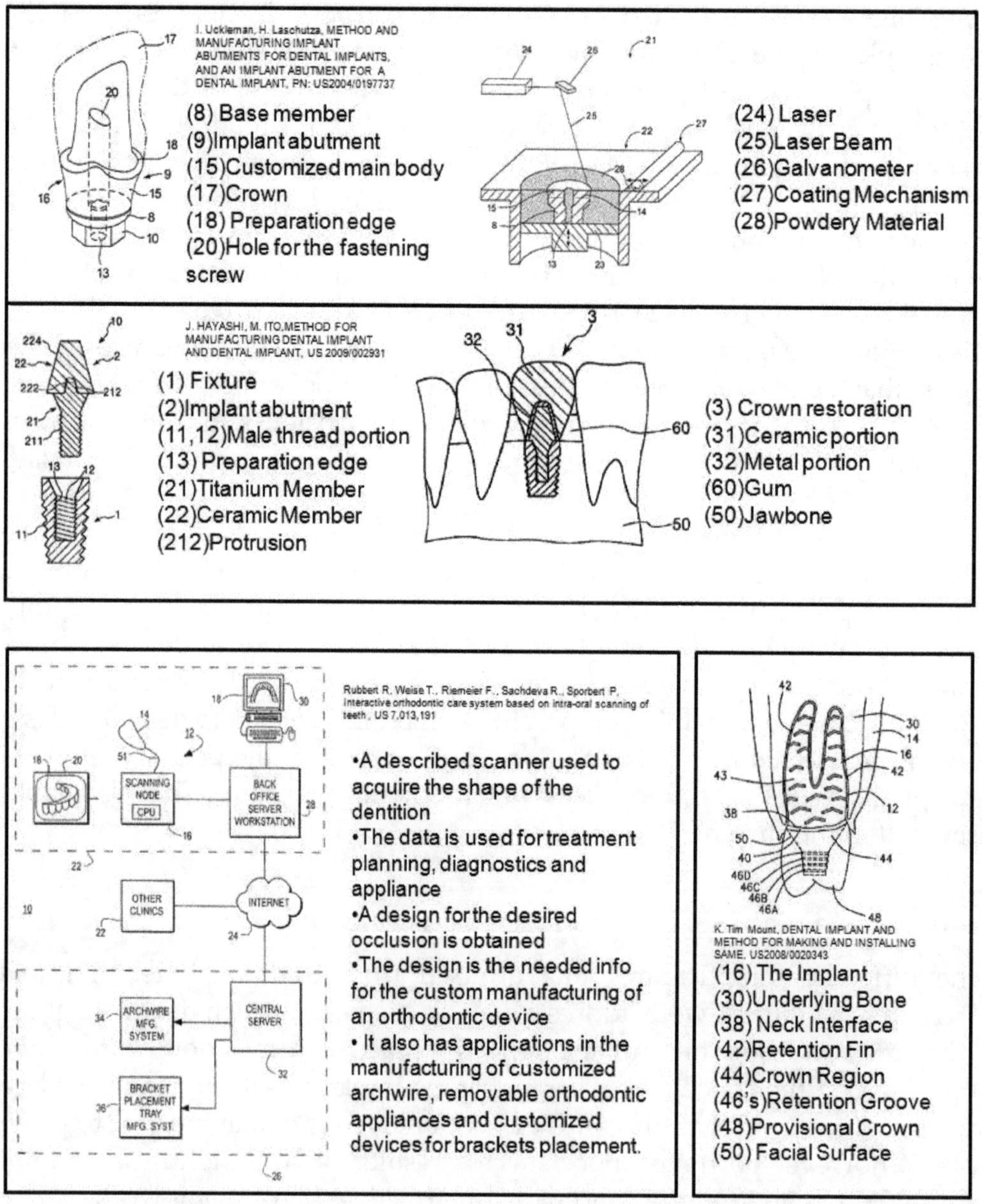

Fig. 2. Different dental implant rationales illustrated by their corresponding patents

An attractive design aspect, which provides a wide range of interest, is the use of porosity on the surface of the implant. In fact, porosity has been proven to improve clinical success by increasing the surface of the contact area (Geng, et al., 2001). In addition, a favorable osteo-blast reaction to the pores is also proven by (Xiropaidis, et al., 2005). One theory suggests that pores provide favorable mechanical conditions for bone growth, which was proven by finite element analysis (Cook, et al., 1982). In addition to porous coatings on the surface, dental implants that are built out of porous materials are also introduced by either additive manufacturing (Laoui, et al., 2006) or the by machining metal foams (NRC, 2005).

Dental implants with damping mechanisms also have been extensively addressed by several concepts, which are believed to provide better load transfer from the bite to the surrounding alveolar bone. Kraut et al. (1993), introduced intra-mobile damping, which employs polyoxymethylene connections, which is found in commercially available IMZ implants (Kanth, 1971; Kirsch, 1983). Patents provided by Ford (1999) and Wagher (1995) also introduced concepts of force distributing, and elastic implants respectively. Despite the several benefits expected from damping capabilities, the mobile aspect of the medical devices introduces failure concerns and maintenance requirement to ensure proper functioning.

3. Rationale of bio-adaptable dental implant

Singularities found in the biomedical field are as frequent as in any biological environment. Every patient has his own characteristics of jawbone density and geometrical aspects of teeth and surrounding biomass. The field of implantology has been limited to certain standards that were adopted due to design and manufacturing limitations. With the advent of digital engineering and its capabilities of designing and producing performance-specific customized parts in a time- and cost-efficient manner, the need of standardized sizes can be eliminated. In contrast of fitting patients' characteristics by means of intrusive and traumatic surgical practices, the implant can be tailored and customized to fit the patient in the least intrusive manner, maximizing benefits and minimizing healthcare cost, which has a positive impact on patient satisfaction and quality of life.

Digital engineering can be defined as the art of using extensive computational power to contribute and ameliorate endeavors in design, manufacturing, and testing. Accordingly, the field unrestrictedly includes: imaging technologies, image processing techniques, reverse engineering, additive manufacturing, and numerical simulation.

The work portrayed in the current chapter discusses the use of the various techniques that constitute digital engineering to design and manufacture a bio-adaptable dental implant that provides high levels of compliance to user-defined needs while abiding to design and functional constraints.

4. Concept

The concept of bio-adaptable dental implants was initially introduced as a customized root-mimicking dental implant (Chahine, et al., 2008; Chahine, et al., 2010). By taking advantage of modern computed tomography (CT) techniques and the subsequent analysis capabilities of the scan data and the generation of three-dimensional computer models, in addition to additive manufacturing (AM) and its ability of producing application-specific parts, a cost and time effective track of designing and producing customized dental implants was devised. A more elaborate approach is discussed in the current section, where the ability of AM to produce highly complex structures is taken to its full extent.

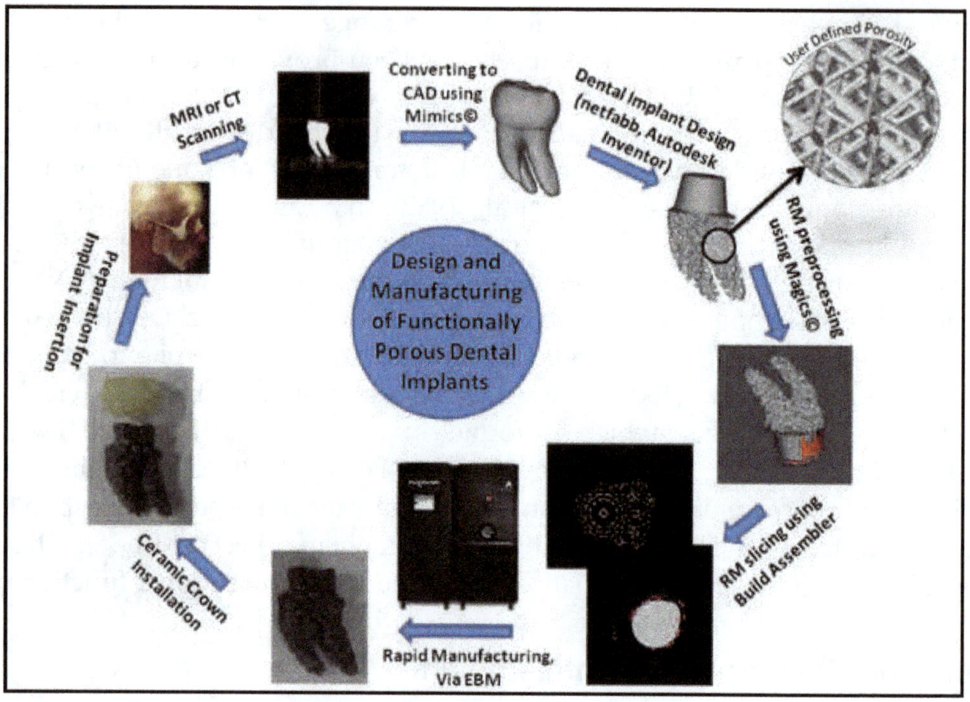

Fig. 3. Design and production of a bio-adaptable dental implant

The main application of the current concept deals with treating decaying posterior teeth by means of immediate implantation after extraction. Fig. 3 displays the design and manufacturing track of a bio-adaptable dental implant. A CT scan of a patient's dentition to be replaced is sufficient to provide enough geometrical data to produce a CAD model of the organ. The model is subsequently used to generate a root-mimicking design along with two main design characteristics: functionally graded porosity (FGP) and advanced abutment design (AAD) which will be discussed in more detail in a subsequent section. The design is then prepared for AM and manufactured. The implant undergoes post-manufacturing processing steps before being sent to the dentist's office before extraction. The lead-time of the entire process is in the range of 24 to 48 hours, enabling the production of the medical device in a time- and cost-efficient manner. Fig. 4 devises the concept of a service center for dental implants, where a the need of several dental clinics treating several patients' needs can be addressed by a single service center by bundling all the different patient-specific dental implants in the building envelope of an AM machine. The development of specialized software to generate bio-adaptable dental implant designs complying with patients' specifics can drastically reduce the already short lead time.

From a clinical concept point of view, the insertion protocol of a bio-adaptable dental implant provides several advantages when compared to the traditional approach. As displayed in Fig. 5, the implantation is executed in one dental visit in contrast to the three-visit protocol discussed earlier. The bio-adaptable implant is customized according to every patient and clinical situation; resultantly it provides optimal function and superior esthetics when compared to stock manufactured implants. In the case where CT scan banks are available, the implant can be ready upon the initial dental visit of the patient where the dentist can atraumatically remove the damaged tooth and insert the implant with minimal to no site preparation. Minimizing trauma will provide with faster healing of the surrounding bone (Misch, et al., 2005). In addition, the immediate placement can provide immediate esthetics and function.

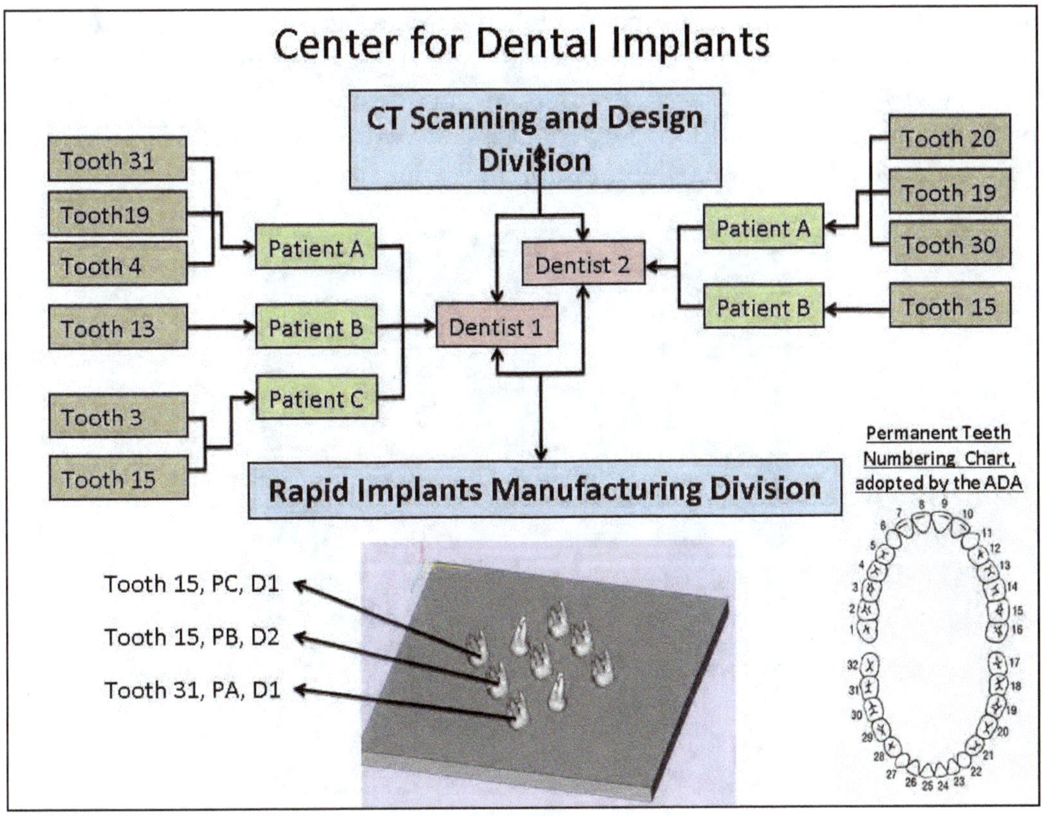

Fig. 4. Mass production Concept of a bio-adaptable dental implant

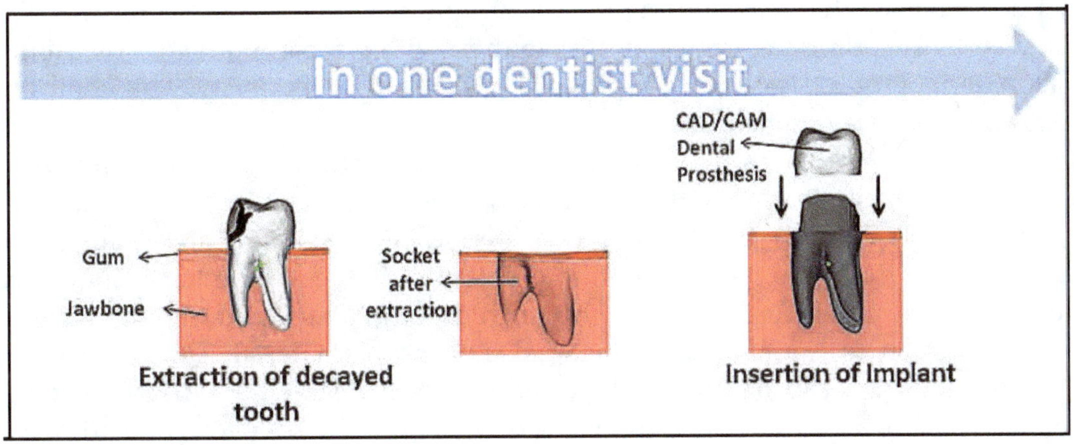

Fig. 5. Clinical concept of a bio-adaptable dental implant as a root-mimicking concept

5. Design and functionality

With the advent of scan analysis techniques and software, surgical pre-planning offers surgeons the ability to visualize and predict the surgical outcome (Stocker, et al., 1992). By analyzing the imaging data obtained from computed tomography (CT) or magnetic resonance imaging (MRI), geometrical models of different organs can be generated and used for a wide range of potential numerical simulation of thermal, bi-mechanical, and biological response. Fig. 6 displays a partial geometry of a patient's jaw that was extracted by CT scan analysis using Mimics®, software developed by Materialise (Leuven, Belgium), where grayscale analysis is employed at every image to separate the different biomaterials (cortical bone, alveolar bone, dentition, periodontal ligament) and produce CAD models of the different bio-components. The first mandibular model displayed in the aforementioned Figure is designated as the dentition to be replaced. Accordingly it is used as the geometrical reference to which a bio-adaptable dental implant would comply.

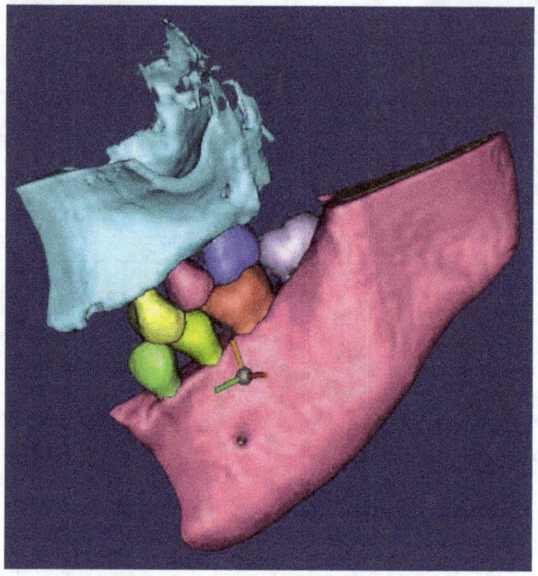

Fig. 6. Geometry of a patient's partial jaw extracted by means of CT analysis

In addition to detecting the geometry of various elements of the bio-environment, grayscale analysis also enables the detection of the anisotropic material properties of the different components. By mapping the grayscale distribution within a component, a distribution of the local material properties can be generated; e.g. elasticity and density. This contributes to a more realistic representation of the domain of interest.

As mentioned earlier, the main functional discrepancy between a dental implant and a dentition is the lack of micromotion, which is also referred to as initial movement. The main reason for the difference is the absence of a periodontal ligament at the implant/bone interface, which surrounds a natural dentition. Actually, a successful implantation is closely dependent on the osseointegration of the surrounding bone, and its mechanical and functional adhesion to the alloplastic material; i.e. the biomaterial. Despite a successful initial retention which can be enforced by macro-topologies at the surface, a long term implantation requires a successful bone reaction on the micro-level. Due to the direct bonding between the rootform area and the surrounding bone, the only approach that can enable crown movement in different directions involves imposing an elastic connection between the dental prosthesis and the anchored rootform.

Fig. 7 displays a preliminary design concept where either a fully porous abutment or an elastic interface can be designed in order to provide the relative micromotion of the crown. A more elaborate concept is shown in Fig. 8, where a thin featured abutment might provide enough flexing to induce micromotion. In contrast to intra-mobile dental implants that are commercially available, the current design approach deviates from the multi-component assembly and converges towards a one-piece dental implant which provides a wide set of functionalities which are provided by locally varying the mechanical properties of the implant.

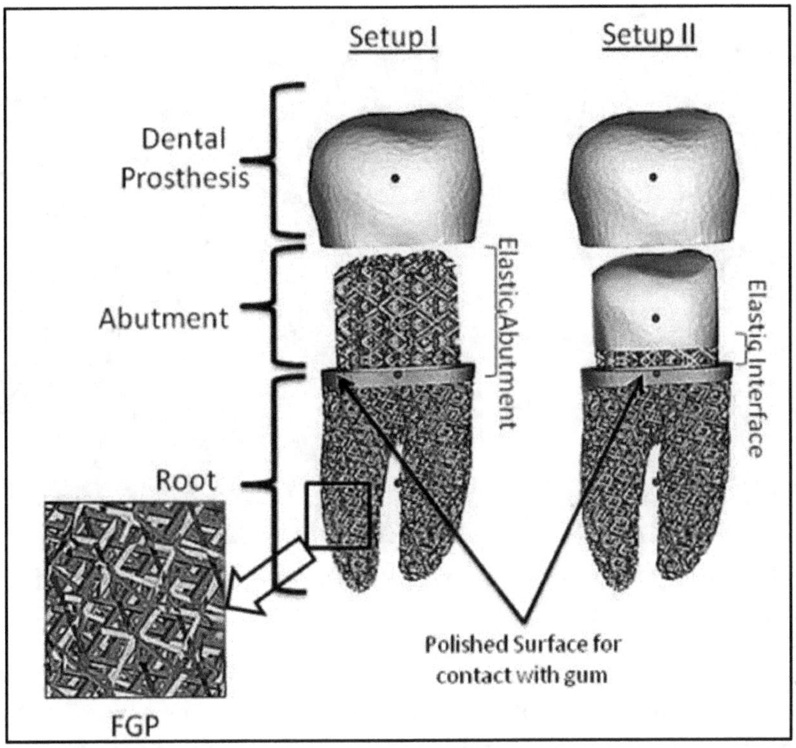

Fig. 7. Rendering of the FGP and AAD design aspects of a bio-adaptable dental implant

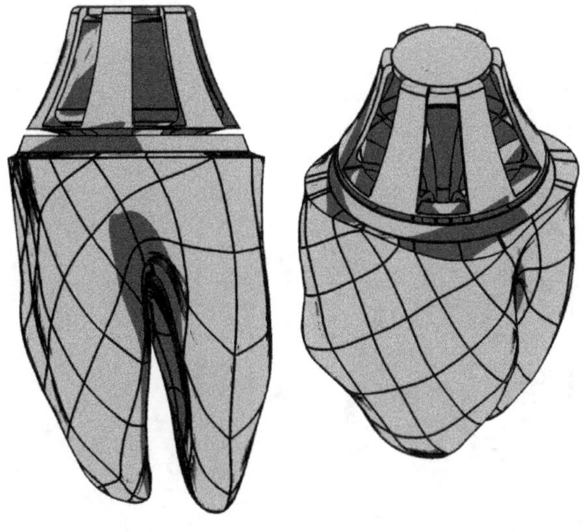

Fig. 8. A rendering of an AAD example

Fig. 9 displays a design example where the abutment rests on an elastic interface that exhibits a porosity corresponding to a desired elasticity. Under loading, the crown will exhibit more elastic behavior in contrast to the conventional case where it is directly anchored to the implant body.

One complication that can be imposed by the current approach of having open gaps in the abutment area is the risk of bacterial infection. A proposed solution involves injecting the cavity by medical polyethylene terephthalate, commonly known by the commercial brand Dacron® which is used in heart valves and internal sutures (Metzger, n.d.). Other candidate materials include medical silicone and polyoxymethylene.

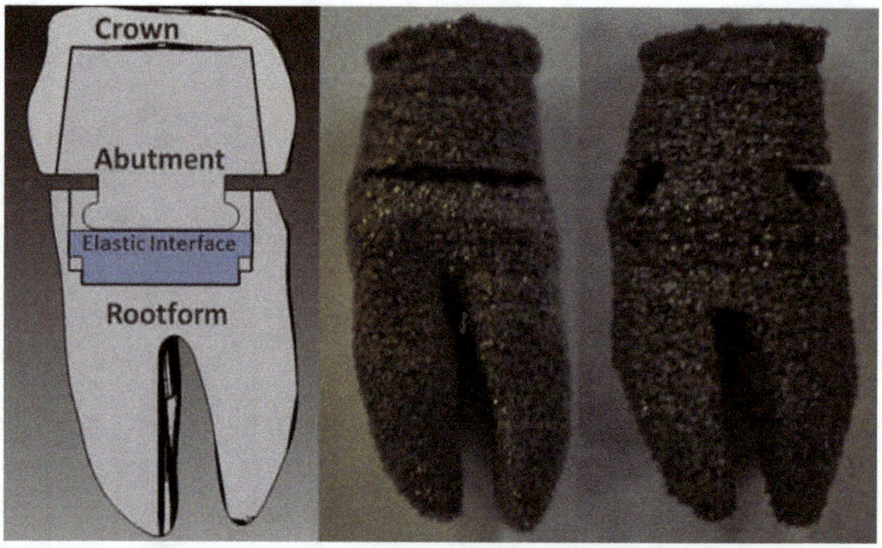

Fig. 9. Bio-adaptable dental implant with AAD (left), built by EBM® (middle), cross-section of the build (right)

The micromotion provided by the AAD, contributes towards a more natural function of the implant, rendering it an improved tooth-replacement. It promotes a more natural bite feel, and an enhanced interaction with the surrounding teeth. In addition, it enables the implementation of fixed bridging supported by a combination of an implant and a tooth, which is traditionally endangered by the discrepancy of the amount of micromotion exhibited by the tooth and the implant. However, perhaps the most prominent advantage of the AAD is minimizing the amount of micromotion transferred from the bite load to the connecting interface between the implant and the surrounding bone, especially in the early stages of implantation where excessive micromotion at the rootform leads to fibrous encapsulation.

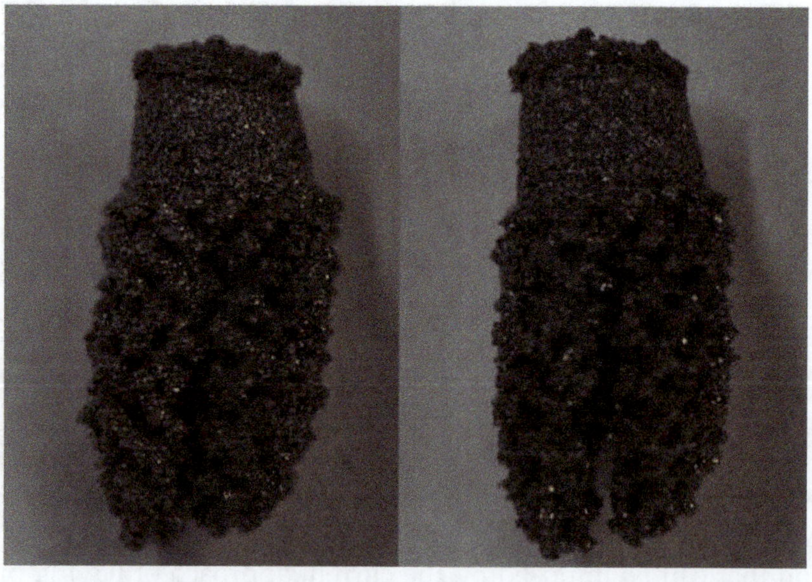

Fig. 10. Two bio-adaptable dental implants with porous rootform built by EBM®

FGP deals with locally varying the geometrical aspects of porosity, inducing locally varying mechanical, physical, and biological properties. FGP is applied at the rootform area of a bio-adaptable dental implant (See Fig. 10) provoking two levels of bone response: a macro-level, and a micro-level. The latter relates to the reaction of bone cells to the micro-topology of the implant's surface. According to Hulbert et al. (1970), a 100 μm pore induces bone ingrowth, while a pore that is larger than 150 μm leads to an osteon formation. Work done by Simmons et al. (1999) discusses how mineralization rates are higher in porous surface when compared to a plasma sprayed texture, which is related to a favorable localized mechanical conditions in the pores. FEM analysis conducted by the same group (Simmons, et al., 2001) proves less severe volumetric and distortional tissue strains at the pores located at the interface of the implant, which provided favorable bone mineralization conditions according to Carter's tissue differentiation law (Carter, et al., 1998). Consequently, a porous surface contributes towards a biological union between the implant and the surrounding bone, leading to a longer lasting and stronger fixation. In fact, studies have shown that metal implants with a rough surface require a larger removal torque when compared to polished implants (Cohen, 1961).

The macro-level of bone response relates to the effect of osseointegration due to the stress induced in the bone. One main function of dental implant is to ensure the compressive bite-load transfer to the surrounding bone, which contributes to maintaining healthy bone levels in the jaw, in contrast to dentures which lead to alveolar ridge resorption. The optimal range of stress in the surrounding bone can be enforced by the development of FGP compliant to the loading conditions and the mechanical properties of the surrounding biomass.

Finally, one important function promoted by the bio-adaptable implant is the preservation of the stress pattern in the surrounding bone, due to the geometrical mimicking of the root of the initial dentition. This fact also reduces the need for orientation adjustments, due to the inert orientation provided by the socket, which otherwise would be calculated by the dentist and provided by a drill guide in the case of traditional implantation.

6. FEM as a design tool

Finite element method (FEM) is a numerical simulation which is used to solve problems in the physical domains of solid mechanics, heat transfer, fluid dynamics, and electromagnetism. Its main functioning deals with solving discretized equations that govern thermal, mechanical, and flow phenomena. During the 1970's, when FEM was initially introduced, it was mostly used in the aerospace industry. Since then, the fields of application have been drastically expanded.

Overviews provided by DeTolla et al. (2000) and Geng et al. (2001) discuss the application of FEM in the field of dental implantology. Compared to in-vivo and in-vitro testing, FEM provides a cost and time effective solution to predicting the clinical outcome of an implantation that is governed by specific variables. Extensive FEM work can be found in the literature that covers the effect of placement and inclination (Akça, et al., 2001; Canay, et al., 1996; Watanabe, et al., 2003), thread design (Eraslan, et al., 2010), implant dimensions (Himmlová, et al., 2004; İplikçioğlu, et al., 2002), occlusal loading position (Eskitascioglu, et al., 2004), and biomaterial (Stegaroiu, et al., 1998) on the surrounding biomasses and organs; i.e. jawbone, periodontal ligament, and neighboring dentition (Ishigaki, et al., 2003; Nagasao, et al., 2002; Nagasao, et al., 2003; Borchers, et al., 1983; Widera, et al., 1976; Akpinar, et al., 2000).

The main approach of implementing FEM into the design of a bio-adaptable dental implant, deals with tailoring the mechanical properties of different elements of the medical device, in order to comply with certain conditions and constraints that are imposed by the implantation. An example is displayed and discussed in the current section.

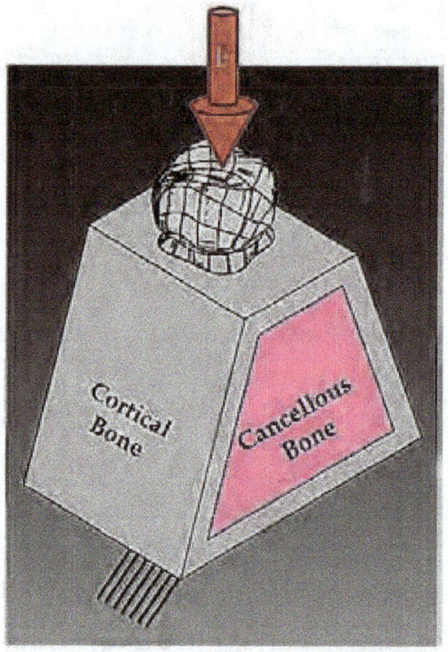

Fig. 11. FEM model, load, and constraints of a bio-adaptable dental implant

The schematic of Figure 11 displays a geometrical model that constitutes of a bio-adaptable dental implant with a solid rootform and elastic interface (See Figure 9) and the surrounding bio-elements; cortical bone, and cancellous bone. The bottom surface is constrained, while a vertical bite load is being applied on the implant. ANSYS® Workbench is used to solve for the stress and strain distribution along the geometrical domain. By employing the DesignXplorer® module provided by the software, the range of different outcomes can be evaluated, depending on user-set variable inputs. In this example the elasticity of the elastic layer is varied between 1-50 GPa, with a bite load ranging from 50-500 N. The plotted outcome is the maximum occlusal displacement of the crown, which related to the micromotion expected to be achieved by implementing AAD in a bio-adaptable dental implant. Figure 12 displays a 3D distribution of the micromotion vs. the two aforementioned inputs. As expected, a lower elasticity and higher bite load produce a higher level of micromotion in the occlusal direction. The range of micromotion that is produced by different combinations of inputs spans from 0.66 to 45.7 microns.
Referring to Table 1, a vertical initial movement of a natural tooth is 28 μm. By evaluating the patient's bite load range, an optimal elasticity of the elastic interface can be selected providing a range of micromotion analogous to that of a natural tooth.

7. Conclusion

The current chapter displayed a detailed description of the novel concept of bio-adaptable dental implants, and the expected clinical and functional advantages that it provides. It employs numerical information obtained from CT scans to produce an implant that provides maximum compliance to patient-specific geometrical and biomechanical constraints, while producing optimized functionality. Design aspects, such as FGP and AAD that display a local tailoring of mechanical properties, take full advantage of additive manufacturing's capability of producing parts with complex geometries. Potential advantages provided by the new concept include:

- Immediate restoration of function and esthetics
- Reduced treatment time
- No to minimally invasive site preparation

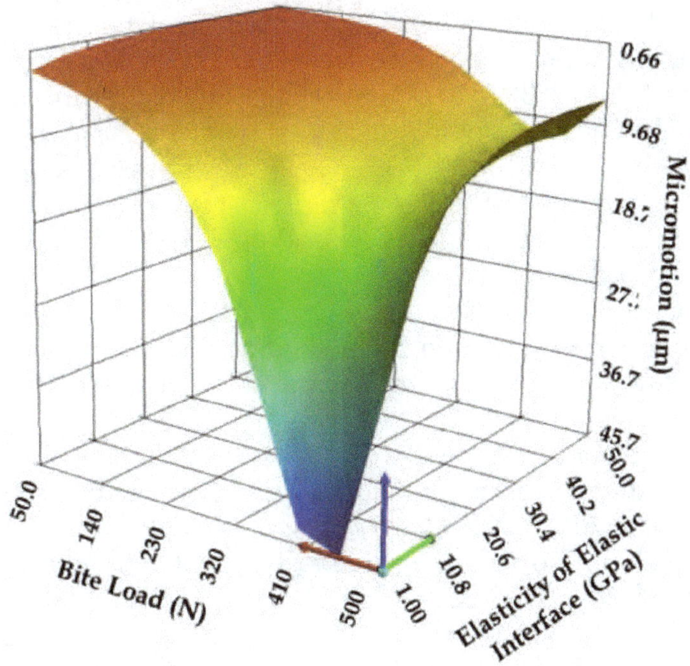

Fig. 12. DOE result of the maximum amount of occlusal micromotion produced by various levels of bite loads and elasticity of the elastic interface

- Better bite feel due to micromotion capabilities
- Enhanced bone response
- Improved patient satisfaction, and quality of life
- Reduced health care cost

The work portrayed discusses a new direction in implantology, where the implant matches the patient, instead of the contrary. This is only possible due to the advent of digital engineering, and the ability of producing customized medical device in a cost and time efficient manner, rendering it economically attractive.

Future work includes in-vivo testing of bio-adaptable dental implants, which depending on the preliminary findings might lead to clinical testing. In addition, with the progression in CT scan and additive manufacturing resolution, more defined features can be designed and produced, and compliance can be achieve at a higher degree.

8. Acknowledgements

The authors would like to acknowledge the contribution and financial support of the Army Research Office with the Research Center for Advanced Manufacturing at Southern Methodist University for the development of the program entitled: "Advanced Precision Supply Parts Manufacturing", Grant No. W911NF-07-2-0056.

9. References

Abe et al., F. (1996). Measurement of Dijet Angular Distributions by the Collider Detector at Fermilab. *Phys. Rev. Lett.*, 77(27), 5336–5341.

Akça, K., & Iplikçioğlu, H. (2001, Sept-Oct). Finite element stress analysis of the influence of staggered versus straight placement of dental implants. *Int J Oral Maxillofac Implants*, 16(5), 722-730.

Akpinar, I., Anil, N., & Parnas, L. (2000, June). A natural tooth's stress distribution in occlusion with a dental implant. *Journal of Oral Rehabilitation*, 27(6), 538-545.

Borchers, L., & Reichart, P. (1983). Three-dimensional Stress Distribution Around a Dental Implant at Different Stages of Interface Development. *J of Dent Res*, 62(2), 155-159.

Brånemark, P.-I., Adell, R., & Breine, U. (1969). Intra-osseous anchorage of dental prostheses.I. Experimental Studies. *Scand J Plast Reconstr Surg*, 3, p. 81.

Brunski, J. B. (1993). Avoid pitfalls of overloading and micromotion of intraosseous implants. *Dent Impantol*, 4, 1-5.

Buser, D., Mericske-Stern, R., Pierre Bernard, J. P., Behneke, A., Bekneke, N., Hirt, H. P., et al. (2002). Long-term evaluation of non-submerged ITI implants. Part 1: 8-year life table analysis of a prospective multi-center study with 2359 implants. *Clinical Oral Implants Research*, 8(3), 161-172.

Canay, S., N., H., Akpinar, I., & Aşik, Z. (1996, September). Comparison of stress distribution around vertical and angled implants with finite-element analysis. *Quintessence Int.*, 27(9), 591-598.

Carter, D. R., Beaupre, G. S., Giori, N. J., & Helms, J. A. (1998, October). Mechanobiology of skeletal regeneration. *Clin Orthop*, (355 Suppl), S41-55.

Chahine, G., Koike, M., Okabe, T., Smith, P., & Kovacevic, R. (2008). The design and production of Ti-6Al-4 customized dental implants. *Journal of Metals*, 60(11), 50-55.

Chahine, G., Smith, P., & Kovacevic, R. (2010). Application of structural optimization in modern rapid manufacturing. International Solid Freeform Fabrication Symposium. Austin Texas.

Cohen, J. (1961, July). Tissue reactions to metals-The influence of surface finish. *J Bone and Joint Surg*, 43(A), 687-699.

Collin, E. W. (1984). The physical metallurgy of titanium alloys. American Society of Metals, 261.

Cook, S. D., Klawitter, J. J., & Weinstein, A. M. (1982). A model of the implant-bone interface, characterics of Porous Dental Implants. *J Dent Res*, 61(8), 1006-1009.

DeTolla, D. H., Andreanna, S., Patra, A., Buhite, R., & Comella, B. (2000). The Role of the Finite Element Model in Dental Implants. *J of Oral Implantol*, 26(2), 77-81.

Eraslan, O., & İnan, Ö. (2010). The effect of thread design on stress distribution in a solid screw implant: a 3D finite element analysis. *Clin Oral Invest*, 14(4), 411-416.

Eskitascioglu, G., Usumez, A., Sevimay, M., Soykan, E., & Unsal, E. (2004, February). The influence of occlusal loading location on stresses transferred to implant-supported prostheses and supporting bone: a three-dimensional finite element study. *Journal of Prosthetic Dentistry*, 91(2), 144-150.

Ford, C. W. (1999, September 21). Patent No. 5,954,505. US.

Geng, J. P., Tan, K. B., & Liu, G. R. (2001). Application of finite element analysis in implant dentistry: A review of the literature. *J Prosthet Dent*, 85, 585-98.

Hayashi, J., & Ito, M. (2009). Patent No. 002931. US.

Himmlová, L., Dostálová, T., Kácovský, A., & Konvičková, S. (2004, January). Influence of implant length and diameter on stress distribution: A finite element analysis. *J of Prost Dent*, 91(1), 20-25.

Hodosh, M., Povar, M., & Shklar, G. (1969). The dental polymer implant concept. *J Prosthet Dent*, 22, 371-380.

Hulbert, S. F., Klawitter, J. J., Talbert, C. D., Young, F. A., Mathews, R. S., & Stelling, F. H. (1970). Potential of ceramics as permanently implantable skeletal prostheses. National Meeting of the American Institute of Chemical Engineers. Atlanta, Georgia.

İplikçioğlu, H., & Akça, K. (2002, January). Comparative evaluation of the effect of diameter, length and number of implants supporting three-unit fixed partial prostheses on stress distribution in the bone. *J of Dent*, 30(1), 41-46.

Ishigaki, S., Nakano, T., Yamada, S., Nakamura, T., & Takashima, F. (2003, February). Biomechanical stress in bone surrounding an implant under simulated chewing. *Clinical Oral Implants Research*, 14(1), 97-102.

Jüngling, M., & Surla, A. (2006, October 12). The Changing World of Dental Implantology, Industrial Overview. Merrill Lynch.

Kanth, L. (1971). The cast (intramobile) screw implant. DDZ, 25(12), 465-467.

Kirsch, A. (1983). The two-phase implantation method using IMZ intramobile cylinder implants. *J Oral Implantology*, 11(2), 197-202.

Kohal, R.-J., Hurzeler, M. B., Mota, L. F., Klaus, G., Caffesse, R. G., & Strub, J. R. (1997). Custom made root analogue titanium implants placed into extraction sockets. An experimental study in monkeys. *Clin Oral Impl Res*, 8, 386-392.

Kraut, R. A., & A., K. (1993). Practical stress absorption by means of modified abutments. *Pract Periodontics Aesthet Dent*, 5, 67-72.

Laoui, T., Santos, E., Oksada, K., Shiomi, M., Morita, M., Shaik, S. K., et al. (2006). Properties of titanium dental implant models made by laser processing. Proceedings of the Institution of Mechanical Engineers, Part C: *Journal of Mechanical Engineering Science*, 220, pp. 857-863.

Metzger, A. (n.d.). Polyethylene Terephthalate and the Pillar™ Palatal Implant:Its Historical Usage and Durability in Medical Applications. Restore Medical Inc.

Misch, C. E. (2008). Comtemporary Implant Dentistry (3rd ed.). Mosby.

Misch, C. E., Suzuki, J. B., Misch-Dietsh, F. M., & Bidez, M. W. (2005). A positive correlation between occlusal trauma and peri-implant bone loss: Literature Support. Implant Dentistry, 14(2), 108-116.

Mount, K. T. (2008). Patent No. 0020343. US.

MRG. (2003, Janurary 3). US market of dental implants 2003. Global Dental Series.

Nagasao, T., Kobayashi, M., Tsuchiya, Y., Kaneko, T., & Nakajima, T. (2002, June). Finite element analysis of the stresses around endosseous implants in various reconstructed mandibular models. *Journal of Cranio-Maxillofacial Surgery*, 30(3), 170-177.

Nagasao, T., Kobayashi, M., Tsuchiya, Y., Kaneko, T., & Nakajima, T. (2003, June). Finite element analysis of the stresses around fixtures in various reconstructed mandibular models–Part II (effect of horizontal load). *Journal of Cranio-Maxillofacial Surgery*, 31(3), 168-175.

NIH. (1988). National Institute of Health consensus development conference statement on dental implants. *J Dent Educ*,(52), 686-691.

NRC. (2005, July 05). Highlights - Dental Porous Titanium Foam Implants: An Idea with Bite. Retrieved from National Research Council Canada: http://www.nrc-cnrc.gc.ca/eng/news/nrc/2005/07/05/dental-titanium-implants.html

Parfitt, G. J. (1960, May-Jun). Measurement of the physiological mobility of individual teeth in an axial direction. *J Dent Res*, (39), 608-618.

Pilliar, R. M. (1991). Quantitative evaluation of the effect of movement at a porous coated immplant-bone interface. (E. J. Davies, Ed.) *University of Toronto Press*, pp. 380-387.

Pilliar, R., Lee, J., & Maniatopoulos, C. (1986, July). Observations on the effect of movement on bone ingrowth into porous-surfaced implants. *Clin Orthop Relat Res*, 208, 108-113.

Pirker, W., & Kocher, A. (2008). Immediate, non-submerged, root-analogues zirconia implant in single root replacement. *Int J Oral Maxillofac Sur*, 37, 293-295.

Poggio, C. E., & Salvato, A. (2002, June). Bonded provisional restorations for esthetic soft tissue support in single-implant treatment. *Journal of Prosthetic Dentistry*, 87(6), 688-691.

Rubber, R., Weise, T., Reimier, F., Sachdeva, R., & Sporbert, P. (2005). Patent No. 7,013,191. US.

Rudd, K. D., O'Leary, T. J., & Stumpf, A. J. (1964). Horizontal Tooth mobility in carefully screened subjects. *Periodontics*, 2, 65-68.

Sadan, A., Blatz, M. B., Salinas, T. J., & Block, M. S. (2004, September). Single-implant restorations: A contemporary approach for achieving a predictable outcome. *Journal of oral and maxillofacial surgery* , 62(Supp 2), 73-81.

Sekine, H., Komiyama, Y., & Hotta H., e. a. (1986). Mobility characteristics and tactile sensitivity of osseointegrated fixture-supporting systems. *Tissue Integration in Oral Maxillofacial reconstruction*.

Simmons, C. A., Meguid, S. A., & Pilliar, R. M. (2001, March). Differences in osseointegration rate due to implant surface geometry can be explained by local tissue strain. *J Orthop Res*, 19(2), 187-194.

Simmons, C. A., Valiquette, N., & Pilliar, R. M. (1999). Osseointegration of sintered porous-surfaced and plasma spray coated implants: an anumal model study of early post-implantation healing response and mechanical stability. *J Biomed Mater Res*, 47(127), 127-138.

Spiekermann, H., & Wolf, H. (1995). *Implantology*. New York: Thieme.

Stegaroiu, R., Kusakari, H., Nishiyama, S., & Miyakawa, O. (1998, Nov-Dec). Influence of prosthesis material on stress distribution in bone and implant: a 3-dimensional finite element analysis. *Int J Oral Maxillofac Implants*, 13(6), 781-790.

Stocker, N. G., Mankovich, N. J., & Valentino, D. (1992, May). Stereolithographic models for surgical planning: Preliminary report. *J of Oral and Maxillofacial Surgery*, 50(5), 466-471.

Szmuckler-Moncler, S., Salama, H., Reingewirtz, Y., & Drubuille, J. H. (1998). Timing of loading and effect of micromotion of bone-dental implant interface: Review of Experimental Literature. *J Biomed Mater Res*, 43, 193-203.

Tatum, O. H. (1988). The Omni Implant System. Alabama Implant Congress.

Touati, B., Guez, G., & Saadoun, A. (1999 , April). Aesthetic soft tissue integration and optimized emergence profile: provisionalization and customized impression coping. *Pract Periodontics Aesthet Dent*, 11(3), 305-14.

Uckleman, I., & Laschutza, H. (2004). Patent No. 0197737. US.

Vaillancourt, H., Pilliar, R. M., & McCammond, D. (1996, May-June). Factors affecting crestal bone loss with dental implants partially covered with porous coating; a finite element analysis. *Int J Oral Maxillofac Implants*, 11(3), 351-359.

Wagher, F. (1995, September 26). Patent No. 5,453,007. US.

Watanabe, F., Hata, Y., Komatsu, S., Ramos, T. C., & Fukuda, H. (2003). Finite element analysis of the influence of implant inclination, loading position, and load direction on stress distribution. *Odontology*, 91(1), 31-36.

Widera, G. E., Tesk, J. A., & Privitzer, E. (1976, July). Interaction effects among cortical bone, cancellous bone, and periodontal membrane of natural teeth and implants. *J Biomed Mater Res*, 10(4), 613-623.

Williams, D. F. (1977). Titanium as a metal for implantation. *J Med Eng Technol*, 1, 195-202, 266-270.

Xiropaidis, A. V., Qahash, M., Lim, W. H., Shanaman, R. H., Rohrer, M. D., Wikesjö, U. M., et al. (2005). Bone–implant contact at calcium phosphate-coated and porous titanium oxide (TiUnite™)-modified oral implants. *Clinical Oral Implants Research*, 16(5), 532-539.

Zimmer Dental. (n.d.). SwissPlus Manual: Implant Design and Specifications.

7

Titanium: A New Allergen

Laurence Evrard
Stomatology and Maxillo-facial Surgery Department
Hopital Erasme – ULB Brussels
Belgium

1. Introduction

Buccal allergies represent a growing problem and often go undiagnosed by health professionals. There is an increase in the prevalence of oral allergies to dental materials, and especially to metals used in dental materials.

Titanium, used in orthopaedic devices and oral implants, although considered an inert material, can actually induce toxicity or allergic type I or IV reactions.

Cases of an allergy to titanium described in the literature reflect the difficulty in the diagnosis of this allergy. In case of a suspected contact allergy, epicutaneous patch tests can be done, which consist of applying the allergens which are to be tested to the patient's back. These tests are known to have a diagnostic efficiency of 75% for metal allergy, and can therefore underdiagnose a titanium sensitization or allergy. Blood tests which can be used for the diagnosis of allergies are based on lymphoblastic transformation. They are more sensitive than patch tests, but sometimes lack specificity.

The occurrence of an allergy to titanium could be responsible for successive unexplained cases of failure of dental implants in some patients (known as "cluster patients"). It has been reported that the risk of an allergy to titanium is increased in patients who are allergic to other metals.

In these patients, an allergy evaluation is recommended, in order to exclude any problem with titanium dental implants.

1.1 Types of allergies

The term "allergy" is used to define a specific immune reaction to one or more exogenic substances (allergens).

Four types of allergies have been described. For a review see Gell and Coombs, 1963.

Type I allergy, known as immediate sensitivity, is characterized by interactions between an allergen and IgE present on the surface of mastocytes inducing histamine and other vasopeptide leakage. This is sometimes associated with atopy. This type of allergy may manifest clinically by acute reaction of anaphylaxis, which can represent a life-threatening condition. Type I allergy also causes urticarial reactions on the skin, in the form of erythematous plaques or papules, accompanied by pruritus or tingling sensations.

Type II allergy, known as cytotoxic, or antibody-dependent hypersensitivity, consists of an autoimmune cytotoxic reaction involving IgG and IgM and is encountered, for example, in acute transplant rejection or autoimmune haemolytic anaemia.

Type III allergy, or immune complex disease, is due to precipitation of immune complex formed by antigen-IgG in the blood vessel walls and can induce vasculitic lesions, manifesting in the form of the Arthus reaction, glomerulonephritis associated with streptococcal throat infection or systemic lupus erythematosus.

Type IV allergy, known as delayed-type hypersensitivity, or cell-mediated immune memory response, antibody-independent or contact allergy, is by far the most frequent type of allergy. It is defined as a cell-mediated delayed sensitization reaction (mediated by Langerhans cells and T-lymphocytes), and occurs after exposure to allergens for between ten days and several years. Type IV sensitization is induced by repeated contact of an allergen with skin or mucosa, and follows several steps (Figure 1). In the first step, a hapten penetrates through the skin or through the epithelium of the mucosa, and combines with endogenous proteins to form an antigenic molecule: the allergen. This allergen is captured by the Langerhans cells, which present it to the T-lymphocytes, which become sensitized and thereafter carry on their surface a specific receptor to the allergen. These lymphocytes are known as "memory lymphocytes", and are able to recognize the allergen. Following another contact, the allergen binds to the specific receptor of the memory lymphocytes, which multiply and produce a set of cytokines. An allergic cellular inflammatory reaction takes place within 48 to 72 hours, and is responsible for the clinical manifestations of type IV allergy (Axell, 2001, Grevers and Röcken, 2002, Gawrodger, 2005). Type IV allergy is more frequently encountered in the skin than in the oral mucosa. This has been explained by the fact that Langerhans cells are about ten times more numerous in the layers underlying the skin than in those underlying the oral mucosa. Another reason is the rich network of capillary vessels which characterizes oral mucosa vascularization and which, in turn, eliminates the allergens more quickly from the area (Forte et al, 2008). Clinically, it may manifest as chronic transplant rejection, or more often as chronic dermatitis (eczema).

Allergy types I, III and IV may manifest in the orofacial region (Axell, 2001, Grevers, 2002, Gawkrodger, 2005).

A hapten penetrates skin or mucosa and combines with endogenous proteins to form an allergen. Langerhans cells capture the allergen, and present it to the T-lymphocytes, which become sensitized and thereafter carry on their surface a specific receptor to the allergen. These lymphocytes are known as "memory lymphocytes".

1.2 Clinical manifestations of an allergy in the orofacial region

Patients with an oral allergy complain of various symptoms such as burning or tingling sensations, with or without swelling, oral dryness or loss of taste (Garhammer et al, 2001, Lygre et al, 2003, Gawrodger 2005), or sometimes more general symptoms such as headache, dyspepsia, asthenia, arthralgia, myalgia (Lygre et al, 2003, Vamnes et al, 2004).

The signs of an oral allergy include erythema of the oral mucosa, labial oedema or purpuric patches on the palate, mouth ulcers, hyperplastic gingivitis, areas of depapillation on the tongue, angular cheilitis, perioral eczematous eruption, or lichenoid reactions localized on the oral mucosa (Alanko et al, 1996, Leigh et al, 2001, Vamnes et al, 2004).

Type I allergy may manifest clinically in the orofacial region, in the acute form by Quincke's oedema, characterized by swelling, which, if it involves the upper respiratory tract, can become life-threatening for the patient. In serious forms, it gives rise to urticarial reactions and/or tingling sensations or pruritus, localized in the oral or pharyngeal cavity (Axell, 2001, Grevers and Röcken, 2002, Gawrodger, 2005).

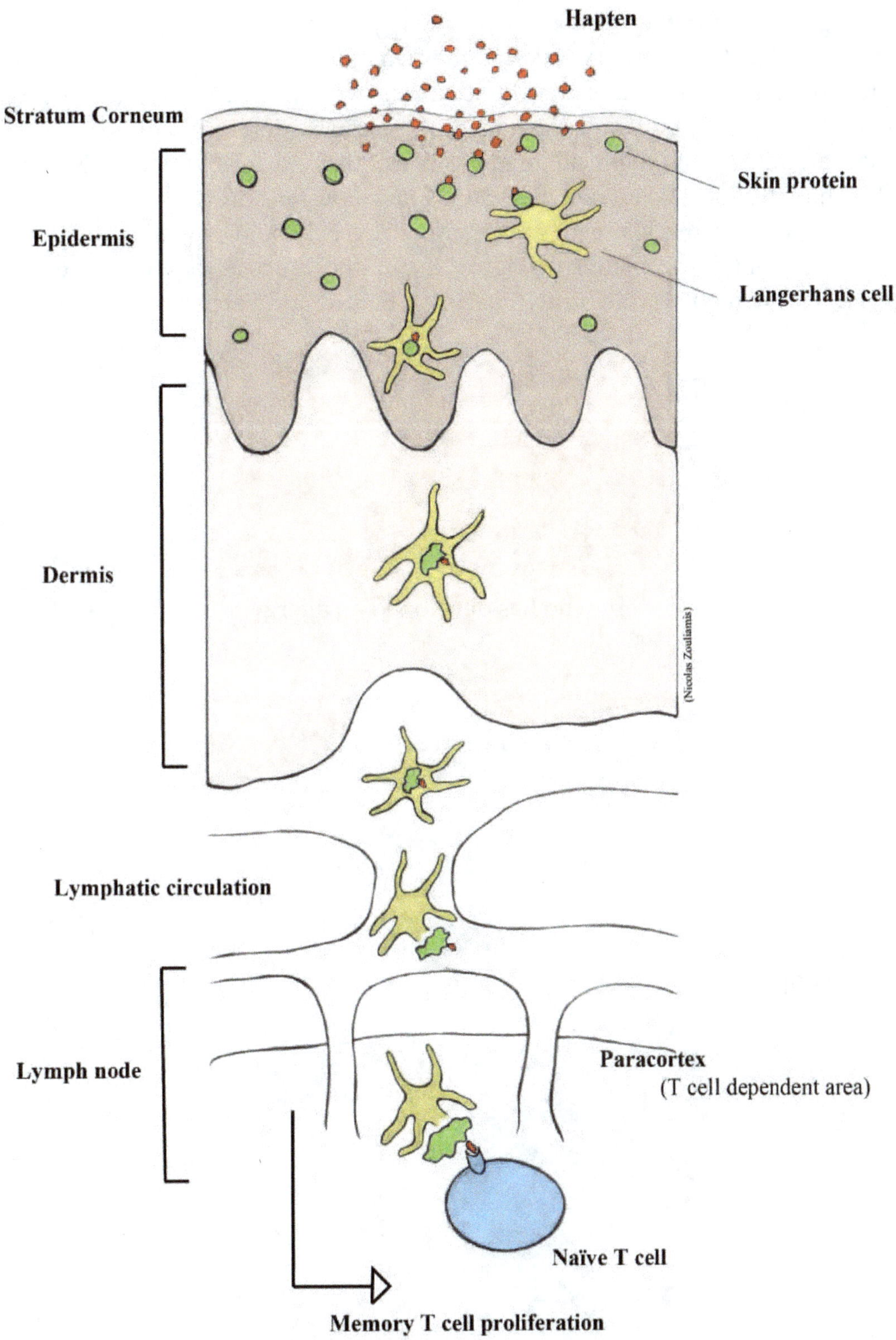

Fig. 1. Development of type IV sensitivity.

Type III allergy in the buccal area can take the form of aphthous ulcerations of the oral mucosa or, in more serious cases, the form of erythema multiforme, with large ulcerations of the oral mucosa found in association with typical skin lesions "en cocarde" (Axell, 2001, Grevers and Röcken, 2002, Gawrodger, 2005).

Type IV allergy is by far the most frequent allergy encountered in the orofacial region (Gawkrodger, 2005). This type IV allergy may manifest clinically by eczema, angular cheilitis, cheilitis (Figure 2), erythema of the oral mucosa, hyperplastic gingivitis (Figure 3), lichenoid reactions of the oral mucosa (Figure 4), perioral dermatitis or a loss of lingual papillae that can mimic "geographical tongue" (Waroquier et al, 2009) (Figure 5) (Vamnes et al., 2004, Leigh et al., 2001, Alanko et al., 1996). Clinical lesions are generally localized next to structures containing the allergen, as illustrated by lichenoid reactions just in front of amalgam fillings containing mercury (Figure 6), or the mucosa of the palate next to a prosthesis containing methacrylate resin (Figure 7) (Evrard and Parent, 2010).

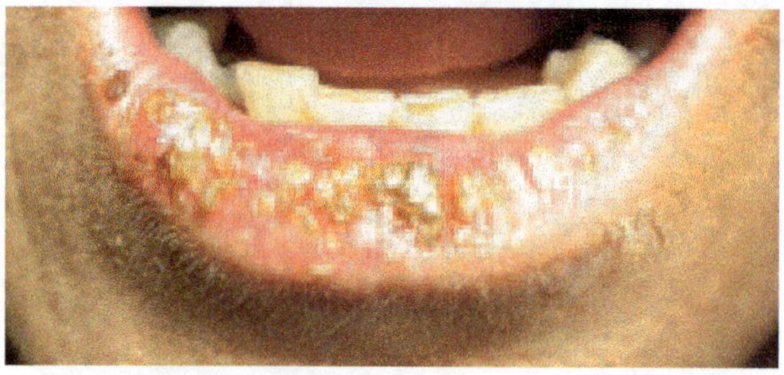

Fig. 2. Contact cheilitis in a patient who has developed an allergy to a component of her lipstick.

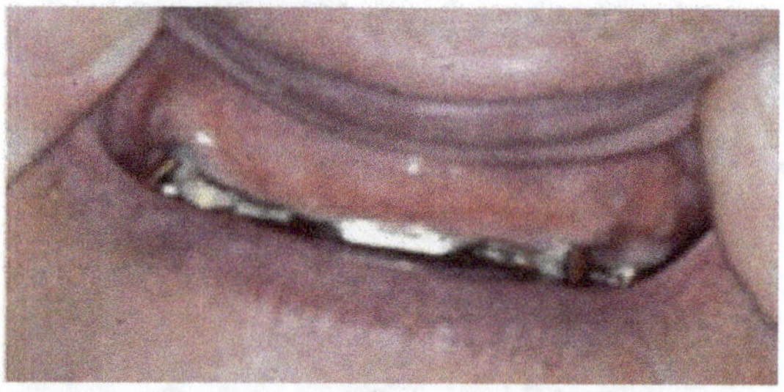

Fig. 3. Hyperplastic gingivitis associated with a contact allergy to gold. There is a prosthetic gold bar in the upper jaw.

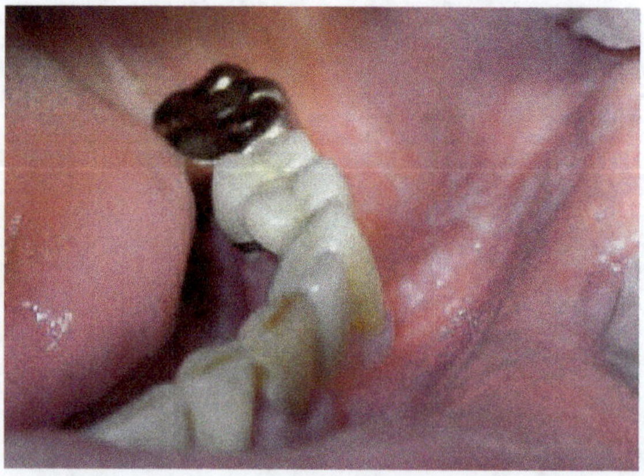

Fig. 4. Lichenoid reaction of the oral mucosa, associated with a contact allergy to gold. The patient has a gold crown on tooth 36.

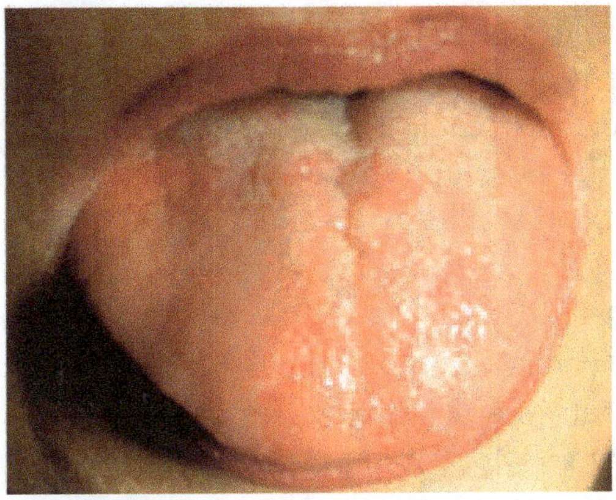

Fig. 5. Depapillation of the tongue, mimicking a geographical tongue, associated with a contact allergy to mercury and gold.

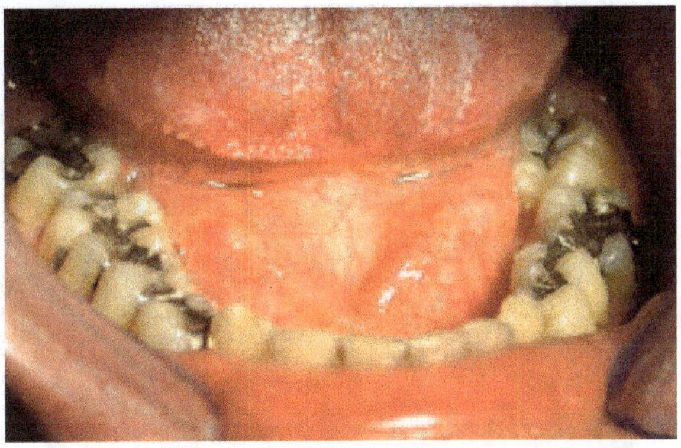

Fig. 6. Lichenoid reactions on the mucosa of the tongue, associated with a contact allergy to mercury. The patient has amalgam filling in his teeth.

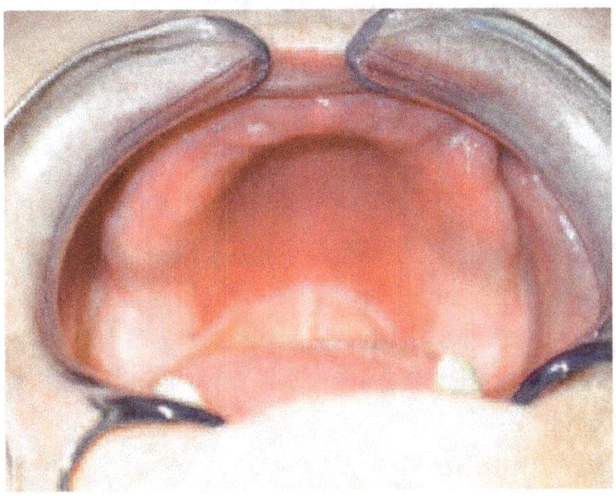

Fig. 7. Erythema of the palate in the area in contact with a resin prosthesis, in association with a contact allergy to methyl methacrylate.

In type IV allergy, patients complain of burning or tingling sensations of the oral mucosa, sometimes of dryness of the mouth, or a metallic taste (Lygre et al., 2003, Gawkrodger, 2005). Burning sensations ("burning mouth") can reach a frequency of 72% in patients with a contact allergy to dental materials (Garhammer et al, 2001, Waroquier et al, 2007). Other causes can give rise to the same signs and symptoms as those found in allergy; in such cases it is necessary, when faced with burning sensations and/or erythematous patches on the oral mucosa, to exclude metabolic causes such as iron, B12 or folate deficiency by doing a blood test, and to rule out the possibility of a fungal infection, taking a swab of the lesion and culturing it, before going on to allergy testing.

1.3 Diagnostic tests for allergy

The diagnosis of a contact/type IV allergy is typically based on the patient's medical record, clinical findings and the results of epicutaneous tests.

Epicutaneous tests are known as "patch tests". The principle is to apply different allergens which are to be tested on the patient's back. The results are read after 48 and 72 hours for most allergens, and also after 10 days for gold testing (because gold can give rise to late reactions). If the test is positive for an allergen, the area of skin corresponding to the tested allergen will show an eczematous reaction: erythema and/or vesicles and pruritus (Alanko et al, 1996, Grevers and Röcken, 2002, Gawrodger, 2005). There is a limit to the utility of patch tests, given their poor sensitivity, which has been shown to be about 75% for type IV metal allergy (Forte et al, 2008). Some authors report a lack of standardization in the patch tests, especially for allergens such as titanium (Fischer, 2008, Forte et al, 2008). According to these authors, patch tests have been validated only for dermal sensitization to allergens, and their relevance for systemic sensitization to allergens such as titanium (mucosal and internal) is limited.

Thus, patch test may underestimate the real prevalence of a metal allergy.

Skin tests (prick tests) help in the diagnosis of a type I allergy. They consist of intradermal inoculation of the antigen (Yamauci et al, 2000). The results are read within 15 to 30 minutes. If the test is positive, there will be a red, papular and/or vesicular reaction of the skin. Prick tests are not routinely done for the diagnosis of an oral allergy to a dental material, because most of the reactions to dental material are Type IV. Nevertheless, prick tests are used in the diagnosis of a food allergy, which may manifest by aphthous lesions of the oral mucosa (Scully, 2004).

A blood test can help in the diagnosis of a type IV allergy. *In vitro* testing with the lymphocyte transformation test (LTT) can detect both dermally and non-dermally (mucosal) sensitizing allergens. It has been used to detect hypersensitivity leading to both local and systemic effects resulting from dental allergies, in particular in the optimized version of LTT known as MELISA (Stjekstal et al, 1994, Muller and Valentine-Thon, 2006). The patient's lymphocytes are exposed to the allergen to be tested. If they have previously been sensitized to the allergen, they will undergo proliferation, which is measured using incorporation of radioactive nucleotides (tritiated thymidine). Some authors have reported that non-relevant proliferation of lymphocytes could happen in non-sensitized patients (Fisher's, 2008), leading to some false-positive results.

It would be valuable in the future to have a test that would respond with good sensitivity and good specificity, thus providing a better diagnostic tool.

2. Allergy to dental materials

There are various dental materials that have been shown to be capable of triggering an allergic reaction in the oral cavity, and contain metals (nickel, cobalt, chromium, gold, palladium, mercury), fragrances (balsam of Peru, fragrance mix, eugenol, cinnamic aldehyde, essential oils), topical medicines (including some synthetic steroids), preservatives, resins, colourings and other products contained in toothpastes (Lesueur and Lannias, 2003, Evrard and Parent 2010).

It has been shown that dental materials can give rise to type I, type III or type IV hypersensitivity. In type IV allergy, which is by far the most frequent type encountered in the oral cavity, signs and symptoms can appear between a few days and several years after the beginning of contact with the allergen (Gawrodger 2005, Vamnes et al, 2004, Garhammer et al, 2001, Lesueur and Yiannias, 2003, Evrard and Parent, 2010).

2.1 Dental metals involved in oral allergy

In the field of dentistry, dental metals are used in precious and non-precious alloys, for producing removable or fixed prostheses, or dental fillings. Titanium is used for its excellent biocompatibility in implantology and maxillo-facial surgery and will be the subject of Chapter 3.

Metals contained in dental alloys may corrode in an electrolytic solution such as saliva. Corrosion will be greater in the case of multiple metals, given the electric potential difference induced following contact between different metals (Messer and Wahata, 2002) (Figure 6).

It has been described that the mercury contained in amalgam dental fillings and gold used in alloys for fixed prostheses can give rise to allergic reactions, in the form of lichenoid reactions of the oral mucosa (Koch and Bahmer, 1999, Yiannias et al, 2000, Laine et al, 1997, Evrard and Parent 2010). In a study on 19 patients with lichenoid reactions of the oral mucosa in the vicinity of amalgam fillings (Koch and Bahmer, 1999), it has been shown that 78.9% of patients proved to be sensitized to mercury and that the removal of dental amalgams allowed healing of the mucosal lesions in 86% of cases. In another study on 46 patients with an oral lichen planus (Yiannias et al, 2000), 14 patients had an epicutaneous test positive to gold. In this study, after removal of gold from the mouth, the oral lichen planus disappeared in 10 patients out of 14. Another study on 118 patients with lichenoid lesions in the mouth (Laine et al, 1997), shows that 80 of them had a contact allergy (type IV allergy) to one or more metals: 78 to mercury, 11 to gold, 17 to nickel, 4 to cobalt, 3 to tin, 2 to palladium and 1 to chromium.

All the authors point out that healing of the lesions takes place in a large number of cases after removal of amalgam dental fillings or prostheses containing gold, in the case of a diagnosed contact allergy to mercury or gold (Lygre et al, 2003, Koch and Bahmer, 1999, Yiannias et al, 2000, Laine et al, 1997, Evrard and Parent 2010).

Cobalt is a metal used in alloys in removable or fixed prostheses, and represents a known allergen giving rise to oral manifestations in the case of an allergy (Forte et al, 2008). In a recent study (Waroquier et al, 2009), it has been shown that the burning sensations and intense pruritus on a geographical tongue were due to the cobalt contained in the hook of a removable resin prosthesis replacing a tooth 51 lost through trauma in a 7-year-old child. In this case, type IV allergy had been diagnosed by a positive patch test to cobalt. After removal of the hook containing cobalt, all the patient's signs and symptoms had disappeared.

Burning sensations represent a frequent complaint in patients allergic to one or more dental metals (Alanko et al, 1996). Our team conducted a pilot study to try and establish the prevalence of oral allergies to dental materials in patients complaining of burning sensations of the oral mucosa (Warroquier et al, 2007). In this study, other causes of burning sensations were excluded by a blood test (in order to rule out a metabolic disturbance such as iron, B12 or folate deficiency), and by swabbing and culture, in order to rule out a fungal infection. Allergy testing revealed that, among that population of 26 "burning mouth" patients, 34.6% were allergic to nickel, 19% to chromium, 11.5% to gold, 11.5% to cobalt and 7.7% to mercury. Only 11.5% of the patients did not display a positive result for an allergy to any of the metals tested. These results are about three times higher than the known percentages of allergies to metals in the general European population, which have been reported to be 20% for nickel, 5.4% for chromium, 6% for gold, 6.5% for cobalt and 2.9% for mercury (Forte et al, 2008).

In a study on 294 patients complaining of both general and local signs (including burning sensations of the oral mucosa), epicutaneous tests have shown an allergy to nickel in 28% of the patients, to gold in 23%, to cobalt in 14%, to palladium in 9% and to mercury in 6% of cases.

All these studies show that the prevalence of allergies to metals in patients presenting signs or symptoms of an oral allergy is higher than the prevalence of allergies in a general European population.

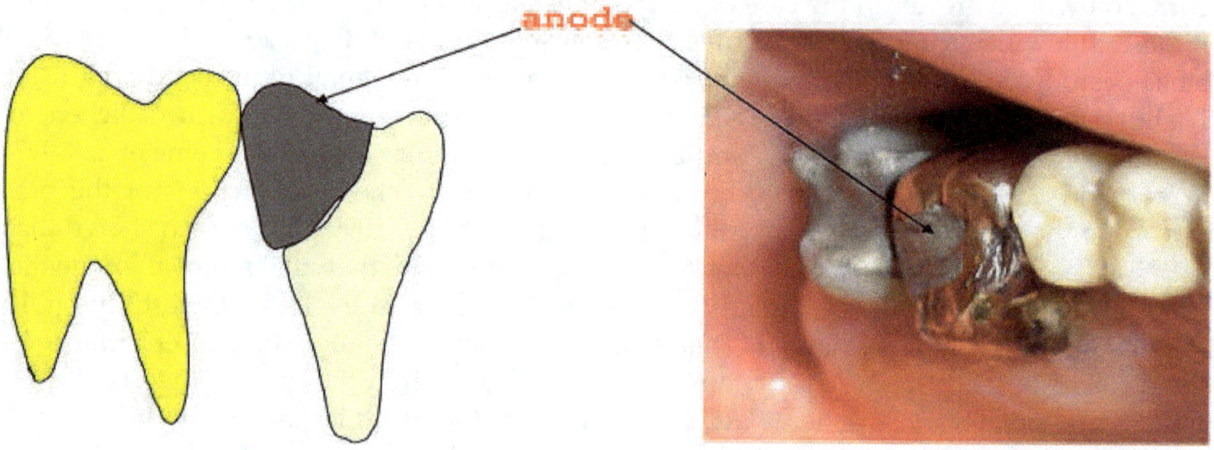

Fig. 6. Multiple metals in contact with each other.

Gold alloy in contact with silver amalgam restoration. The silver amalgam represents the anode pole, and gold alloy the cathode pole. There is an electric potential difference, and electrolytic corrosion within the electrolytic saliva solution may occur.

3. Titanium: a metal allergen of growing significance

Titanium is a metal used in medical and dental fields, because of its properties of strength, corrosion resistance behaviour and excellent biocompatibility due to the formation of an oxide layer on its surface (Steinemann, 2000). In oral and maxillofacial surgery, titanium alloys are used for ostheosynthesis plates used in traumatology or maxillofacial surgery, and for dental implants. In implantology, titanium is used most often in the form of "commercially pure" titanium (cpTi: grade I to IV alloys). CpTi contains trace elements (N, C, H, Fe, O, Al, V), that can represent 1% of its volume, and can enhance its mechanical properties and resistance to fracture (Steinemann, 2000, Messer and Wahata, 2002, Geetha et al, 2009). In implantology, titanium is used also in the form of an alloy (grade V titanium): Ti-6Al-4V, Nitinol (Ti-Ni), Ti-Co (Geetha et al, 2009) or titanium-zirconium, especially in cases where narrow implants are recommended (Evrard and Atash, 2009).

The insertion of titanium dental implants can cause internal exposure, and it has been proved that concentrations of 100-300 ppm titanium can be observed in tissues surrounding implants, as well as in regional lymph nodes and pulmonary tissue (Wennerberg et al, 2004). Under unfavourable conditions: acidic pH occurring in a peri-implantitis for example, or excessive mechanical forces on the implant, or close contact of the implant with another metal (amalgam, gold alloy), titanium may corrode and release titanium ions or microparticles of titanium in the area of bone surrounding the implant, which can induce inflammation in affected tissues (Messer and Wataha, 2002). It has been suggested that this mechanism may play a role in loosening orthopaedic endoprostheses (Nakashima et al, 1999), but it has not yet been demonstrated as a factor in the failure of dental implants. Titanium has also been reported to activate macrophages, which may secrete cytokines involved in various disease processes (Muller and Valentine-Thon, 2006). Titanium has a high affinity for proteins, and titanium ions (haptens) released by corrosion may combine with endogenous proteins to form antigenic molecules, captured by Langerhans cells, presented to T-lymphocytes, which in turn can cause the patient to be sensitized to titanium. People are exposed to titanium through environmental sources. Numerous devices such as watches, jewellery and spectacle frames are made of titanium alloy. Most environmental exposure to titanium results from exposure to TiO2 (E171), which is used in cosmetics such as sunscreens, make-up and deodorants, and in food, medicines or toothpaste. It has been shown that our body can contain a concentration of 50 ppm of titanium (Forte et al, 2008). From then on, sensitization to titanium is possible, through environmental sources, and not necessarily from previous contact with dental implants.

3.1 Allergy to titanium

The first cases in which delayed sensitivity to titanium was suspected, with a local granulomatous reaction, have been described in patients wearing a cardiac pacemaker (Peeters et al, 1984, Yamauchi, 2000). In these cases, the diagnosis of a titanium allergy was made with, respectively, a positive patch test with a little square of the pacemaker placed in artificial perspiration (Peeters et al, 1984), and a positive intra-dermal reaction to an eluate of the surface of the pacemaker (Yamauchi et al, 2000).

More recently, a well documented case of type IV allergy to titanium contained in an osteosynthesis plate inserted for a fracture of the hand was described. The patient had developed eczema on the hand within a few weeks of the insertion of the plate, and an absence of bone healing. A lymphoblastic transformation blood test (LTT) proved positive, although the patch test for TiO2 was negative. Following the removal of the plate, the LTT gave negative results and the eczema disappeared (Thomas et al, 2006).

Admittedly, it may be difficult to extrapolate results in cases of dental and orthopaedic implants. The skin and the oral mucosa behave differently regarding their potential to develop an allergic reaction (the number of Langerhans cells is greater in skin, the vascular network is more highly developed in the oral mucosa, and the latter is less permeable to antigens). Moreover, implant prosthetic abutments are coated in the mouth with glycoproteins which act as a protective barrier hampering contact between the metal and the mucosa, and the intraosseous contact surface is smaller in dental implants than in orthopaedic ones (Fischer, 2008). In orthopaedic allergy cases, biopsies generally reveal a granulomatous reaction, with numerous macrophages in the vicinity of the prosthesis. This is not the case with dental implants, and different immunological mechanisms may be involved in the two cases (Messer and Wataha, 2002, Nakashima et al, 1999, Muller and Valentine-Thon, 2006).

The case of a patient with facial eczema suggestive of type IV allergy to titanium following the placement of a mandibular dental implant has been reported (Egusa et al, 2008). In this case, an allergy to titanium was diagnosed by the combination of clinical signs (appearance of eczema within a few weeks of implant placement), and a positive blood test (LTT). The diagnosis of allergy to titanium was confirmed by the disappearance of eczema following removal of the implants.

More recently, it has been demonstrated that clinically-relevant hypersensitivity to titanium can occur following exposure to titanium (Muller and Valentine-Thon, 2006). In that study, 56 patients had developed severe health problems (muscle and joint pain, chronic fatigue syndrome, neurological problems, depression, or acne-like facial inflammation) after receiving Ti-based dental implants, orthodontic braces or endoprostheses. The authors used the MELISA test, which had proved effective in the diagnosis of hypersensitivity to metals (Stejskal et al, 1994), as well as patch tests. Of the 56 patients tested with MELISA, 37.5% were positive, 28.5% ambiguous and 33.9% negative to titanium. Among the 33.9% negative to titanium, 57.9% showed lymphocyte reactivity to nickel or other metals. All 54 patch-tested patients were negative to titanium. Following removal of the implants, a remarkable clinical improvement was noticed and among the 15 retested patients this clinical improvement correlated with normalisation of MELISA reactivity.

In a prospective study over a three-year period (Sicilia et al, 2008), 1500 patients with dental implants were monitored. In that study, an allergy to titanium was diagnosed on the basis of clinical signs of an allergy appearing following implant placement, or on the basis of an unexplained failure of the implant, and a patch test positive for titanium, tested in the form TiO2, or for a titanium metal powder in aqueous solution. The results of this study show that 0.6% (1/800) of patients with dental implants have a patch-test positive for titanium, but 0% (0/35) of the patients without implants have this result. The epicutaneous tests are positive in 50% (8/16) and 62.8% (5/8) of the patients who show signs, respectively, of an allergy following implant placement, and unexplained early failure of one or more implants. In patients having allergies to one or more metals (nickel, chromium, cobalt, gold or mercury), 5.3% (1/19) have a patch test positive for titanium. It should be noted that the authors do not report the characteristics of the titanium in their patients (titanium alloy or commercially pure titanium?). The rate of corrosion is higher with titanium-aluminium-vanadium implants, which may have an influence on the prevalence of allergic reactions.

All these reports reflect the difficulty in evaluating suspected titanium hypersensitivity. It is known that the epicutaneous tests used in the diagnosis of an allergy to titanium are still not very sensitive, and there is no standardized valid patch-test preparation for this. Moreover, the lack of concordance between the results of patch-tests and blood tests (MELISA) is illustrated in the above study (Muller and Valentine-Thon, 2006). Given the difficulties of diagnosing a titanium allergy, studies probably underestimate the true prevalence of titanium allergies in patients having dental implants.

3.2 Diagnosis of a titanium allergy

The above studies demonstrate that titanium can induce clinically relevant hypersensitivity and other immune dysfunctions in certain patients chronically exposed to this metal. Titanium should no longer, therefore, be considered biologically inert. In implantology, it is reasonable to say that allergy testing for titanium is indicated in some cases.

3.2.1 Before implant placement

It has been shown that many patients suffer from multiple allergies (Forte et al, 2008), and that people with a history of allergy to metals or jewellery have a greater risk of developing a hypersensitivity reaction to a metal implant (Hallab et al, 2001).

Furthermore, although titanium allergy has a low prevalence rate, for patients with a previous history of allergies, it may be advisable to carry out a metal allergy assessment and allergy testing before placing permanent implants, in order to avoid a failure of the implant due to an allergic reaction to titanium.

3.2.2 After implant placement

The failure of implants has been widely studied, and the main causes of dental implant failure are infection and overload (Esposito et al, 1999a, 1999b, 1999c). However, some failures are difficult to explain, such as spontaneous rapid exfoliation of the implant, or the successive failure of implants in the same patients, known as "cluster phenomenon", without any infection or overload risk factor identified. Authors agree that in these cases, there must be a systemic determinant of failure that has not been identified or understood (Wood and Vermilyea, 2004, Chuang, 2005).

An allergic reaction can be reasonably suspected after dental implant placement, on the basis of signs or symptoms associated with allergy, such as rash, urticaria, pruritus, swelling in the orofacial region, oral or facial erythema, eczematous lesions of the cheeks, or hyperplastic lesions of soft tissue (the peri-implant mucosa) (Mitchel et al, 1990). In these cases, allergy testing should be performed.

3.2.3 Tests available for the diagnosis of an allergy to titanium

As described in chapter 3.2, there is no consensus on how a sensitization and/or allergic reaction to titanium should be explored. It is also difficult to compare the results from different studies related to titanium allergies, because some refer to the use of patch tests, while others use prick tests and/or blood tests (LTT, MELISA) (Sicilia et al, 2008, Valentine-Thon et al, 2006).

To date, no standard patch test for titanium has so far been developed, and positive reactions to titanium have only rarely been demonstrated with skin testing (Forte et al, 2008).

The sensitivity of patch tests has been shown to be about 75% for type IV metal allergy. Some authors have suggested that 0.1% and 0.2% titanium sulphate solution and 0.1% and 0.2% titanium chloride are successful reagents for the skin-patch tests and could be a valuable alternative to the titanium oxide normally used for patch testing (Okamura et al, 1999), but so far no study related to dental implants allergies has used the method.

The MELISA test has been validated to detect sensitization to titanium and other metals (Sjekstal et al, 1999, Muller and Valentine-Thon 2006), but there can be some lack of specificity in lymphocyte proliferation.

It would be valuable to have a sensitive and specific test that could help in the diagnosis of titanium sensitization or allergy.

3.2.4 Future prospects in the diagnosis of sensitization or allergy to titanium

Interleukin-17 and Interleukin-22 are produced by a subset of a recently defined T-cell line, known as Th-17. IL-17 has been associated with many inflammatory diseases in humans, including rheumatoid arthritis, organ rejection and asthma. It has been showed that the number of Th-17 cells and the expression of IL-17 was significantly increased in positive patch test biopsies, regardless of the nature of the antigen (Oboki et al, 2008, Zhao et al, 2009, Larsen et al, 2009).

IL-22 is a critical mediator in mucosal host defence, which has complex pro-inflammatory and anti-inflammatory and autoimmune effects. It has been shown that patients with contact dermatitis to nickel had a significantly higher IL-22 blood level, compared with control (Ricciardi et al, 2009), indicating a possible involvement of IL-22 in the pathogenesis of human allergic contact dermatitis.

It would be interesting to develop a blood test, based on the measurement of the production of IL-17 and/or IL-22 by lymphocytes, in order to be able to diagnose with certainty a sensitization to titanium.

Our team is currently trying to develop a technique, using flow cytometry, for the purpose of detecting the activation of lymphocytes stimulated by a metal, and measuring different mediators (cytokines, inflammatory mediators) released in response to the metal.

4. References

Alanko K., Kanerva L., Jolanki R., Kannas L. & Estlander T. *Oral mucosal diseases investigated by patch testing with a dental screening series.* Contact Dermatitis, 1996; 34 (4):263-267.

Axell T. *Hypersensitivity of the oral mucosa: clinics and pathology.* Acta Odontol. Scand.2001, 59:315-319.

Chuang S., Cai T., Douglass C., Wei L. & Dodson T. *Frailty approach for the analysis of clustered failure time observation in dental research.* J.Dent Res., 2005; 84: 54-58.

Egusa H., Ko N., Shimazu T. & Yatani H. *Suspected association of an allergic reaction with titanium dental implants: a clinical report.* J. Prosthet Dent. 2008, 100: 344-7.

Esposito M., Hirsch J., Lekholm U. & Thomsen P. *Differential diagnosis and treatment strategies for biologic complications and failing oral implants: a review of the literature.* Int J. Oral Maxillofac. Impl. 1999; 14: 473-90.

Esposito M., Lausmaa J;, Hirsch J; & Thomsen P. *Surface analysis of failed oral titanium implants.* J. Biomed. Mater res. 1999; 48: 559-68.

Esposito M., Thomsen P., Ericson L. & Lekholm U. *Histopathologic observations on early oral implant failures.* Int J Oral Maxillofac Impl. 1999, 14: 798-810

Evrard L. & Atash R. *Restauration de l'édentation complète mandibulaire dans le cas d'une crête osseuse fine, à l'aide de deux implants de faible diamètre en alliage Titane-Zircone stabilisant une prothèse en résine par l'intermédiaire de deux attachements Locator.* Dentist News, 2009, 19: 14-19

Evrard L., Waroquier D. & Parent D. *Allergies to dental metals. Titanium: a new allergen.* Rev. Med. Brux. 2010, 31: 44-9

Evrard L. & Parent D. *Oral allergies to dental materials. Review of the literature and report of three cases.* Bull. Group Int Rech Stomatol. Odontol., 2010; 49: 14-19

Fischer 's. *Allergy.* Eds. Spinger-Verlag. 2008: 684-5.

Forte G., Petrucci F. & Bocca B. *Metal allergens of growing significance: epidemiology, immunotoxicology, strategies for testing and prevention.* Inflammation and Allergy, 2008, 7: 1-18

Garhammer P., Schmalz G., Hiller K., Reitinger T. & Stolz W. *Patients with local adverse effects from dental alloys: frequency, complaints, symptoms, allergy.* Clin. Oral Invest. 2001;5:240-249.

Gawkrodger D J. *Investigation of reactions to dental materials.* Br. J. Dermatol.2005; 153:479-485.

Geetha M., Singh AK., Asokamani R. & Gogia AK. *Ti based biomaterials, the ultimate choice for orthopedic implants – A review.* Prog Mater Sci, 2009, 10: 1-29

Gell P. & Coombs R., *The classification of allergic reactions underlying disease.* In: R.R.A. Coombs and P.G.H. Gell, Editors, *Clinical Aspects of Immunology,* Blackwell Science (1963).

Grevers G. & Röcken M. *Atlas de poche d'allergologie.* 2002. Flammarion Médecine-Sciences.

Axell T. *Hypersensitivity of the oral mucosa: clinics and pathology.* Acta Odontol. Scand.2001;59:315-319.

Hallab M., Mikecz K., Vermes C., Skipor A. & Jacobs J. *Differential lymphocyte reactivity to serum-derived metal-protein complexes produced from cobalt-based and titanium-based implant alloy degradation.* J. Biomed Mater. Res. 2001; 56: 427-36.

Koch P. & Bahmer F. *Oral lesions and symptoms related to metals used in dental restorations: A clinical, allergological, and histological study.* J. Am. Acad. Dermatol. 1999; 41:422-430.

Laine J., Kalimo K. & Happonen RP. *Contact allergy to dental restorative materials in patients with oral lichenoid lesions.* Contact Dermatitis. 1997;36:141-146.

Larsen J., Bonefeld C., Poulsen S. & Geisler C. *IL-23 and IL-17-mediated inflammation in human allergic contact dermatitis.* J Allergy Clin Immunol. 2009; 123: 486-492

Leigh AS., Fowler JR., Morgan W. & Looney SW. *Dental metal allergy in patients with oral, cutaneous and genital lichenoid reactions.* Am. J. Contact Dermatitis. 2001;12 (3):146-150.

LeSueur BW. & Yiannias AJ. *Contact stomatitis.* Dermatol. Clin 2003;21:105-114.

Yiannias JA., el-Azhari RA., Hand JH., Pakzad SY. & Roger RS. *Relevant contact sensitivities in patients with the diagnosis of oral lichen planus.* J. Am Acad. Dermatol. 2000;42:177-182.

Lygre G. B., Gjerdet N. R., Grönningstraeter A. G. & Björkman L. *Reporting on adverse reactions to dental materials: intraoral observations at a clinical follow-up.* Community Dent Oral Epidemiol. 2003;31:200-206.

Messer & Wahata. *Dental materials: biocompatibility. In Encyclopedia of Materials: Science and Technology.* 2002. ISBN: 0-08-043152-6. pp 1-10

Müller K. & Valentine-Thon E. *Hypersensitivity to titanium: clinical and laboratory evidence.* Neuro Endocrinol Lett, 2006, 27: 31-35

Nakashima Y., Sun D., Trindade M., Maloney W., Goodman S. & Schurman D. *Signaling pathways for tumor necrosis – a and interleukin-6 expression in human macrophages exposed to titanium alloy particulate debris in vitro.* J Bone Joint Surg. 1999; 81: 603-15.

Oboki K., Ohno T., Saito H. & Nakae S. *Th17 and allergy.* Allergology International. 2008; 57: 121-134

Okamura T., Morimoto M,. Fukushima D. & Yamane G. J Dent res. 1999; 78: 1135.

Peeters MS., Schroeter AL., Van Hale HM., Broadbent JC. *Pacemaker contact sensitivity.* Contact Dermatitis, 1984, 11:218-218

Ricciardi L., Minciullo P., Saitta P., Trombetta D., Saija A. & Gangemi S. *Increased serum levels of IL-22 in patients with nickel contact dermatitis.* Contact Dermatitis. 2009; 60: 57-58

Scully C. *Oral and Maxillofacial Medicine.* Ed Elsevier, Edinburgh; 2004, ISBN 0723610746, PP194-204.

Sicilia A., Cuesta S., Coma G., Guisasola C., Ruiz E. & Maestro A. T*itanium allergy in dental patients: a clinical study on 1500 consecutive patients.* Clin. Oral Implants Res; 2008, 19: 823-35.

Steinemann S. *Titanium – the material of choice?* Periodontology; 2000; 17: 7-21.

Stejskal V., Cederbrant K., Lindvall A., Forsbeck M. &MELISA- *An in vitro tool for the study of metal allergy.* Toxicol in vitro. 1994; 8: 991-1000.

Thomas P., Brandl W., Majer S., Summer B. &, Przybilla B. *Hypersensitivity to titanium osteosynthesis with impaired fracture healing, eczema and T-cell hyperresponsiveness in vitro: case report and review of the literature.* Contact Dermatitis, 2006, 55: 199-202.

Vamnes J., Lygre G., Grönningstraeter A. & Gjerdet N. *Four years of clinical experience with an adverse reaction unit for dental biomaterials.* Comm. Dent. Oral Epidemiol. 2004;32:150-157.

Waroquier D., Evrard L., Nelis M. & Parent D. *Allergic contact dermatitis presenting as geographical tongue with pruritus.* Contact Dermatitis. 2009; 60: 106-119.

Waroquier D., Evrard L., Flamme M. & Parent D. *Apport des tests épicutanés dans la mise au point des stomatodynies.* Bull du GERDA, 2007

Wennerberg A., Ide-Ektessabi A., Hatkamata S., Sawase T., Johansson C., Albrektsson T., Martinelli A., Sodervall U. & Odelius H. *Titanium release from implants prepared with different surface roughness.* 2004. Clin. Oral Impl. Res. 15: 505-512.

Wood M., Vermilyea S. *A review of selected dental literature on evidence-based treatment planning for dental implants: reports of the committee on research in fixed prosthodontics of the academy of fixed prosthodontics.* J Prosthetic Dentistry. 94: 447-462.

Yamauchi R., Morita A., Tsuji T. *Pacemaker dermatitis from titanium.* Contact Dermatitis, 2000, 42: 52-53

Zhao Y., Balato A., Fishelevich R., Chapoval A., Mann D. & Gaspari A. *Th17/Tc17 infiltration and associated cytokine gene expression in elicitation phase of allergic contact dermatitis.* British J Dermatol; 2009, 161: 1301-1306

8

Soft Tissue Biology and Management in Implant Dentistry

Yeung Stephen C H
Faculty of Dentistry, University of Sydney, Sydeny,
Westmead Centre for Oral Health, Westmead Hospital, Westmead,
Australia

1. Introduction

Implant Dentistry has been the fastest growing treatment modality in dentistry for the past 20 years. The success in using dental implant to support dental restorations and reconstructions has been underpinned by the predictable formation of a bone-to-titanium interface (osseointegration) after the insertion of a titanium implant into the human jaw bone. As a result, the titanium implant becomes a rigid extension of the jaw and can be utilised as a stable foundation to support dental restorations and enable normal function of mastication to be carried out by the patient in comfort over long periods of time. The longevity of the dental implant treatment is therefore dependent upon the stability of the bone-to-implant interface. This interface is a dynamic situation subject to the influence of bone metabolism and turnover as well as bone remodelling according to functional demand. It is therefore reasonable to assume that successful implant treatment and implant supported prostheses can be maintained over long periods of time in the absence of bone metabolic diseases or disturbance.

The reporting of peri-implantitis as a significant threat to implant survival in the jaw bone (Roos Jansåker, Lindahl et al. 2006; Lindhe and Meyle 2008) has dramatically changed our perception of the expected trouble-free service life of dental implants in patients, particularly in those who have had a history of periodontal disease in the past. It also brought into focus a number of known risk factors associated with the bacteria-related breakdown of osseointegration and raised concerns about how best to address these risks. It is now apparent that maintaining a competent seal of the "gingival cuff" surrounding dental implants or abutments has an important role to play in achieving long term complication-free service of dental implant restorations/reconstructions(Berglundh, Lindhe et al. 1991). This Chapter will review all relevant biological and clinical aspects of our current knowledge of the peri-implant gingival tissue and the management of this tissue to achieve long term clinical success of implant treatment.

In the anterior aesthetic zone, the restorative dentist is often faced with a challenge to restore not only the missing teeth but also the missing volume of gingival tissue surrounding them. In augmented implant sites, the recreated volume of gingival tissue must have a healthy appearance and be in harmony with the gingival tissue surrounding adjacent teeth. Furthermore, this tissue should be stable and remain unchanged in volume and appearance over time. This demand in aesthetic outcome for dental treatment in the anterior region is often at odds with the known biological events in soft tissue healing and remodelling after surgical wounding. In clinical practice, it is therefore critically important for the dentist to understand all the biological events associated with wound healing and to have the knowledge and skill to perform procedures of augmentation that are evidence based. Equally important, the patient should be encouraged to have only "realistic" expectation in terms of aesthetic outcome in any dental reconstruction in the anterior region. This Chapter will also review some surgical procedures that had been shown to yield reliable results.

2. Biological basis for soft tissue healing around dental implants

2.1 Gingival shrinkage around dental implants

During the healing phase following implant placement surgery (stage 1 surgery) or the trans-mucosal surgery for abutment connection (stage 2 surgery), the soft tissue re-organises itself according to the new environment (namely, surrounding a metallic implant). Noting the histologic observation made by Berglundh (Berglundh, Lindhe et al. 1991)and other investigator groups (regarding the orientation of the collagen fibre groups in the peri-implant gingival tissue) it is easy to appreciate why the peri-implant gingival tissue appears to shrink during the early stage of wound healing. The longitudinal arrangement of the major collagen fibre groups amplifes the process of collagen fibril contraction (as part of collagen maturation) in the vertical direction. Clinically, this process is observed as marginal gingiva shrinkage. In the anterior aesthetic zone, the amount of gingival shrinkage can be crucial to the success or failure of a case. Therefore when planning such a case, it is important to take into account the position and structural integrity of the labial bone wall which forms form the support base for the labial gingiva.

2.2 Peri-implant soft tissue seal

In a dog study(Berglundh, Lindhe et al. 1991), Berglundh and co-workers compared the similarities in the peri-implant soft tissue to that of the gingival tissue around teeth. In both cases, the soft tissue consisted of a junctional epithelium component and a connective tissue component. In both situations, the epithelium adhered to the tooth or titanium surface in similar fashion. However, in the connective tissue compartment there were notable differences. The peri-implant tissue had a higher fibre content (and hence a lower cellular content) than that of gingiva around teeth. In addition, the collagen fibres were arranged parallel to the titanium surface(Çomut, Weber et al. 2001) in contrast to that of the gingiva which tended to be arranged perpendicular to the cementum surface of the tooth root with other fibre groups arranged in various patterns elsewhere in the marginal gingiva. Some of these fibres had previously been observed to be inserted and embedded into the cementum layer forming Sharpey's fibers(Garant and Cho 1979). Because the study animals were subjected to plaque control regime for 8 weeks prior to sacrifice, there was little or no inflammatory cell infiltrates observed in either the gingiva or peri-implant tissues. The authors thus concluded that a satisfactory seal had been formed around the implant/abutment and that this seal was capable of maintaining tissue health (provided plaque control is practiced).

Since the time when the Berglundh's group described the pattern of collagen fibre bundles running parallel along the titanium surface (Berglundh, Lindhe et al. 1991), others had reported various fibre bundles organized in different fashions either obliquely to the titanium surface or circumferential to it(Buser, Weber et al. 1992; Ruggeri, Franchi et al.

1994; Piattelli, Scarano et al. 1997; Çomut, Weber et al. 2001; Schupbach and Glauser 2007). The precise significance of these observations was unclear. There were speculations that these fibre groups fulfil structural support and defensive role of the peri-implant soft tissue. In one recent report, controversial claims were made that "functionally" oriented fibre bundles were found lying perpendicular to the TiUnite surface of Branemark implants(Rocci, Martignoni et al. 2003). The significance of this finding was also not clear as no follow up study was done. Nevertheless, implants with roughened surface (up to the collar) are now available for clinical use, on the basis that such implant design could enable faster osseointegration and allow the formation of a durable soft-tissue cuff even on roughened titanium surface. This concept has not received general support among dental practitioners partly because of the lack of good clinical data to support its use, and partly because of concern about the potential for accelerated loss of osseointegration should this roughened surface becomes uncovered and exposed to the oral environment(Cosyn, Sabzevar et al. 2007).

This anatomical feature of soft tissue around titanium implant was found to be consistent for titanium surfaces irrespective of the type of implant system used(Abrahamsson, Berglundh et al. 1996). Furthermore, the surface roughness of the titanium had no bearing on the adherence of the soft tissue(Abrahamsson, Zitzmann et al. 2002). Neither was the clinical protocol used in implant placement (one-stage as versus 2 stages protocol)(Abrahamsson, Berglundh et al. 1999). Despite these observations, the clinical performance of this seal in protecting against bacterial ingression and thus peri-implant infection remained untested. Indirect evidence from human clinical studies which generally reported very low incidence of peri-implantitis and peri-implant mucositis suggested that indeed, the soft tissue cuff around titanium implant/abutment could provide comparable protection as gingiva around teeth. The importance of this physical seal notwithstanding, for long term peri-implant health, the presence of bacteria, bacterial plaque and biofilm will also need to be kept at a minimum. It is therefore crucial that restorations supported by implants should have built-in access channels or space for hygiene practice, and the patient should be educated in an effective method of plaque control. The failure to do so are seen too frequently as heavy plaque and calculus build-up around dental constructions as well as abutment or even implant surfaces when significant gingival recession has uncovered these implant components.

2.3 The keratinized gingival zone

The controversy about the need for a keratinized (attached) gingival zone around implant supported restorations is an interesting one. Based on the data from long term implant success and implant survival studies, there appeared to be little or no difference in the success rate for implants to be placed in oral mucosa zone or keratinized gingival zone(Jemt, Chai et al. ; Brånemark, Svensson et al. 1995; Lindquist, Carlsson et al. 1996; Buser, Mericske stern et al. 1997; Mericske-Stern 1998). It was therefore argued that there was no convincing evidence to support the clinical obsession of placing dental implants in keratinized gingival zone only or to re-create this soft tissue band after implant placement(Carmichael, Apse et al. 1989). In a recent systemic review, Esposito and colleagues concluded that there was insufficient evidence to suggest any surgical technique or approach was superior to another although they did note that flapless approach tended to result in less post-operative discomfort and pain. They also found no case to recommend that increasing the "keratinized tissue" band around dental implants as a preferred method of tissue management(Esposito, Murray-Curtis et al. 2007). Nevertheless, the common clinical observation of frequent plaque accumulation associated with mobile mucosal tissue around implant restorations and the subsequent soft tissue inflammation (and hence patient complaints) often lead to the demand for clinical intervention (figure 1). Clearly, the amount of peri-implant mucosal tissue movement during function is influenced by a number of physical variables and is difficult to measure. Until there is a reliable and accurate way of clinically assessing soft tissue movement during function, for many clinicians there is a case for routinely providing a keratinized gingival band around implant restorations in order to facilitate plaque control and hence reduce the incidence of plaque-related peri-implant disease. In a recent publication in the International Journal of Oral & Maxillofacial Implants, in a Current Issues Forum, the editor posted the question "To minimize complications, is it essential that implant abutments be surrounded by keratinized tissue?"(Krygier, Glick et al.). The consensus of opinions expressed by the authors participating in this debate was in general, supportive of the clinical practice of providing a keratinized gingival band around implant restorations where possible and practical. Another recent study reported a 5-year observation provided further data to support that keratinized gingival band of > 2 mm promotes better gingival health around dental implant/restorations(Schrott, Jimenez et al. 2009). In a systemic review, Cairo and others concluded that in some clinical situations soft tissue augmentation is warranted(Cairo, Pagliaro et al. 2008). A more recent review also concluded that "the functional need for attached gingiva around implants has not been established but its aesthetic value has been widely accepted.(Mehta and Lim 2010)

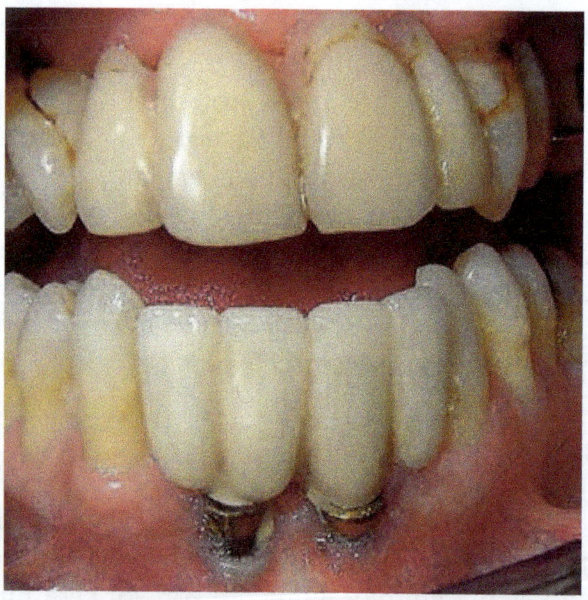

Fig. 1. Common situation encountered where poor oral hygiene resulted in the breakdown of mucosal tissue around implant/abutment.

2.4 Peri-implant tissue thickness and biological width

The dimension of the soft tissue attachment to the implant/abutment surface was considered important for the maintenance of peri-implant health and for the overall aesthetics of the final restoration. For many years, the concept of a biological width was used to explain the clinical observation of a constant dimension of dento-gingival junction around teeth and dental restorations(Gargiulo, Wentz et al. 1961). Berglundh and Lindhe demonstrated that in a dog model, similar constancy of gingival dimension was observed in

peri-implant tissue as well(Berglundh and Lindhe 1996). In an elegant experiment, the authors showed that by surgically reducing the thickness of the gingival flap prior to suturing, a corresponding crestal bone remodelling will subsequently occur allowing for the re-establishment of the "biological width" of the peri-implant soft tissue to its original dimension at the expense of reduced crestal bone height. This situation is analogous to the surgical procedure used in " crown lengthening" on natural teeth –an attempt to surgically position the gingival margin more apically and thus allow for an increased restorative space either for aesthetic reasons or for increasing the ferrule of coronal structure to improve on the retention of the planned restoration. This finding had great clinical implications because it provided a rationale for the careful placement of the soft tissue at the "correct" and stable position for the final peri-implant tissue finish. It also explained, at least in part, why it was important to maintain the alveolar crest in order to support the over-lying soft tissue.
Further studies comparing one-stage and two-stage procedures (submerged versus non-submerged) (Buser, Weber et al. 1992; Weber, Buser et al. 1996), loaded or unloaded non-submerged implants (Cochran, Hermann et al. 1997), different implant systems (Abrahamsson, Berglundh et al. 1996), different material surfaces (Arvidson, Fartash et al. 1996) and different level of placement of the implant-abutment junction (micro-gap) (Hermann, Cochran et al. 2001) failed to demonstrate any difference in peri-implant tissue dimension (thickness) under these variable conditions. Taken together, these observations confirmed that the concept of biological width of the gingiva around natural teeth was equally applicable to peri-implant soft tissues. These data further validated the need for a suitable implant design that allow for optimal soft-tissue attachment in order to achieve good soft tissue stability. It also provided a useful reminder to the clinicians that careful attention should be paid to the soft tissue finish when planning implant treatment cases.

2.5 The 3-dimensional relationship between alveolar bone and the overlying gingiva

If the biological width concept does indeed accurately describe the natural phenomenon of the inter-dependency of these two tissues (alveolar bone and gingiva), a corollary of the biological width concept would then state that a fixed thickness of gingiva will follow the position and contour of the underlying alveolar bone crest. Indeed, clinical observation of the remodelling of alveolar ridge, such as that following tooth extraction, does appear to confirm this concept. It is therefore important that when planning an implant placement in an extraction site, the dentist is able to predict and anticipate where the remodelled bone will be in future, and hence where the gingival margin will lie in relation to the dental restoration supported by the implant(Khoury and Happe 2000; Grunder, Gracis et al. 2005). Unfortunately, it is not always possible to accurately predict the extent of bone resorption during the remodelling process. In an animal model, Araujo and colleagues described in detail the pattern of alveolar remodelling following tooth extraction(Araujo and Lindhe 2005) and following implant placement(Araújo, Sukekava et al. 2005). Cumulative clinical experience suggests that bulky alveolar process (thick biotype) shows greater dimensional stability during remodelling compared with less bulky alveolar process (thin biotype). It was theorised that in thick biotype, the presence of lamina bone adjacent to the outer cortical plate of the alveolus provides the foundation for metabolic support of the cortical bone, and hence its stability and sustainability. In thin biotype, where the lamina bone is scarce or absent, the cortical bone is subjected to rapid resorption by osteoclastic type cells present in the healing bone wound (such as an extraction socket). Although the relationship between bone repair and the host genotype is not entirely clear at the moment, the above theory does go some way in explaining the clinical observation in alveolar ridge remodelling following tooth extraction.

2.6 Does the presence of implant help to preserve bone?

The placement of a dental implant in a fresh extraction socket (immediate placement) does not appear to interrupt the healing process of the socket wound(Botticelli, Berglundh et al. 2004; Araújo, Sukekava et al. 2005; Araújo, Sukekava et al. 2006; Araujo, Wennstrom et al. 2006). It is therefore, possible to extract a tooth (or teeth) and place dental implants in the same visit. The proponents and supporters of this clinical protocol of immediate implant placement have argued that the presence of a dental implant helps to preserve the height of the surrounding bone. Animal studies and human clinical studies have not yield evidence to support this notion(Wyatt and Zarb 2002; Covani, Cornelini et al. 2003; Covani, Bortolaia et al. 2004). In a single-tooth implant situation, the stability of the interseptal bone appears to be influenced by the periodontal ligament level of the adjacent teeth, rather than the level of bone-titanium interface. The labial bone plate is not supported by any neighbouring teeth and therefore can undergo rapid resorption and remodelling once its "host tooth" has been extracted. In patients with thin biotype, a rapid remodelling and disappearance of the labial bone crest can often result in disastrous clinical outcome where implants were placed immediately into extraction sockets. It is now clear that this clinical technique can yield unpredictable results and therefore should be attempted only with great caution. Drawing from our current understanding of the sequence of biological events in bone repair after tooth extraction, and in particular, the remodelling of the labial bone plate, it is not surprising to find that many immediately placed implants in the aesthetic zone ended up with disastrous results.

3. Managing the soft tissue around implants

3.1 Implant placement in the "correct" anatomical position

Based on our understanding of the constancy of gingival tissue thickness overlying alveolar bone surrounding teeth or dental implants and our knowledge of the healing behaviour of peri-implant soft tissue after wounding, it is possible to estimate the "final position" of the healed tissue around restorations placed on dental implants. The ability of the clinician to accurately forecast the final position of the healed tissue will underpin the long term success of any implant restoration (figures 2a and 2b). On the other hand, unrealistic expectation of reconstituting lost tissues by placing gingival tissue a greater distance from the underlying alveolar bone, such as in the case when the implant is placed apically relative to the adjacent teeth, will inevitably lead to future complications. This scenario can arise when the implanted site has been compromised by previous extraction or exposed to infection of long standing. In these situations, bone augmentation should be considered as part of the treatment plan if a stable soft tissue result is to be achieved. (Figure 3 a and b)

3.2 Important considerations during case planning

During the treatment planning stage of dental implant treatment, special attention should be given to assessing the proposed implant site as well as other systemic factors that may influence the performance and survival of the implant. Implant site assessment should include:

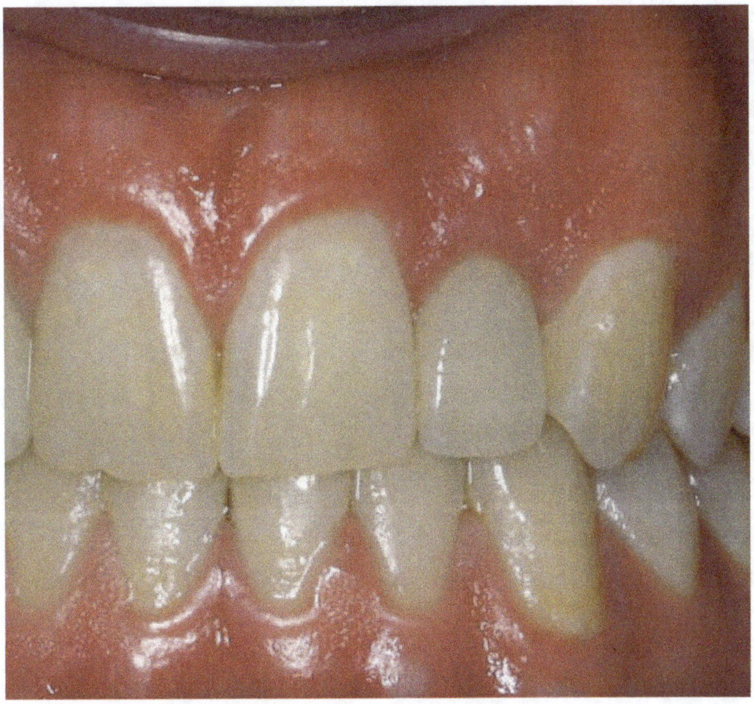

Fig. 2a. Stable gingival position with adequate bone support

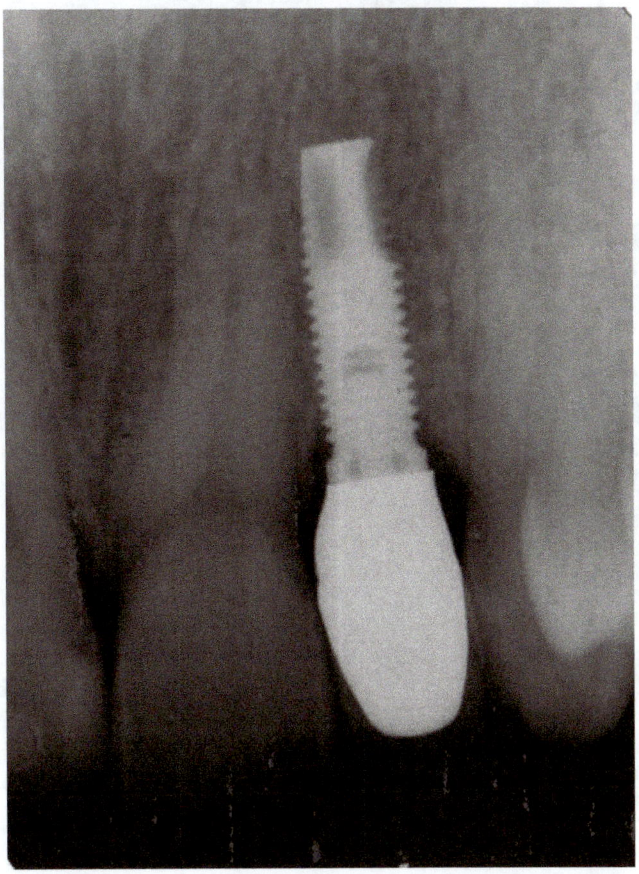

Fig. 2b. Radiograph showing the position of the dental implant relative to the adjacent teeth

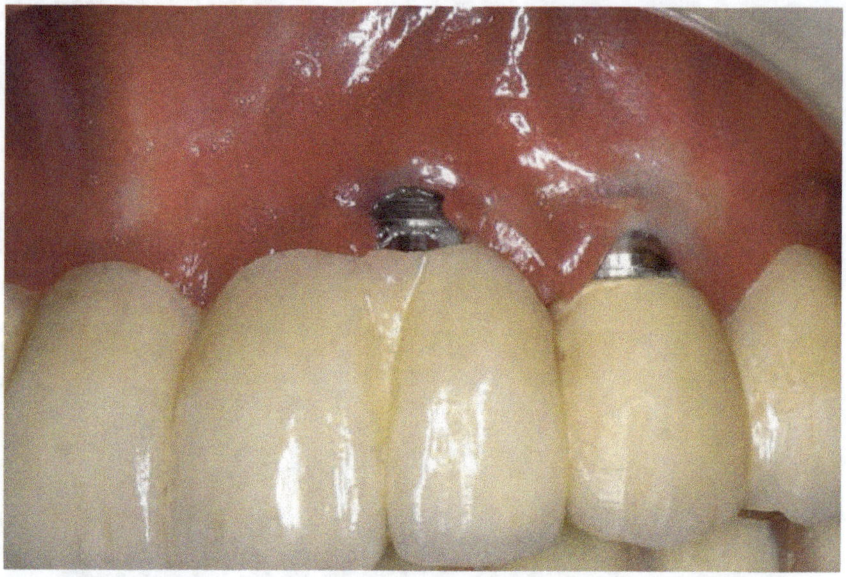

Fig. 3a. Gingival recession due to missing bone underneath

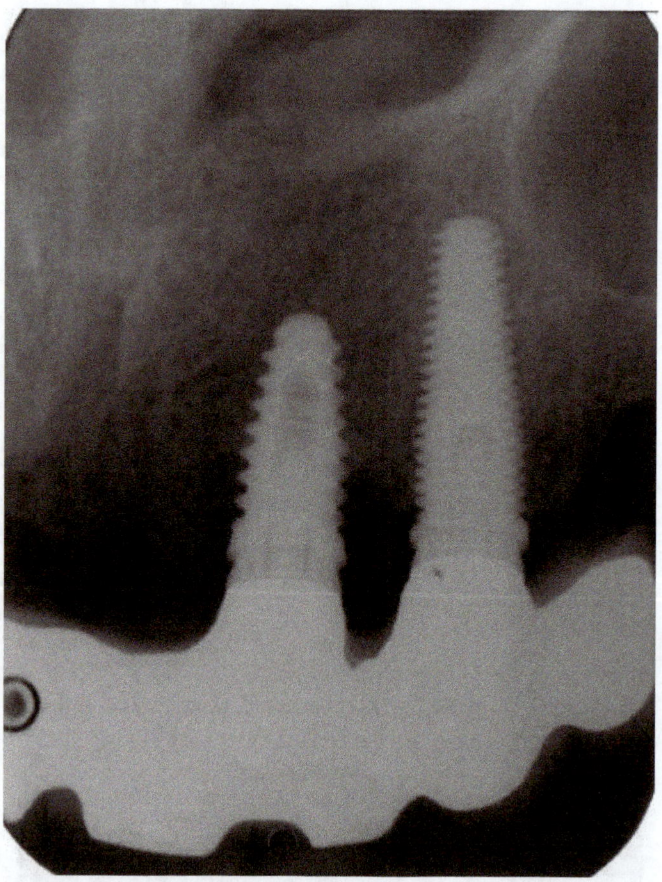

Fig. 3b. Radiograph of the same patient in figure 2a

- Checking for pre-existing pathology - such as chronic and persistent granulomatous lesions associated with the extracted tooth, non-healing abscesses, dentigerous cysts etc
- Evaluating the anatomical defect at the site - such as extreme ridge resorption following extraction
- Determining the biotype of the patient especially when the treatment site is in the aesthetic zone
- Deciding on the appropriate time for the implant placement in relation to the time of extraction

The systemic factors that require special attention are the important "risk factors" associated with implant complications and failures such as past history of periodontal disease and a smoking habit.

3.3 Surgical techniques

There had been numerous publications in the dental literature describing various surgical techniques suitable for augmenting the implant sites. Most of these procedures aim at adding bulk and thickness to the soft tissue surrounding dental implant restorations. Others aim at increasing the width of the attached gingival band surrounding these restorations. The interchangeable use of the term "keratinized gingiva" and "attached gingiva " had led to some confusion among dentists. From the current data available, there is no conclusive evidence to suggest that keratinized gingiva is essential in maintaining health of the peri-implant soft tissue(Carmichael, Apse et al. 1989). Paradoxically, most clinicians comment that attached gingiva around implant restorations will provide longer term stability and comfort and acceptance by the patient(Cairo, Pagliaro et al. 2008; Schrott, Jimenez et al. 2009). It may well be that the "immobilisation" of the soft tissue band is important for oral hygiene maintenance and stability and health of the tissue, and not so much the type of epithelial cells covering this soft tissue band.

By far the most popular surgical technique for augmenting the soft tissue at implant sites utilises autogenous graft from the same patient either in the form of subepithelial gingival graft (connective tissue graft)(Langer and Langer 1985) or gingival graft (free gingival graft)(Miller Jr 1982; Miller Jr 1985; Miller Jr 1993). These grafts are usually harvested from the palatal vault of the same patient and transferred to the recipient site. In the aesthetic zone it is usually necessary to provide a band of keratinized gingiva in order to harmonise with those surrounding the adjacent natural teeth. Under this circumstance, a connective tissue graft with a collar of epithelium attached will achieve the desired result. (Figure 4)

In a systemic review of surgical procedures for soft tissue augmentation, all autogenous tissue graft procedures were found to be effective in increasing tissue volume. No one technique was found to be superior to others (Thoma, Beni et al. 2009). It would therefore appear that treatment success is not a function of the choice of a surgical technique and the choice of a specific surgical technique is not as important as the adherence to sound biologic principles (such as those listed earlier in this chapter) if good clinical outcome is to be achieved.

4. Future research

The advancement in implant dentistry in the past 20 years has been rapid. Studies in the biological sciences have provided us with a clearer understanding of the wound healing events following tooth extraction as well as following dental implant placement in the

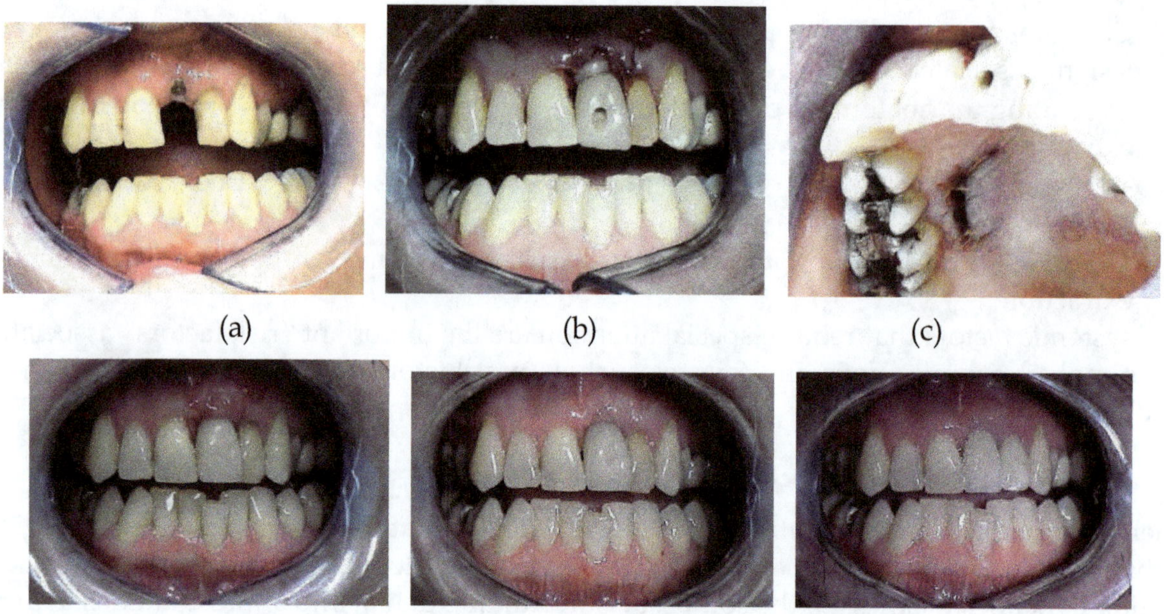

(a) (b) (c) (d) (e) (f)

Fig. 4. Connective tissue grafting was used to repair tissue deficit as a result of implant mal-positioning. a) positioning of dental implant (too labially placed and too palatally angled) and showing a lack of labial gingiva; b) connective tissue graft placed at the time when the temporary crown was issued; c) donor site on the palatal vault where the graft tissue was harvested from; d) healing at 1 week; e) at 1 month and f) at 1 year.

human jaws. This in turn drove the implant industry to seek to improve on the surface characteristics of implants to enhance early healing. The introduction of the "roughened" surface did show reduced time for osseointegration and establish clinical stability to enable earlier loading. However, the concept of immediate implant placement after extraction had not demonstrated universal success mainly due to bone remodelling complications. The research in "biological factors" to enhance the speed and quality of osseointegration has shown some promise and is continuing. The release into the market place of two dental implants with "bioactive" surface has not met with resounding success.(Cooper, Zhou et al. 2006; Schwarz, Herten et al. 2007; Junker, Dimakis et al. 2009). Clearly, the industry-driven effort in improving the engineering aspect of implant development will continue at a rapid pace. On the other hand, we have not made as much progress in the biological advances in the clinical science of implant therapy. We have used biomechanical refinement on the engineering of implant to cope with "softer" bone, such as implant thread design, implant body design, and implant surface design. To date, we have not explored the possibility of modifying the bony trabecular pattern and density in order to change a "type 4 bone" to a "type 3 bone", or from a "type 3 bone" to a "type 2 bone" etc. Equally important, we have not harnessed the adaptive property of living bone to respond to the presence of a loaded dental implant nor have we attempted to influence the metabolic activity of bone tissue to ensure that the dynamics of the osseointegration interface is maintained throughout the life of the implant. Last, but not the least, we have not paid enough attention to the complication of peri-implantitis - how to prevent it, how to treat it and how to repair the defect it creates. Future research in these two important areas of biology and clinical practice is urgently needed.

5. References

Abrahamsson, I., T. Berglundh, et al. (1999). "Peri-implant tissues at submerged and non-submerged titanium implants." Journal of clinical periodontology 26(9): 600-607.

Abrahamsson, I., T. Berglundh, et al. (1996). "The peri implant hard and soft tissues at different implant systems. A comparative study in the dog." Clinical Oral Implants Research 7(3): 212-219.

Abrahamsson, I., N. Zitzmann, et al. (2002). "The mucosal attachment to titanium implants with different surface characteristics: an experimental study in dogs." Journal of clinical periodontology 29(5): 448-455.

Araujo, M. G. and J. Lindhe (2005). "Dimensional ridge alterations following tooth extraction. An experimental study in the dog." Journal of clinical periodontology 32(2): 212-218.

Araújo, M. G., F. Sukekava, et al. (2005). "Ridge alterations following implant placement in fresh extraction sockets: an experimental study in the dog." Journal of clinical periodontology 32(6): 645-652.

Araújo, M. G., F. Sukekava, et al. (2006). "Tissue modeling following implant placement in fresh extraction sockets." Clinical Oral Implants Research 17(6): 615-624.

Araujo, M. G., J. L. Wennstrom, et al. (2006). "Modeling of the buccal and lingual bone walls of fresh extraction sites following implant installation." Clinical Oral Implants Research 17(6): 606.

Arvidson, K., B. Fartash, et al. (1996). "Histological characteristics of peri implant mucosa around Brånemark and single crystal sapphire implants." Clinical Oral Implants Research 7(1): 1-10.

Berglundh, T. and J. Lindhe (1996). "Dimension of the periimplant mucosa." Journal of clinical periodontology 23(10): 971-973.

Berglundh, T., J. Lindhe, et al. (1991). "The soft tissue barrier at implants and teeth." Clinical Oral Implants Research 2(2): 81-90.

Botticelli, D., T. Berglundh, et al. (2004). "Hard tissue alterations following immediate implant placement in extraction sites." Journal of clinical periodontology 31(10): 820-828.

Brånemark, P. I., B. Svensson, et al. (1995). "Ten year survival rates of fixed prostheses on four or six implants ad modum Brånemark in full edentulism." Clinical Oral Implants Research 6(4): 227-231.

Buser, D., R. Mericske stern, et al. (1997). "Long term evaluation of non submerged ITI implants. Part 1: 8 year life table analysis of a prospective multi center study with 2359 implants." Clinical Oral Implants Research 8(3): 161-172.

Buser, D., H. Weber, et al. (1992). "Soft tissue reactions to non-submerged unloaded titanium implants in beagle dogs." Journal of Periodontology 63(3): 225.

Cairo, F., U. Pagliaro, et al. (2008). "Soft tissue management at implant sites." Journal of clinical periodontology 35: 163-167.

Carmichael, R., P. Apse, et al. (1989). "Biological, microbiological and clinical aspects of the peri-implant mucosa." The Branemark Osseointegrated implant. Chicago: Quintaessence.

Cochran, D. L., J. S. Hermann, et al. (1997). "Biologic width around titanium implants. A histometric analysis of the implanto-gingival junction around unloaded and loaded nonsubmerged implants in the canine mandible." Journal of Periodontology 68(2): 186.

Çomut, A. A., H. P. Weber, et al. (2001). "Connective tissue orientation around dental implants in a canine model." Clinical Oral Implants Research 12(5): 433-440.

Cooper, L. F., Y. Zhou, et al. (2006). "Fluoride modification effects on osteoblast behavior and bone formation at TiO2 grit-blasted cp titanium endosseous implants." Biomaterials 27(6): 926-936.

Cosyn, J., M. M. Sabzevar, et al. (2007). "Commentary: Two-Piece Implants With Turned Versus Microtextured Collars." Journal of Periodontology 78(9): 1657-1663.

Covani, U., C. Bortolaia, et al. (2004). "Bucco-lingual crestal bone changes after immediate and delayed implant placement." Journal of Periodontology 75(12): 1605-1612.

Covani, U., R. Cornelini, et al. (2003). "Bucco-lingual bone remodeling around implants placed into immediate extraction sockets: A case series." Journal of Periodontology 74(2): 268-273.

Esposito, M., L. Murray-Curtis, et al. (2007). "Interventions for replacing missing teeth: different types of dental implants." Cochrane database of systematic reviews (Online)(4): CD003815.

Garant, P. R. and M. I. Cho (1979). "Autoradiographic evidence of the coordination of the genesis of Sharpey's fibers with new bone formation in the periodontium of the mouse." Journal of Periodontal Research 14(2): 107-114.

Gargiulo, A. W., F. M. Wentz, et al. (1961). "Dimensions and relations of the dentogingival junction in humans." J Periodontol 32(3): 261-267.

Grunder, U., S. Gracis, et al. (2005). "Influence of the 3D bone-to-implant relationship on esthetics." Restorative Dent 25: 113-119.

Hermann, J. S., D. L. Cochran, et al. (2001). "Biologic Width around one and two piece titanium implants." Clinical Oral Implants Research 12(6): 559-571.

Jemt, T., J. Chai, et al. "A 5-year prospective multicenter follow-up report on overdentures supported by osseointegrated implants." The International journal of oral & maxillofacial implants 11(3): 291.

Junker, R., A. Dimakis, et al. (2009). "Effects of implant surface coatings and composition on bone integration: a systematic review." Clinical Oral Implants Research 20: 185-206.

Khoury, F. and A. Happe (2000). "Soft tissue management in oral implantology: a review of surgical techniques for shaping an esthetic and functional peri-implant soft tissue structure." Quintessence international (Berlin, Germany: 1985) 31(7): 483.

Krygier, G., P. Glick, et al. "To minimize complications, is it essential that implant abutments be surrounded by keratinized tissue?" The International journal of oral & maxillofacial implants 12(1): 127.

Langer, B. and L. Langer (1985). "Subepithelial connective tissue graft technique for root coverage." Journal of Periodontology 56(12): 715-720.

Lindhe, J. and J. Meyle (2008). "Peri implant diseases: Consensus Report of the Sixth European Workshop on Periodontology." Journal of clinical periodontology 35: 282-285.

Lindquist, L., G. Carlsson, et al. (1996). "A prospective 15 year follow up study of mandibular fixed prostheses supported by osseointegrated implants. Clinical results and marginal bone loss." Clinical Oral Implants Research 7(4): 329-336.

Mehta, P. and L. P. Lim (2010). "The width of the attached gingiva--Much ado about nothing?" Journal of dentistry 38(7): 517-525.

Mericske-Stern, R. (1998). "Treatment outcomes with implant-supported overdentures: clinical considerations." The Journal of Prosthetic Dentistry 79(1): 66-73.

Miller Jr, P. (1982). "Root coverage using a free soft tissue autograft following citric acid application. Part 1: Technique." The International journal of periodontics & restorative dentistry 2(1): 65.

Miller Jr, P. (1985). "Root coverage using the free soft tissue autograft following citric acid application. III. A successful and predictable procedure in areas of deep-wide recession." The International journal of periodontics & restorative dentistry 5(2): 14.

Miller Jr, P. (1993). "Root coverage grafting for regeneration and aesthetics." Periodontology 2000 1(1): 118.

Piattelli, A., A. Scarano, et al. (1997). "Histologic aspects of the bone and soft tissues surrounding three titanium non-submerged plasma-sprayed implants retrieved at autopsy: a case report." Journal of Periodontology 68(7): 694.

Rocci, A., M. Martignoni, et al. (2003). "Histology of retrieved immediately and early loaded oxidized implants: light microscopic observations after 5 to 9 months of loading in the posterior mandible." Clinical implant dentistry and related research 5: 88-98.

Roos Jansåker, A. M., C. Lindahl, et al. (2006). "Nine to fourteen year follow up of implant treatment. Part II: presence of peri implant lesions." Journal of clinical periodontology 33(4): 290-295.

Ruggeri, A., M. Franchi, et al. (1994). "Histologic Ultrastructural Findings of Gingival Circular Ligament Surrounding Osseointegrated Nonsubmerged Loaded Titanium Implants." International Journal of Oral and Maxillofacial Implants 9(6): 636-643.

Schrott, A. R., M. Jimenez, et al. (2009). "Five year evaluation of the influence of keratinized mucosa on peri implant soft tissue health and stability around implants supporting full arch mandibular fixed prostheses." Clinical Oral Implants Research 20(10): 1170-1177.

Schupbach, P. and R. Glauser (2007). "The defense architecture of the human periimplant mucosa: a histological study." The Journal of Prosthetic Dentistry 97(6): S15-S25.

Schwarz, F., M. Herten, et al. (2007). "Bone regeneration in dehiscence type defects at chemically modified (SLActive®) and conventional SLA titanium implants: a pilot study in dogs." Journal of clinical periodontology 34(1): 78-86.

Thoma, D. S., G. I. Beni , et al. (2009). "A systematic review assessing soft tissue augmentation techniques." Clinical Oral Implants Research 20: 146-165.

Weber, H., D. Buser, et al. (1996). "Comparison of healed tissues adjacent to submerged and non submerged unloaded titanium dental implants. A histometric study in beagle dogs." Clinical Oral Implants Research 7(1): 11-19.

Wyatt, C. C. L. and G. A. Zarb (2002). "Bone level changes proximal to oral implants supporting fixed partial prostheses." Clinical Oral Implants Research 13(2): 162-168.

9

Bone Biology for Implant Dentistry in Atrophic Alveolar Ridge - Theory and Practice

Jeong Keun Lee
Ajou University School of Medicine
Republic of Korea

1. Introduction

It's a common experience for dental clinicians to note that the edentulous alveolar ridges always become atrophic as time goes by. It was late in the 19th century that Doctor Wolff first mentioned that form follows function (Wolf, 1892, as cited in Bilezikian et al., 2002). He described the individual capacity of morphological adaptation to a specific function as an "ontological adaptation" against the gravity through a daily locomotion or other daily mechanical duties (Fig.1-a). As a dentist I may illustrate the "dental compensation" in an Angle's class III malocclusion as a morphological adaptation to a masticatory function (Fig. 1-b), which itself is an example of the Wolff's "ontological adaptation."

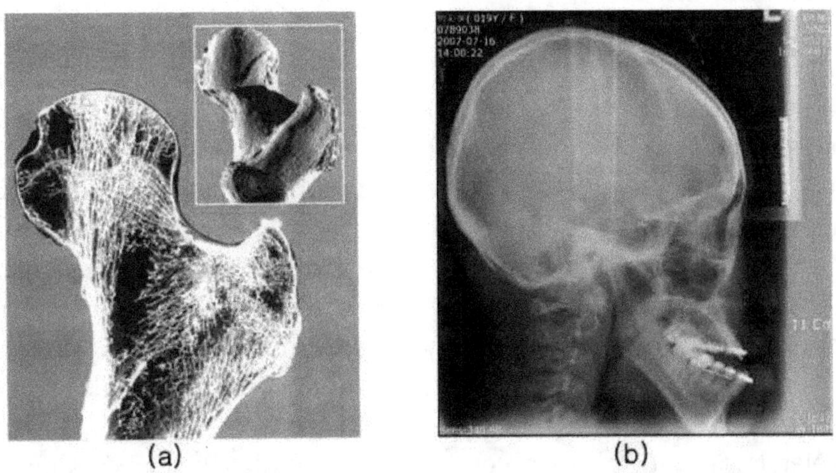

(a) (b)

Fig. 1. Form as determined by function.
(a) As an orthopaedic surgeon, Dr. Wolff mentioned ontological adaptation on observing the morphological adaptation against gravity. The trabecular pattern of the trochanter reflects the functional loading against gravity through a daily locomotion or other daily mechanical duties.
(b) As dentists, we may exemplify the dental compensation as Dr. Wolff's ontological adaptation. Upper incisors are labially tipped in accordance to everyday masticatory function.

There's a tendency for Angle's class II patients to have new symptoms of temporomandibular disorder (TMD) after orthognathic surgery. In contrast, there's no definite relationship of Angle's class III patients to postoperative development of TMD. It was deduced that altered biomechanical situation after orthognathic surgery was the causative factor for the new TMD symptoms in Angle's class II patients after orthognathic surgery (De Clercq et al., 1995). De Clercq compared the trabecular bone pattern of the Angle's class II and III patients to show that those of the former usually have less compact trabecular pattern than those of the latter. He conceived that this natural sparse trabecular pattern of the Angle's class II patients was brought about by the less functional loading subject to the mandibular condyle during mastication. And it was the increased masticatory stress after changed biomechanical circumstances that, in his opinion, was related to the newly-developed TMD after orthognathic surgery. It's a good example of the observation that "form follows function."

The author intended this chapter into two parts; the matter of why in the basic aspect and the matter of what to do for the clinician's perspective. First I will address the matter of why. Why does the unloaded bone go atrophic? Not exactly can we answer this question yet but current opinion pertaining to this problem will not only encourage current clinical treatment such as the principle of orthodontic tooth movement, but also implicate the future development of treatment outcome such as the complete regeneration of the alveolar bone loss of the periodontal pathologic origin. Next part will be on clinical aspect to assist in improving the implant site. Current treatment rationale, principles, and techniques for site improvement will be discussed with emphasis on autogenous bone graft using bone blocks. Additionally I will address the treatment strategy for the edentulous maxillary posterior alveolar ridge which is of main concern to many dental practitioners planning implant treatment in this troublesome region.

2. Why does the unloaded bone go atrophic?

2.1 Mechanotransduction

Solutions to the problem of atrophic alveolar bone begin with understanding why unloaded bone goes atrophic. Nobody can exactly depict why alveolar ridge goes atrophic after extraction of teeth. Efforts have been made to elucidate the scientific basis for the observation that the integrity of the skeletal tissue has something to do with mechanical usage. Frost has evolved the concept of the mechanostat (Frost, 1996) which he himself proposed as a new paradigm of understanding the mechanical-usage-dedicated message traffic routes between the skeletal tissue and the circumstances in which it is tuned. He argued the mechano-biologic negative feedback mechanisms would adjust skeletal architecture under the control of a subject's mechanical usage (Fig. 2).

Nowadays the secret of skeletal adaptation is more and more unveiling since around the opening of the 21st century. Doctor Burger hypothesized mechanotransduction as a main cause of the skeletal adaptation to a given functional loads (Burger & Klein-Nulend, 1999). She suggested that strain-derived fluid flow transduces the strain information to stimulate bone metabolism as a cellular response to a given load by the annular porosity produced by the osteocytes and their lacuno-canalicular hollow (Fig. 3). Osteocyte, the most abundant cell in our skeletal tissue was at first known as just a terminal stage cell of the osteoblastic lineage. But evidences are accumulating concerning its role as orchestrating skeletal adaptation to given functional loads. Orchestration of the cellular function is presumed earlier to be performed by the osteocytic syncitium through gap junctions (Moss, 1997). Evolving technology of current molecular biology has revealed many aspects of scientific evidences for this sophisticated orchestration of the skeletal tissue.

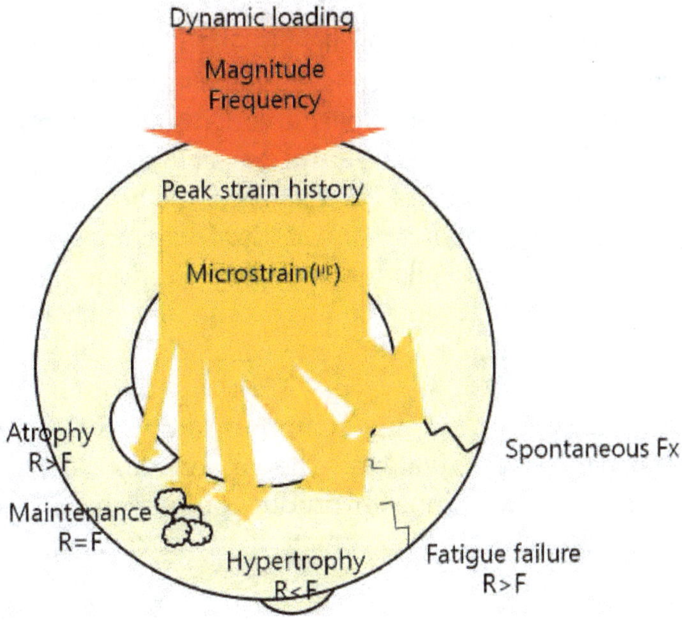

Fig. 2. The concept of the mechanostat.
Mechanostat hypothesis by Frost is schematically presented. Skeletal tissue has its loading history by dynamic loading which is remembered as a microstrain.
(1) If the strain is too small value, resorption dominates formation of bone tissue and the bone goes atrophic.
(2) If the strain is adequate, resorption balances formation and the bone maintains its volume.
(3) If the strain is adequately high value, formation at last dominates resorption and the bone goes hypertrophic.
(4) If the strain value is high by the overloading outreaching the range of physiological limitation, the strain is accumulated in the bone tissue causing microdamage leading to fatigue failure.
(5) Finally, if the strain value over the limit of yield strength the bone goes spontaneous fracture.

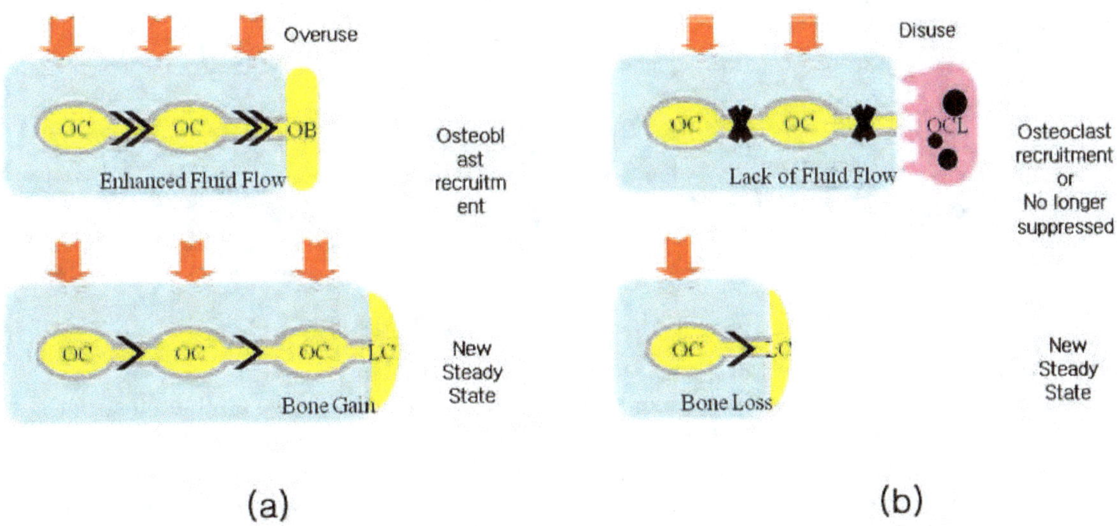

Fig. 3. Schematic diagram of mechanotransduction.
Mechanical information indicating the change of the external loading (red block arrows) is transduced by the strain-derived fluid flow (thin black arrowheads) to deliver biological information for the surrounding osteocytes to initiate bone metabolism for either (a) bone gain (overuse hypertrophy), or (b) bone loss (disuse atrophy). OC, osteocyte; OB, osteoblast; LC, bone lining cell; OCL, osteoclast.

2.1.1 Gap junction

Gap junction is the connection of the 2 hemichannels of each neighbouring cells which permits nanomolecular exchange of these cells. Hemichannel, in other words connexon is composed of six connexins switching from closed to open state depending upon the external stimulation (Fig. 4-1). Fluid shear stress stimulates cell to increase the production of connexin, an amino acid sequence that has 4 transmembrane domains with its two terminals in the cytoplasm (Fig. 4-2). Freely floating on the lipid bilayer, the connexons are able to dock with hemichannels of adjacent cells forming gap junctions (Fig.4-3). Gap junction is known to be restrictively permissive to intercellular mediators such as nitric oxide, Ca^{2+}, and prostaglandin (PG) E_2 (Bakker et al., 2001; Jørgensen et al., 2003; Siller-Jackson et al., 2008) or secondary messenger such as cAMP, IP_3 or cADP ribose (Civitelli, 2008). Connexons can work even without coupling with apposing connexons letting the PG E_2 or ATP out of the cell in response to mechanical stimulation (Cherian et al., 2005). External mechanical stimulus is thought to increase the connexin production, which will promote exchange of the biochemical information through the formation of new gap junctions (Cheng et al., 2001).

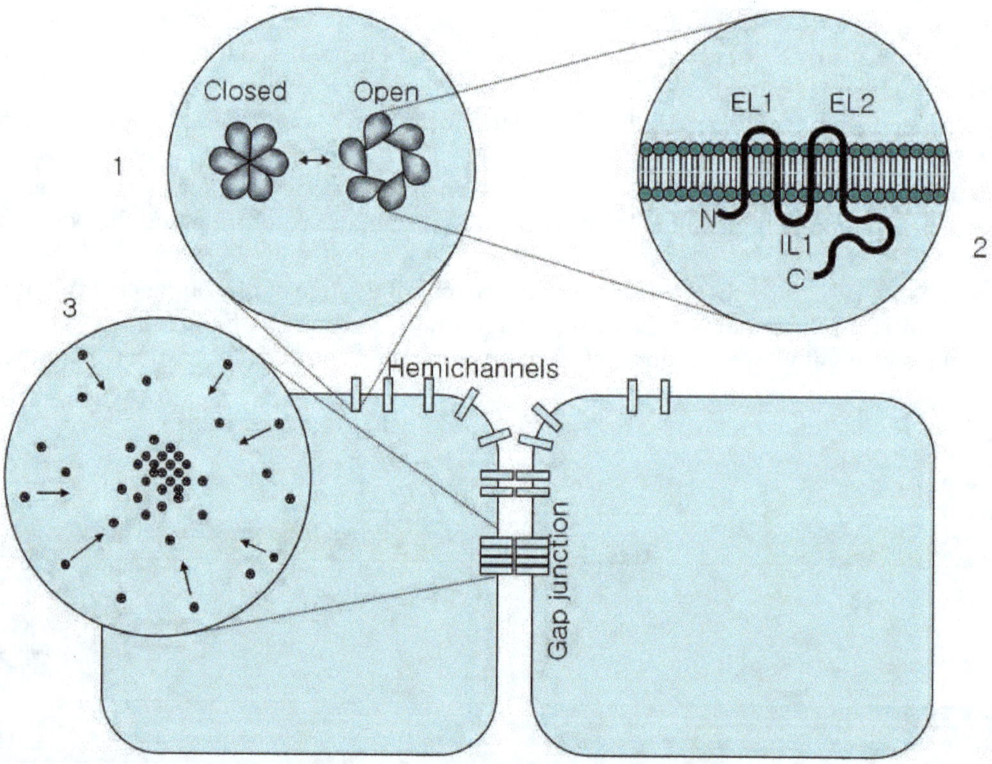

Fig. 4. Schematic diagram of the gap junction and hemichannel.
Hemichannels are selectively permissive pore of nanomolecular size staying free on the cell surface or docking with a hemichannel at sites of cell-cell contact to form a gap junction channel. Gap junction channels may cluster to form a gap junction plaque. 1: En face view of the hemichannels which are at a steady-state between two conformational states (open and closed). 2: Connexin topology at the plasma membrane. 3: En face view of a growing gap junction plaque.

2.1.2 Ionic mechanotransduction

The main mechanical stimulus which evokes mechanotransduction in bone cells is shear stress caused by the fluid flow. Stretch-activated channels open their gate in response to external mechanical stimuli via this shear stress caused by fluid flow. The net results are increase of the intracellular concentration of the divalent ionic molecules such as calcium ion. These calcium ions are propagated to the neighbouring cells via the gap junctions, which is called slow intercellular calcium waves. On the other hand, intercellular calcium waves can occur by activation of purinergic receptors by extracellular nucleotides, resulting in fast intercellular calcium waves. Ionic mechanotransduction is through both of these mechanisms in human bone cells (Jørgensen et al., 2003). Activation of G-proteins also induces fluid-induced PG E_2 production in osteoblasts (Reich et al., 1997). As a kind of intercellular mediators of bone cells, PG E_2 mediates bone anabolic effect via prostaglandin receptor EP_4 (Machwate et al., 2001).

2.1.3 Mechanical mechanotransduction

Other than ionic mechanotransduction, hypothetical genomic control mechanism was postulated involving transmembrane protein integrins (Huang et al., 2004). Integrins are thought to form focal adhesions against the extracellular matrix to sense the external mechanical loading. Transduced mechanical signals are relayed to the nucleus mechanically via nuclear junctions. Thus genomic activity in response to external mechanical stimuli is postulated to encourage biochemical change in mechanical cellular devices, which is called mechanical mechanotransduction. Cell-cell junctions can also be mechanically involved to inform the signal to the neighbouring cells. But there is no direct evidence supporting this hypothesis until now.

2.1.4 Established model for cell mechanotransduction

Mechanical adaptation is one of the determining factors for regulating bone mass along with calcium and sex steroids (Harada and Rodan, 2003). Many efforts in the area of the molecular biologic cell study have revealed the details of mechanotransduction in all areas of the biological sciences. We now have a schematic depiction on mechanotransduction in cellular level (Jaalouk and Lammerding, 2009) although it is still lacking much (Fig 5). Up to now, mechanotransductive pathways are known to be activated via stretch-activated ion channels, G-protein coupled receptors, and transmembrane protein integrins which sense the shear stresses caused by the extracellular fluid flows. This mechanotransduction model is currently evolving according to cutting-edge knowledge lead by prominent molecular biological work.

2.2 Dynamic alveolar bone

Bone is a dynamic tissue as a kind of supporting structure for our body. Systemically controlled under the influence of calcium and phosphate metabolism, it is under tight control of local physical influence sensitive to surrounding mechanical conditions (Harada & Rodan, 2003). Alveolar bone, the most labile structure of the 4 periodontium, is more active in bone metabolism as much as 10 times that of the long bones, which makes the alveolar bone more sensitive to external mechanical stimuli.

Bisphosphonate is one of the anti-osteoporotic drugs on worldwide sales nowadays. One of the most widely used bisphosphonate is Fosamax and a newer drug, Fosamax Plus D, which had worldwide sales of more than \$23.8 billion from 1999 to 2009, according to IMS Health, a health information company that tracks drug sales (Singer, 2010). Since the first report (Marx, 2003), bisphosphonate-related osteonecrosis of the jaw (BRONJ) has been a matter of

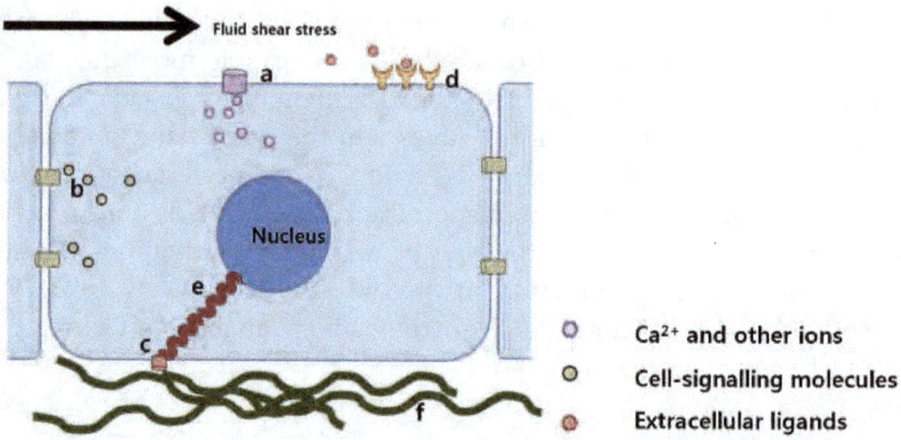

Fig. 5. Schematic depiction of mechanotransduction
a. Stretch-activated ion channels in the plasma membrane. b. Gap junctions for nanomolecular exchanges. c. Extracellular matrix (ECM)–cell focal adhesions to probe their environments. d. Cell surface receptors for autocrine and paracrine signalling molecules which are altered by compression of the intercellular space. Additionally, changes in G-protein-coupled receptors, lipid fluidity and even mitochondrial activity have been proposed as mechanosensors. e. The nucleus itself as proposed to be a mechanosensor. f. Mechanotransductive signalling outside the cell as given by force-induced unfolding of ECM proteins, such as fibronectin.

debate. Its pathogenesis is also still obscure but there is some clue. Osteonecrosis of the jawbone is caused not only by bisphosphonate but also by Denosumab, a monoclonal antibody to osteoclastogenetic factor, RANKL (Aghaloo et al., 2010; Taylor, et al., 2010). Upon this observation, pathogenesis of BRONJ is presumed to be delayed bone turnover resulting from osteoclastic inactivation. The jawbone is the only bone to be necrotised among the whole skeletal system that is complicated by the anti-osteoporotic bisphosphonate drugs, which is known as a BRONJ. Detailed information on BRONJ will be addressed elsewhere in this book.

2.3 Bone remodelling and sclerostin

Sensitive bone reaction is performed by the bone remodelling procedure encompassing bone resorption by osteoclast and bone redeposition by osteoblast. Microdamage to the bone tissue accumulates by mechanical overloading, and causes osteoclastic resorption of the damaged bone tissue. After osteoblastic transition which is marked by switching from bone resorption to formation, functional bone adaptation to a given loading is completed. One of the most dramatic advances in the study of the osteocyte is its orchestrating function on the bone remodelling procedure, the key protein of which is the recently discovered sclerostin.
Sclerostin is a gene product of the SOST and secreted by the osteocytes into the extracellular matrix reaching a steady concentration gradient. As a functioning glycoprotein it inhibits the osteoblast development and bone formation via Wnt signalling pathway (van Bezooijen et al., 2007). Adequate concentration gradient of the sclerostin enables the maintenance of the normal bone mass responding to a given functional loading. Adequate mechanical stimulation increases bone mass via a downregulation of the osteocytic production of the sclerostin. Irritable overloading affords the osteocytes focal microdamage, which renders reduced concentration of the sclerostin around the focal damage site. Soon the recruitment of the osteoclastic lineage cells is commenced to resorb the focal site, followed by the influx of osteoblastic precursor cells to build a new bone tissue. Generally bone remodelling is accomplished according to the change of local mechanical stress.

3. What can I do for atrophic bone to be prepared for dental implant?

3.1 Characteristics of the bone tissue

Bone is a distinctive tissue in that it undergoes regeneration rather than a repair procedure in the healing process after surgical trauma. The result is that it is always replaced by the same parenchymal structure, i.e. bone, and not by the scar tissue formation. The most important aspect for the adequate regeneration process is the close contact and rigid fixation of the graft bone to the recipient bed. We will discuss the aspect of wound healing of the skeletal tissue in the implications from the fracture healing (See 3.3)

Developmentally there are two types of bone formation, intramembranous and intracartilagenous ossification, with the resultant two types of bone tissues, membranous and endochondral bone, respectively. Cranial bone underwent progressive evolutionary adaptation to be composed of neurocranium and viscerocranium (Park, 2005). The combination of these two classification systems yield four types of cranial bone; membranous neurocranium, cartilaginous neurocranium, membranous viscerocranium, cartilaginous viscerocranium (MacKinnon & Morris, 1990) (Fig. 6). Alveolar bone belongs to membranous viscerocranium and has different developmental origin from iliac bone which belongs to endochondral bone. It is my clinical experience that donor bone block from the mandibular ramus is rather hard and difficult to manage in drilling and fixating with screws on the recipient bone bed in alveolar bone reconstruction. But the clinical result after bone graft is fairly good without so much resorption. Contrast to it, iliac bone block relatively offers little difficulty in surgical manipulation with some degree of bone resorption after alveolar bone reconstruction procedure.

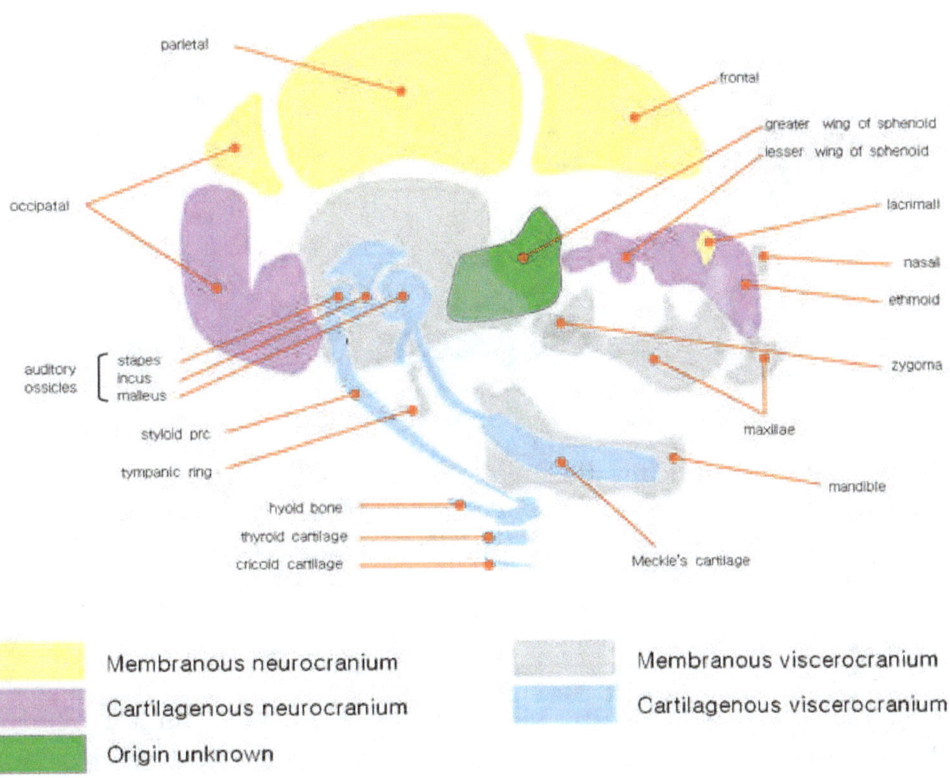

Fig. 6. Head and neck bone tissue.

Cranial bone is classified into four types; membranous neurocranium, cartilaginous neurocranium, membranous viscerocranium, cartilaginous viscerocranium.

3.2 What is going on in there?

Contrasted to the previous issue, an atrophic alveolar bone which is a matter of why, selection of the bone augmentation method is a matter of choice. Adequate selection of the graft material is based upon correct understanding of the biology pertaining to bone graft. Regeneration after bone graft is well studied in autogenous bone graft, which is the gold standard of the bone grafting procedures. Free-graft bone must be replaced with new bone of the recipient site origin, which is called osteoconduction. It functions as a scaffold for osteoprogenitor cells to reside in, and adequate remodelling process is essential because timely activation of osteoclastic function must be preceded before full blown osteoblastic cells begin to build new bone tissue. In addition to osteoconduction, osteoinduction is also an important mechanism of autogenous bone graft repair. Bone morphogenetic protein (BMP) is a potent skeletal mesodermal inducer, which blocks all the other pathways from mesenchymal stem cell but to the osteoblastic commitment. Bone formation can also be accomplished by the bone cell of donor origin, which is called osteogenesis. This is the predominant mechanism for new bone growth in vascularised bone grafts.

3.3 Implications from the fracture healing

Management principle of the bony injuries is close contact of the fractured segments and undisturbed healing without movement or infection (Lavery, 1994). So the most important aspect of the fracture healing is firm immobilization after adequate reduction and the same rule applies to bone graft.

3.3.1 Direct healing

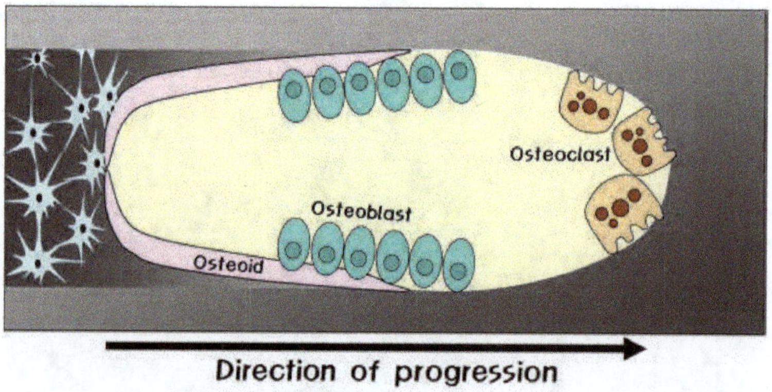

Fig. 7. Schematic diagram of basic multicellular unit (BMU).
Histologically the BMU consists of 1) osteoclastic front or osteogenic front, 2) reversal phase mononucleocytes, 3) osteoblastic layer. It is observed in the Haversian system of the cortical bone which is under the physiological loading such as the masticatory function. The osteoblasts are exclusively intraosseous Haversian system osteoblasts reacting to the load.

3.3.1.1 Contact healing

Contact healing occurs when the fracture segments are held firm within the interfragmental distance of 100 μm (Shapiro, 2008). Histologically it is mediated mainly by the intraosseous Haversian system osteoblasts (Fig. 7). Bone repair occurs bridging the minimal gap with osteoprogenitor cells crossing in the same direction of the Haversian system. It seems like that the osteoclastic front feels no barrier on its way across the gap. (Fig. 8).

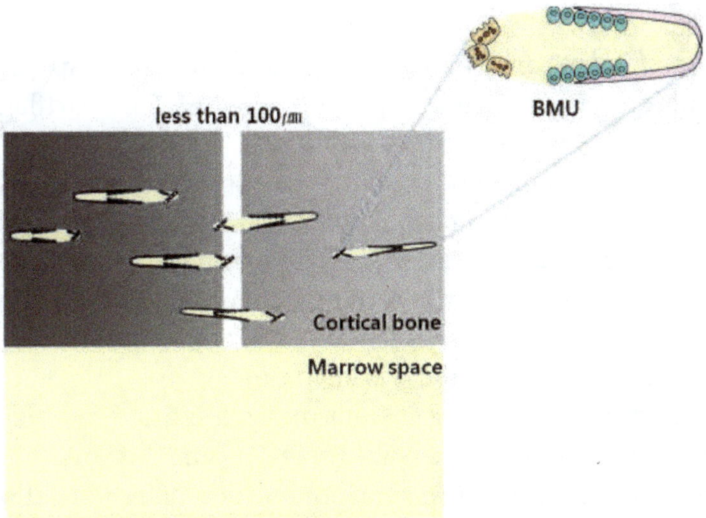

Fig. 8. Schematic diagram of the contact healing.
When the fracture segments are held firm within the interfragmental distance of 100 ㎛, the shape of the osteones in the cortical bone does not change when crossing the fracture or osteotomy. The direction of the lamellar bone is parallel to the long axis of the bone from osteoprogenitor cells in the Haversian longitudinal vessels.

3.3.1.2 Gap healing

If the fracture is reduced and rigidly fixated but the gap is over 100 ㎛, it goes gap healing procedure. Reduced segments are stable but the distance is too far for the Haversian longitudinal osteogenic front to cross. New bone begins to form in the marrow laid to the pre-existing rim of lamellar cortical bone at right angles to the long axis of the bone. After the gap is filled with this mechanism, the osteogenic fronts of the original pre-existing fracture segments find their ways to cross the filled gap (Fig 9).

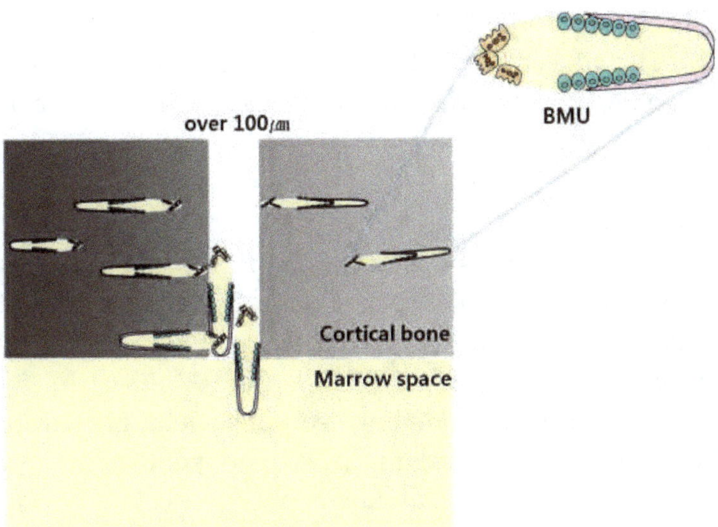

Fig. 9. Schematic diagram of the gap healing.
When the interfragmental distance is over 100 ㎛ under the stable rigid fixation, gap healing commences. Osteoprogenitor cells from Haversian longitudinal vessels cannot cross the gap anymore, and instead those of bone marrow origin will creep on the segmental surfaces to fill the gap at right angles to the long axis of the bone. At last osteoclastic cutting cone from the original cortex begins to cross the filled gap to realign the lamellar bone parallel to the longitudinal axis.

3.3.2 Indirect healing

Failed anatomic repositioning or mobility across the fracture gap gives rise to indirect healing. Indirect healing occurs by callus formation followed by cartilage formation. Initial hematoma under hypoxic circumstances is gradually replaced by the granulation tissue, which in turn forms a fibrocartilagenous callus in the condition of hydrostatic pressure. With minimal strength but having the tolerance to the deforming forces in the interfragmentary zone, granulation tissue helps attenuate interfragmentary movement. Decreased interfragmentary movement in tern aids laydown of the fibrous tissue. Stabilised bone segments further permits fibrocartilagenous callus to form. Bridging the gap across the fracture segments the callus shades into the bone tissue.

The type of force healing bone experiences determines the tissue type the healing bone will be. It's a general agreement that the tensile force favours intramembranous ossification, while compressive stress encourages the pluripotent mesenchymal cells into chondrocytes. Continuous hydrostatic compression incurs cartilage formation whereas intermittent compressive stress gives intracartilagenous ossification (Carter et al., 1998).

3.4 Healing process after bone graft

3.4.1 Initial phase

At the beginning of the bone graft healing, cells with bone forming potential must be recruited to the graft site to construct a new bone tissue. This is done in two weeks after bone graft, which is called the initial phase. It is the most important period although there is no actual bone formation because the osteoblast can lay down mineralized tissue only in their adjacent area.

3.4.2 Phase 1 bone regeneration

Actual mineralization ensues following 4 weeks in which period new bone is formed as a woven bone type. There is no orientation of bone trabeculae irrespective of surrounding mechanical stress. Designated as a phase 1 bone regeneration, it is finished by 6 weeks after the bone grafting, followed by mechanical stress-sensitive period, phase 2 bone regeneration.

3.4.3 Phase 2 bone regeneration

It reaches a peak around 3 to 4 months after bone grafting when bone remodelling occurs in accordance with the mechanical demand. Functional loading guides the existing woven bone into a lamellar type of new bone which is suitable for supporting the mechanical stress within a functional range.

Bone remodelling differs from bone modelling seen in skeletal growth period, in which the bone resorption and formation are accomplished independently in concert with bone growth. On the contrary, the osteoclastic and osteoblastic effects are coupled tightly in bone remodelling which is well demonstrated histologically in the temporary anatomical structure, basic multicellular unit (BMU) (Frost, 1963, as cited in Robling et al., 2006)(Fig. 7). The time with which the BMU travels through tissue space is called sigma (σ). In human cortical bone, it would take approximately 120 days to complete one σ, consisting of roughly 3weeks of osteoclastic phase, 10days of reversal phase, and 3months of osteoblastic phase (Robling et al., 2006).

3.5 Autogenous block bone graft in alveolar defect of height and/or width problems

Edentulous alveolar ridges must be prepared for dental implant treatment. Autogenous bone block can be harvested from diverse sites (Fig. 10) which have their own advantages and disadvantages. Small defects such as those caused by periodontitis can be prepared using small bone blocks from intraoral donor origin. Two intraoral sites are outstanding; the external oblique ridge-ramal area of mandible, and the chin cortex. Of these, I prefer an external oblique ridge-ramal bone, for approaching to chin bone possibly risks the incisive branches of the mental nerve, which is very annoying. Large defects over the basal bone as a result of radical resection of the large head and neck tumours or major trauma can be rehabilitated with reconstructive surgery with extraoral large donor bone block such as iliac bone or fibula. I prefer iliac free bone graft but free vascularised osteocutaneous fibular graft can also be of use.

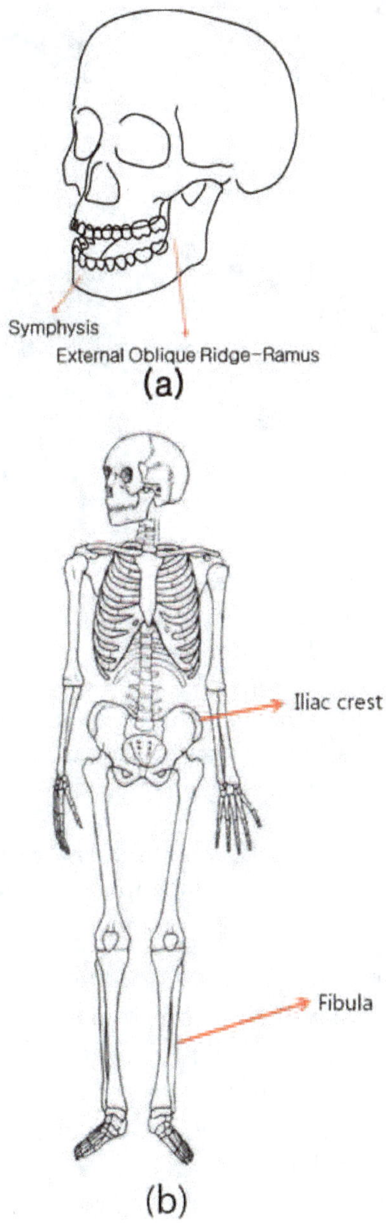

Fig. 10. Favoured donor sites for autogenous alveolar bone reconstruction with bone block. Many parts can be donor site for autogenous alveolar bone reconstruction but the author favours these arrow-indicated sites; (a) intraoral, and (b) extraoral donor sites.

3.5.1 Reconstruction with external oblique ridge-ramal bone block

Fifty six years old female patient resorted to our clinic with the chief complaint of lost anterior upper teeth. Her problem was not only the lost dentition, but also the lost alveolar ridge revealed as in Fig. 11-a. External oblique ridge-ramal area of the mandible was selected as a donor site and harvested for augmentation of the depressed alveolar bone as in Fig. 11-b. Harvested bone was placed and secured in the recipient site as in a Fig. 11-c and waited 4 months for dental implant fixture installation. Immediate before fixture installation we evaluated the bone graft area with CT scan, which revealed good integration of the graft (Fig. 11-d).

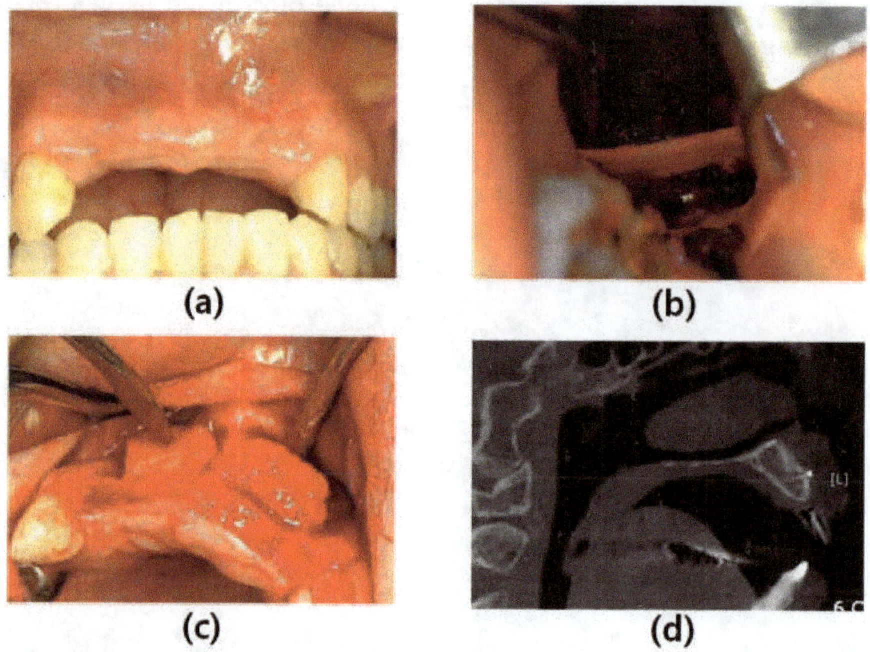

Fig. 11. Alveolar bone augmentation with ramal bone block.

(a) Preoperative figure shows depressed anterior maxillary wall due to lost alveolar bone accompanying loss of maxillary anterior 4 teeth.

(b) As an augmentation source for donor bone, both external oblique ridge-ramal area of the mandible were approached and 2 pieces of bone blocks were harvested.

(c) Harvested bones were well adapted in the depressed recipient area which were fixated with adequate miniscrews.

(d) Graft area was evaluated with CT scan four months after the graft procedure, which showed adequate healing ready for installation of the dental implant fixtures. One of miniscrews was evident on this CT slice.

After instillation of local anesthetics with 2% lidocaine and 1:100,000 epinephrine, previously augmented site was approached, which showed acceptable augmentation as in Fig. 11-e. Fixation screws were retrieved before dental implant fixtures were installed as in Fig. 11-f, and zirconia abutments were used because the aesthetic consideration was important in maxillary anterior region (Fig. 11-g). Clinical appearance after the completion of final prosthesis was good as in Fig. 11-h although slight loss of interdental papilla was observed.

3.5.2 Reconstruction with chin bone block

This 56 years old male patient was diagnosed as total maxillary insufficiency precipitated by long duration of periodontal diseases (Fig.12-a). Implant was planned for implant-

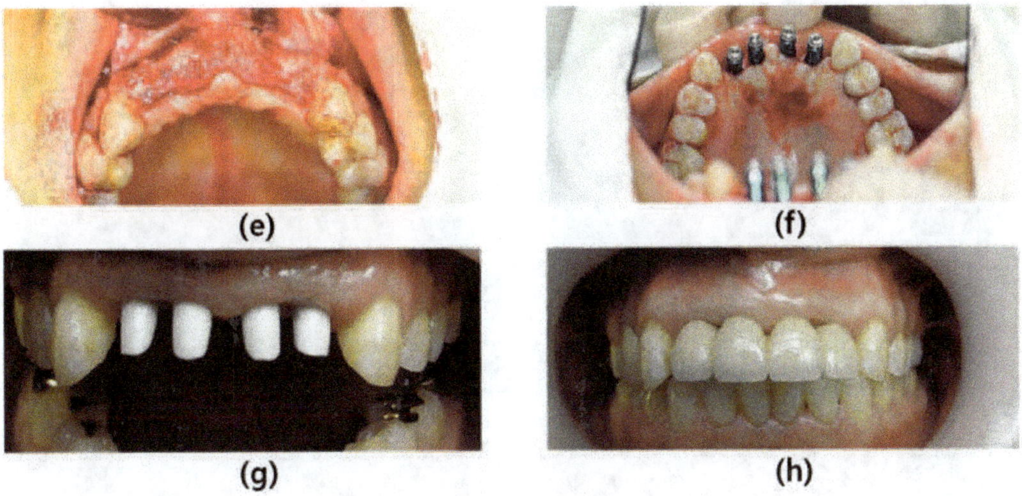

Fig. 11. (continued). Alveolar bone augmentation with ramal bone block.
(e) Maxillary anterior area of the same patient was re-entered 4 months later to find acceptable appearance of the graft site for implant fixture installation.
(f) Fixtures were installed after retrieval of the fixation screws.
(g) Zirconia abutment was selected for cosmetic consideration.
(h) Minimal aesthetic problem was detected after final prosthodontic rehabilitation.

supported overdenture and total height- and width problem was identified (Fig. 12-b). Ideally iliac bone graft was recommended but the patient refused general anesthesia and finally multiple event of minor augmentation procedure under local anesthesia was accepted as an alternative method. Insufficient alveolar bone was recovered with bilateral sinus graft and lateral wall augmentation along with anterior subapical block bone augmentation. Fig. 12-c shows insufficient anterior maxillary wall inadequate for dental implantation. Both mandibular ramal bone blocks were utilised as the donor for both lateral maxillary wall augmentation, and still we need another bone block for anterior maxillary alveolar ridge. In spite of the possible numbness after donor bone harvesting, chin bone was unavoidable choice (Fig. 12-d). Along with autogenous bone block, allogenic bone powder was accepted for filling the gap between the graft and recipient bed (Fig. 12-e). Fig. 12-f shows clinical picture after successful dental implantation 4 months after the bone graft.

3.5.3 Reconstruction with free iliac bone block

Initial diagnostic panoramic view of forty nine years old male with severe chronic periodontitis showed many hopeless teeth on maxillary anterior and right posterior areas (Fig. 13-a). After scheduled periodontal treatment with extraction of many hopeless teeth diagnostic CT scan revealed compromised areas of the maxillae on the anterior (Fig. 13-b) and right posterior region (Fig. 13-c).
Free iliac bone graft was done under general anesthesia, in which operation inner medial cortical bone was harvested with cancellous bone and marrows leaving the outer cortical bone intact (Fig. 13-d). Maxillary alveolar bone was augmented with harvested cortical block for future dental implant treatment (Fig. 13-e). Prosthodontic treatment was done with excellent treatment outcome as in Fig. 13-f and g.

3.5.4 Microsurgical reconstruction with free vascularised fibular bone

Young man resorted to our clinic with the chief complaint of painless lower facial swelling and preoperative panoramic findings revealed multiple radiolucencies all around the mandible

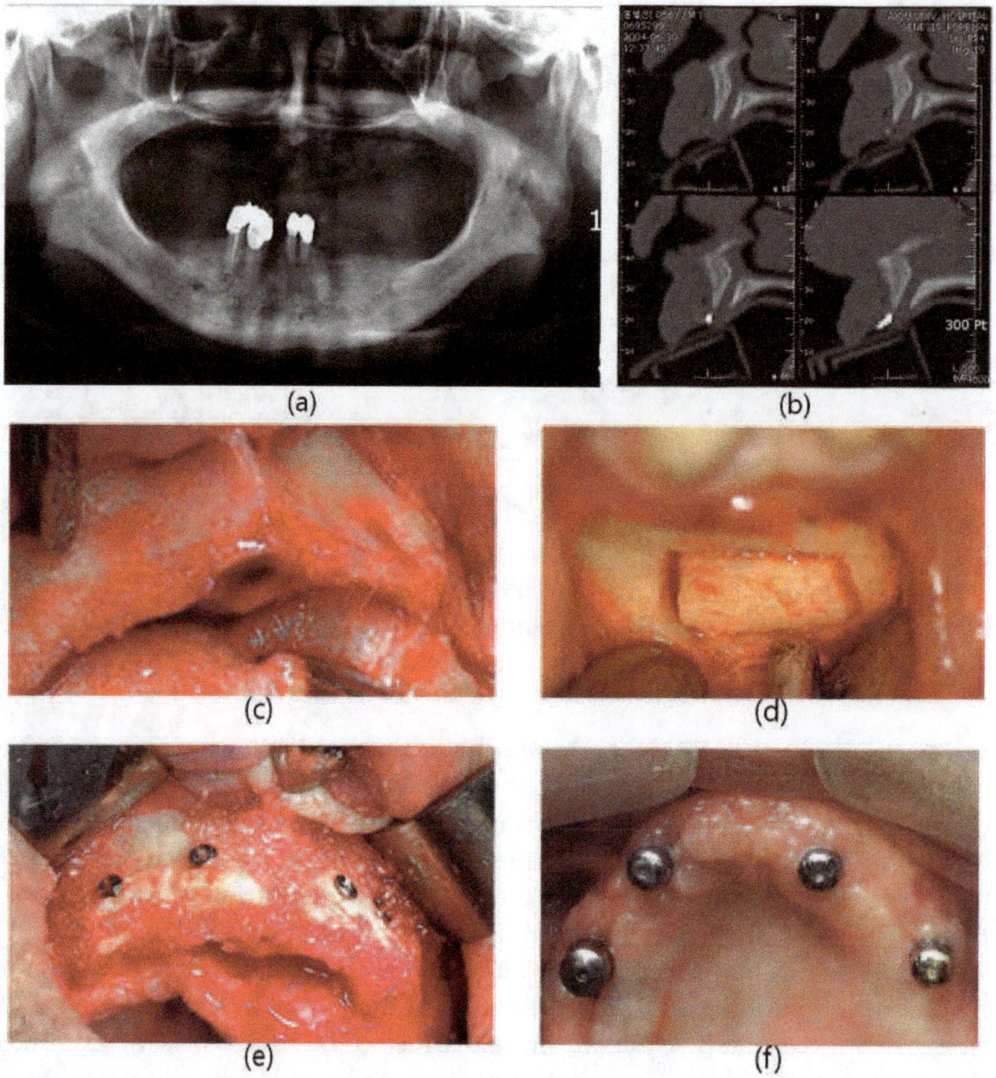

Fig. 12. Alveolar bone augmentation with chin bone block on anterior maxillary defect.
(a) General bone resorption is identified on preoperative panoramic view.
(b) Dentascan on anterior maxillary region revealed large space for nasopalatine neurovascular bundle and poor bone bed for dental implant.
(c) Reflection of the flap revealed thin alveolar process on the anterior maxillary edentulous area. Note large nasopalatine foramen hindering fixture installation on #11 and #21 site.
(d) Dense labial cortex of the chin bone was found after careful dissection, which was harvested for augmentation of the thin anterior maxillary alveolar process.
(e) Bone blocks from the chin cortex were fixated with miniscrews and the remaining gaps were filled with commercially available allogeinic bone powder.
(f) Four fixtures were installed 4 months after the bone graft on the strategic sites.

(Fig. 14-a). Biopsy of the lesion confirmed the diagnosis of ameloblastoma and the mandible was extensively removed using segmental resection ranging total body area anterior to both antegonial notches. Mandibular reconstruction plate was utilised immediately as a bridging plate for the maintenance of the mandibular continuity. Six months later when no evidence of recurrence was confirmed, free vascularised fibular reconstruction was done with microsurgical technique utilising peroneal artery as a feeding artery (Fig. 14-b). Four months later when successful reconstruction was identified (Fig 14-c), six fixtures were installed (Fig. 14-d), followed by hybrid type overdenture treatment (Fig. 14-e).

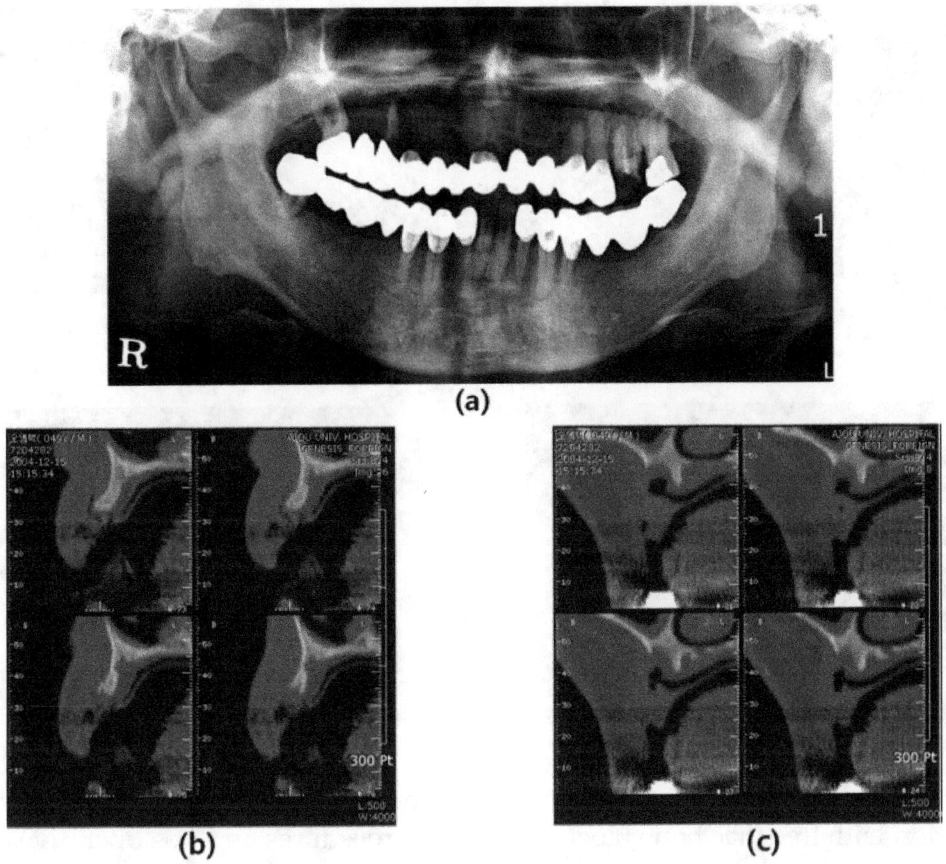

Fig. 13. Alveolar bone augmentation and additional maxillary basal bone reconstruction with free iliac bone block-Preoperative diagnostic imaging.

(a) Severe periodontal disease were evident in preoperative panoramic view in which all maxillary anterior teeth and maxillary right posterior teeth were scheduled to be extracted and periodontally treated with surgical intervention.

(b) Diagnostic CT scanning was inevitable after extraction of all poor teeth and scheduled periodontal surgery was finished, where width problem was evident in anterior maxillary region.

(c) CT also revealed both width and height problems in right maxillary region.

3.6 Treatment strategy for the edentulous maxillary posterior alveolar ridge

Dental implantation on the atrophic posterior maxillary alveolar ridge is always challenging because both quantity and quality of the bone are poor in this area. Maxillary posterior alveolus exhibits poor bone quality, for anatomically maxillae consists almost of cancellous bone and biomechanically posterior teeth are subject to three times more occlusal forces than anterior teeth. Usually the quality of the bone in this region is classified as D3 or D4 in Misch's classification which is composed of fine trabecular bone with thin cortical bone or even finer trabecular bone with almost no cortical bone (Misch, 1990, as cited in Misch, 2008). The amount of available alveolar bone is usually deficient because of the dual resorption inside and outside of the sinus floor, because of pneumatisation and alveolar resorption, respectively. Frequently this area needs bone augmentation to allow an implant-supported prosthesis.

Alabama implant meeting held at Birmingham in 1976 was the first meeting that Tatum presented a surgical technique involving the maxillary sinus (Tatum, 1986). It was several years later that the first publication on this technique was reported by Boyne and James

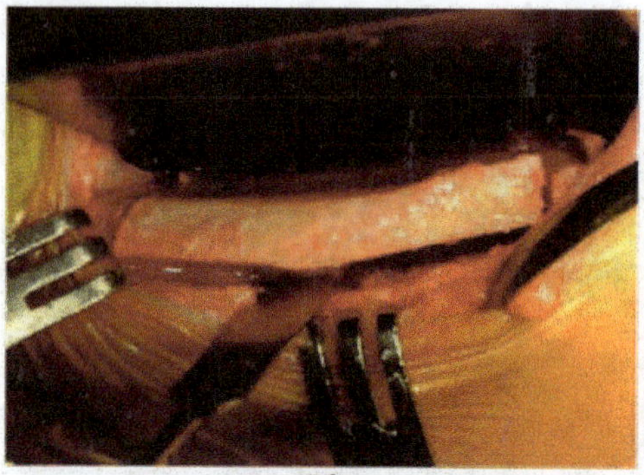

(d)

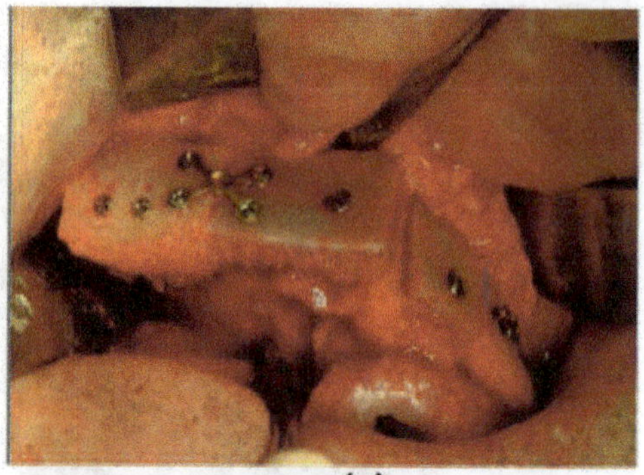

(e)

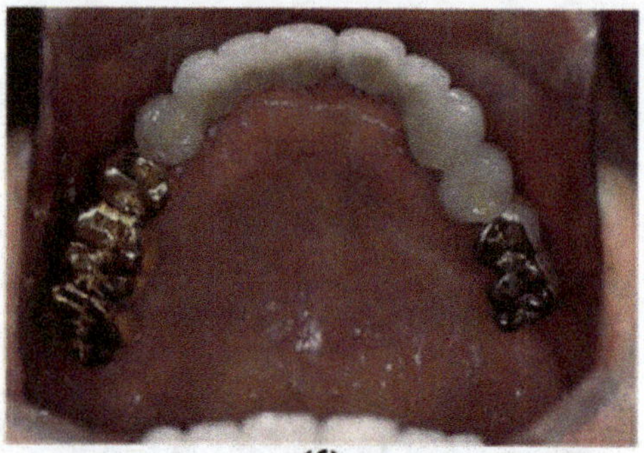

(f)

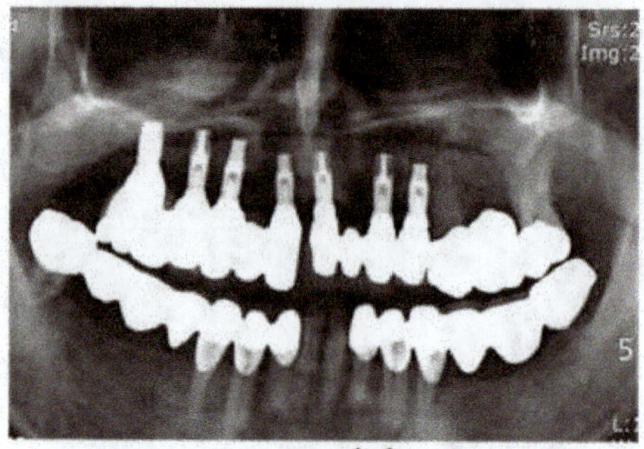

(g)

Fig. 13. (continued). Alveolar bone augmentation and additional maxillary basal bone reconstruction with free iliac bone block-Operative procedures and postoperative results.
(d) Harvesting of the free iliac bone. Cancellous bone and marrows along with inner medial cortex were harvested leaving the outer cortical bone intact for reduction of postoperative complication.
(e) Insufficient maxillary alveolar bone was augmented with the harvested iliac bone.
(f) Complete prosthodontic rehabilitation was possible after dental implant fixture was osseointegrated to successfully augmented graft bone.
(g) Panoramic view taken after the completion of the dental implant treatment.

(Boyne & James, 1980). They introduced infracture technique with upper hinge in the lateral wall of the maxilla. Consensus meeting on sinus surgery held in 1996 at Babson College, Willesley City, MA was remarkable in that it was the first meeting that reaches an agreement on terminology on the sinus surgery for dental implantation. Sinus augmentation is generally considered a good method for edentulous maxillary posterior alveolar bone to allow an implant-supported prosthesis. Some modifications are available involving hydraulic elevation of the sinus floor via crestal approach (Vitkov et al., 2006) or outfracture of the lateral maxillary window (Lee, 2010).

Evaluation of bone graft is based on the clinical evidence of fixture survival and functioning final prosthesis. However strict criteria for success are based upon the histological evidence of a microscopic activity conducted by vital bone tissue. It can be evidenced by bone remodelling, which means the viable osteoclast and osteoblast is available by the bone grafting procedures. It is therefore one of the criteria for bone graft materials to be incorporated in the bone remodelling procedure. The determinant factor for success of sinus bone graft however is known to be not related to the kind of a graft bone but to the remaining alveolar bone height. Actually many graft materials used in the sinus floor augmentation demonstrate an acceptable success rate irrespective of their nature. It is because that the sinus cavity is compartmentalised and has a natural housing for the graft materials to be stabilized, which is a specific anatomical advantage of the sinus cavity.

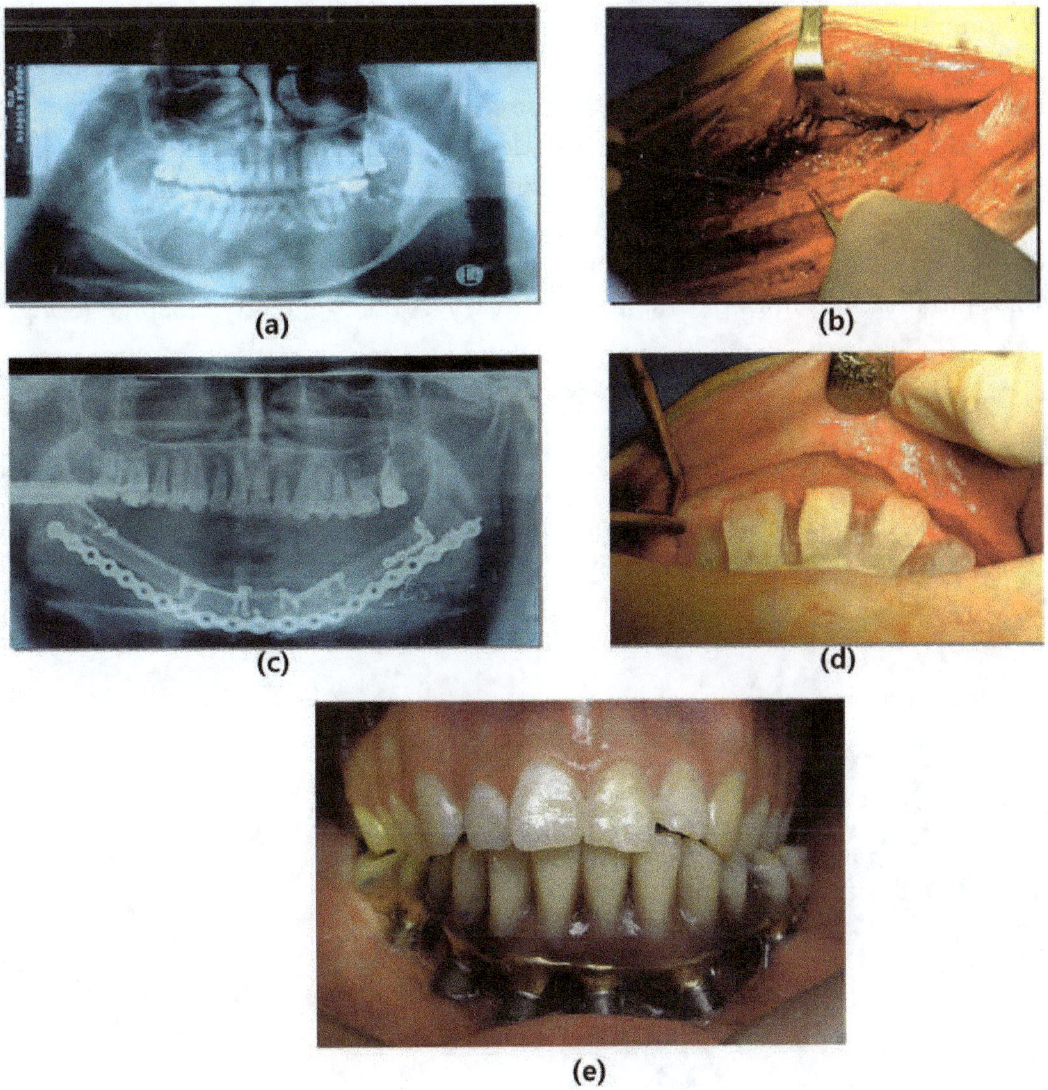

Fig. 14. Mandibular reconstruction utilising microvascular free fibular graft.
Preoperative panoramic view showing multiple large radiolucencies all around the mandibular body area (a), which was segmentally resected for radical treatment diagnosed as multicystic ameloblastoma. Confirming no evidence of recurrence at 6 months later, patient's fibula was utilised as in (b) for reconstruction of the basal part of the mandibular body. Four months later when stable reconstruction was identified (c), dental implant fixtures were installed on strategic positions in the fibula as in (d). This fibula was only for the basal part of the mandible and the final denture was designed as a hybrid type as in (e) to facilitate the oral hygiene procedures.

3.6.1 Outfracture osteotomy sinus graft technique for posterior maxillary edentulous ridge concomitant with dental implantation.

The original method of Tatum first presented in the Alabama implant meeting (Tatum, 1986) adopted a trapdoor design which involved inward opening of the lateral bony window with a top hinge. It was a methodological revolution for it was a pushing back the frontiers of a prosthodontic treatment by surgical measure. But it has its own limitations in anatomical considerations in cases with a sinus septum or a thick lateral sinus wall in the operation field. These limitations were overcome by modifying window opening method form inward to outward direction. Outfracture osteotomy sinus graft technique was introduced utilising readaptation of the outfractured bony window segment after sinus floor augmentation (Lee, 2010). It involves routine window opening on the lateral maxillary wall as in Fig. 15-a. Completion of the outfracture of the bony window segment (Fig. 15-b) is followed by the elevation of the Schneiderian membrane and floor augmentation using the space created by the membrane elevation (Fig. 15-c). Outfractured bony segment was placed back into the original position and secured without any screws or plates (Fig. 15-d). The success rate with the outfracture osteotomy sinus graft technique was reported as 97.2 % in 113 cases through August 2004 to July 2009 in Department of Dentistry, Ajou University Hospital (Song, 2009).

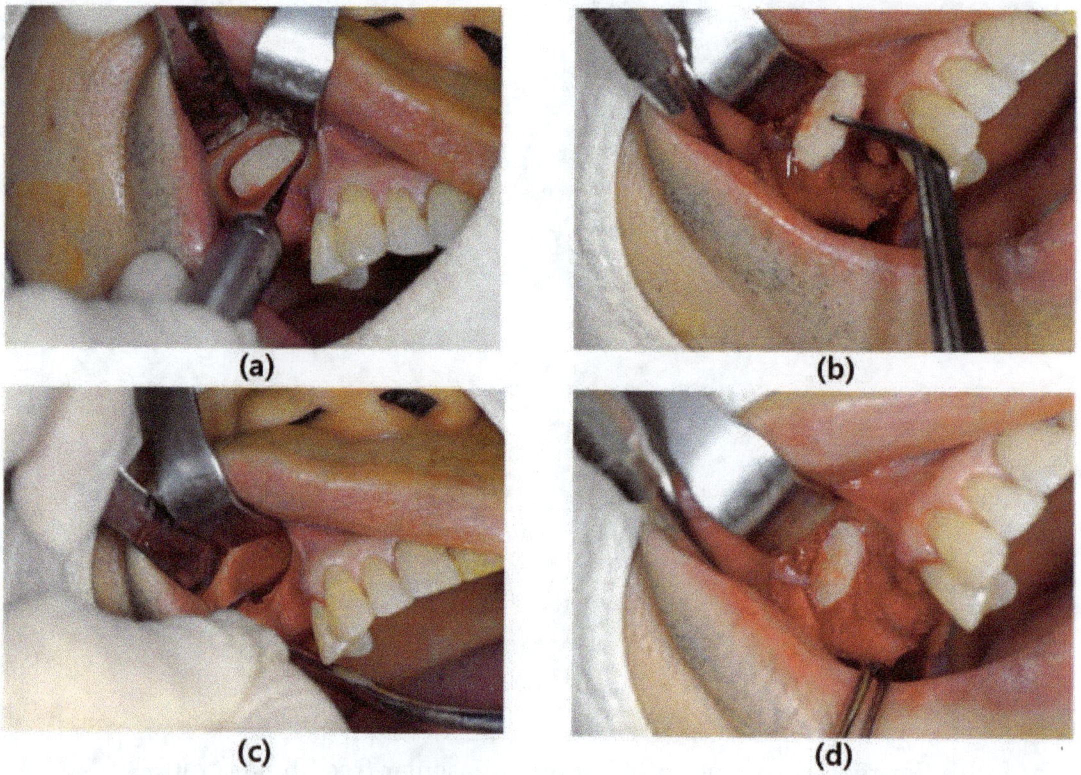

Fig. 15. Outfracture osteotomy sinus graft technique.
(a) Osteotomy of the lateral maxillary wall is done as routine.
(b) Outfractured bony window is shown, which is to be preserved in normal saline solution during Schneiderian membrane elevation.
(c) Schneiderian membrane is elevated via bony aperture created by the osteotomy.
(d) Repositioned bony segment is secured without a screw or plate.
Courtesy by Lee JK in J Oral Maxillofac Surg 68:1639-1641 (2010).

3.6.2 Dental implant treatment in severely compromised posterior maxillary edentulous ridges

Fifty nine years old female resorted to our clinic with a chief complaint of chewing difficulty owing to complete loss of teeth. Several years of ill-fitting denture was very annoying to her and doing without this ill-fitting denture inevitably caused her severe alveolar resorption. She agreed with mandibular removable denture but insisted on fixed type maxillary prosthesis. Prosthesis design for the mandible was an implant supported overdenture but maxillary alveolar bone must be augmented for dental implant treatment. Anterior maxillary wall was planed to be augmented with external oblique ridge-ramal bone block from both sides of the mandible. Both maxillary sinuses were examined with dental CT showing that double resorption inner and outer sides of the sinus floor due to pneumatisation and alveolar bone resorption, respectively (Fig. 16-a and b). The CT showed resultant minimal alveolar bone heights with maximum thickness of 2 mm in these areas. Maxillary sinus floor augmentation was done utilising outfracture osteotomy sinus graft technique (Fig. 16-c and d) on both sides. She was very satisfied with maxillary fixed-type prosthesis along with removable-type mandibular overdenture (Fig. 16-e). Radiographic finding after final prosthodontic treatment demonstrated excellent treatment results Fig. 16-f).

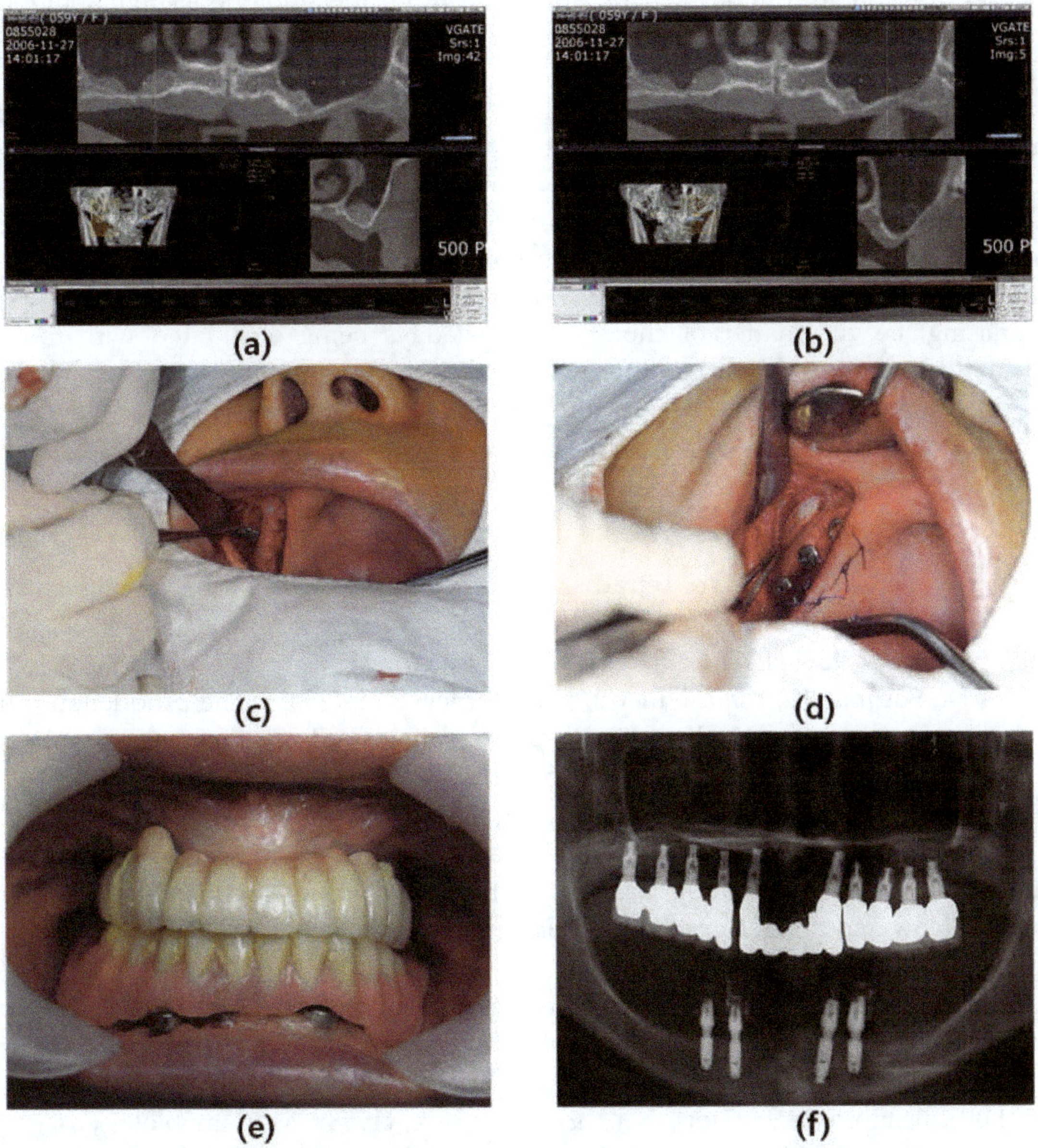

Fig. 16. Sinus graft and dental implant treatment with fixed type bridges.
Preoperative CT showed severe pneumatisation and alveolar bone loss leaving only thin cortex of 2 mm thickness or less on both sides of the floor of the maxillary sinus (a and b). Sinus graft utilising outfracture osteotomy technique was done on right maxillary antrum (c and d). The same procedure was repeated on the contralateral sides later. Clinical photograph (e) and panoramic radiograph (f) of final prosthesis showed good function without any complication.

4. Conclusion

Treatment strategy for the dental implant-supported prosthesis in atrophic edentulous alveolar ridge is one of the most difficult tasks for dental clinicians. As a rule, autogenous bone is a gold standard of bone graft and has rated better treatment score than any other types of bone. Clinically available autogenous donor bone was exemplified by respective clinical cases with the theoretical background based upon the basic bone biology. In severe cases such as the defect involving not only an alveolar bone but also a basal part of the jaw bone, harvesting a donor bone was not a minor oral surgery anymore requiring microsurgical techniques under general anaesthesia. But the sinus floor augmentation was possible under local anaesthesia even in the severe cases with the remaining floor thickness only 2 mm or less (Fig. 16).

Dental implant treatment is a powerful option in the treatment choice for edentulous ridge and is now replacing many parts of the traditional prosthodontic treatment. In general losing teeth is accompanied by atrophic alveolar ridge, which compels dentists into complete understanding of the biology of bone augmentation to maximize the benefit of the patients. Ever accumulating medical information and technologies have been increasing the quality of life of many patients. Although still obscure many aspects of the biology of the bone grafting; i.e. the matter of choice, are nowadays being elucidated with molecular biological advancement. What is more, what makes the edentulous bone atrophic; i.e. the matter of why, is unveiling its secret through unwearying enthusiasm of the many brilliant scientists. Having a long way to go, we're still on the road.

5. References

Aghaloo, T.L., Felsenfeld, A.L., & Tetradis, S. (2010). Osteonecrosis of the jaw in a patient on Denosumab. *Journal of Oral and Maxillofacial Surgery,* Vol.68, No.5, (May 2010), pp.959-963, ISSN 0278-2391

Bakker, A.D., Soejima, K., Klein-Nulend, J., & Burger, E.H. (2001). The production of nitric oxide and prostaglandin E(2) by primary bone cells is shear stress dependent. *Journal of Biomech*anics, Vol.34, No.5, (May 2001), pp.671-677, ISSN 0021-9290

Bilezikian, J.P., Raisz, L.G., & Rodan, G.A. (2002). *Principles of Bone Biology*(2nd ed.), Academic Press, ISBN 0-12-098652-3, London, UK

Boyne, P.J. & James, R.A. (1980). Grafting of the maxillary sinus floor with autogenous marrow and bone. *Journal of Oral Surgery,* Vol.38, No.8, (August 1980), pp.613-616, ISSN 0022-3255

Burger, E.H. & Klein-Nulend, J. (1999). Mechanotransduction in bone-role of the lacuno-canalicular network. *FASEB J,* Vol.13, No.Suppl, (May 1999), pp.S101-112, ISSN 0892-6638

Carter, D.R., Beaupré, G.S., Giori, N.J., & Helms, J.A. (1998). Mechanobiology of skeletal regeneration. *Clinical Orthopedics and Related Research,* Vol.355, No.Suppl, (October 1998), ppS41-55, ISSN 0009-921X

Cheng, B., Zhao, S., Luo, J., Sprague, E., Bonewald, L.F., & Jiang, J.X. (2001). Expression of functional gap junctions and regulation by fluid flow in osteocyte-like MLO-Y4 cells. *Journal of Bone and Mineral Research,* Vol.16, No.2, (February 2001), pp.249-259, ISSN 0884-0431

Cherian, P.P., Siller-Jackson, A.J., Gu, S., Wang, X., Bonewald, L.F., Sprague, E. & Jiang, J.X. (2005). Mechanical strain opens connexin 43 hemichannels in osteocytes: a novel mechanism for the release of prostaglandin. *Molecular Biology of the Cell*, Vol.16, No.7, (July 2005), pp.3100–3106, ISSN 1059-1524

Civitell, R. (2008). Cell–cell communication in the osteoblast/osteocyte lineage. *Archives of Biochemistry and Biophysics*, Vol.473, No.2, (May 2008), pp.188-192, ISSN 0003-9861

De Clercq, C.A., Abeloos, J.S., Mommaerts, M.Y., & Neyt, L.F. (1995). Temporomandibular joint symptoms in an orthognathic surgery population. *Journal of Craniomaxillofacial Surgery*, Vol.23, No.3, (June 1995), pp.195-199, ISSN 1010-5182

Frost, H.M. (1996). Perspectives: a proposed general model of the "mechanostat" (suggestions from a new skeletal-biologic paradigm). *Anatomical Record-Advances in Integrative Anatomy and Evolutionary Biology*, Vol.244, No.2, (February 1996), pp. 139-147, ISSN 1932-8486

Harada, S. & Rodan, G.A. (2003). Control of osteoblast function and regulation of bone mass. *Nature*, Vol.423, No.6937, (May 2003), pp.349-355, ISSN 0028-0836

Huang, H., Kamm, R.D., & Lee, R.T. (2004). Cell mechanics and mechanotransduction: pathways, probes, and physiology. *American Journal of Physiology-Cell Physiology*, Vol.287, No.1, (July 2004), pp.C1-C11, ISSN 0363-6143

Jaalouk, D.E. & Lammerding, J. (2009). Mechanotransduction gone awry. *Nature Reviews Molecular Cell Biology*, Vol.10, No.1, (January 2009), pp63-73, ISSN 1471-0072

Jørgensen, N.R., Teilmann, S.C., Henriksen, Z., Civitelli, R., Sørensen, O.H., & Steinberg, T.H. (2003). Activation of L-type calcium channels is required for gap junction-mediated intercellular calcium signaling in osteoblastic cells. *Journal of Biological Chemistry*, Vol.278, No.6, (February 2003), pp.4082-4086, ISSN 0021-9258

Lavery, K.M. (1994). Basic principles of treatment, In: *Rowe and Williams' Maxillofacial Injuries*, Williams, J.Ll., pp.51-64, Churchill Livingstone, ISBN 0 443 04591 7, Edinburgh, UK

Lee, J.K. (2010). Outfracture osteotomy on lateral maxillary wall as a modified sinus graft technique. *Journal of Oral and Maxillofacial Surgery*, Vol.68, No.7, (July 2010), pp.1639-1641, ISSN 0278-2391

Machwate, M., Harada, S., Leu, C.T., Seedor, G., Labelle, M., Gallant, M., Hutchins, S., Lachance, N., Sawyer, N., Slipetz, D., Metters, K.M., Rodan, S.B., Young, R., & Rodan, G.A. (2001). Prostaglandin Receptor EP_4 Mediates the Bone Anabolic Effects of PGE_2. *Molecular Pharmacology*, Vol. 60, No. 1, (July 2001), pp.36-41, ISSN 0026-895X

MacKinnon, P.C.B. & Morris, J.F. (1990). *Oxford Textbook of Functional Anatomy*. Vol.3, Oxford University Press, ISBN 0-19-261519-X, London, UK

Marx RE. (2003). Pamidronate (Aredia) and zolendronate (Zometa) induced avascular necrosis of the jaws: a growing epidemic. *Journal of Oral and Maxillofacial Surgery*, Vol.61, No.9, (September 2003), pp. 1115-1117. ISSN 0278-2391

Misch, C.E. (2008). *Contemporary Implant Dentistry* (3rd ed.), Mosby, ISBN 978-0-323-04373-1, St. Louis, MO

Moss, M.L. (1997). The functional matrix hypothesis revisited. 2. The role of an osseous connected cellular network. *American Journal of Orthodontics and Dentofacial Orthopedics,* Vol.112, No.2, (February 1997) pp.221-226, ISSN 0889-5406

Park, H.W. (2005). *Human Embryology*(3rd ed.), Koonja Publishing Co., ISBN 89-7089-534-5, Seoul, Korea

Reich, K.M., Mcallister, T.N., Gudi, S, & Frangos, J.A. (1997). Activation of G Proteins Mediates Flow-Induced Prostaglandin E2 Production in Osteoblasts. *Endocrinology,* Vol. 138, No. 3, (March 1997) pp.1014-1018, ISSN 0013-7227

Robling, A.G., Castillo, A.B., & Turnern, C.H. (2006). Biomechanical and molecular regulation of bone remodeling. *Annual Review of Biomedical Engineering,* Vol.8, No.1, (January 2006) pp.455-498, ISSN 1523-9829

Shapiro, F. (2008). Bone development and its relation to fracture repair. The role of mesenchymal osteoblasts and surface osteoblasts. *European Cells and Materials,* Vol.15, No.1, (April 2008) pp.53-76, ISSN 1473-2262

Siller-Jackson, A. J., Burra, S., Gu, S., Xia, X., Bonewald, L.F., Sprague, E., & Jiang, J.X. (2008). Adaptation of Connexin 43-Hemichannel Prostaglandin Release to Mechanical Loading. *Journal of Biological Chemistry,* Vol.283, No.39, (September 2008) pp.26374-26382, ISSN 0021-9258

Singer, N. (November 10, 2010). Drug Suits Raise Questions for Doctors, and Juries, In: *the New York Times,* January 10, 2010, Available from: http://www.nytimes.com/2010/11/11/health/11bone.html?_r=1&ref=merckandcompany

Song, S.I., Jeong, H.R., Kim, H.M., & Lee, J.K. (2009). Clinical investigation on the feasibility of outfracture osteotomy sinus graft technique. *Journal of Korean Association of Oral and Maxillofacial Surgery,* Vol.35, No.5, (October 2009), pp.367-371, ISSN 1225-1585

Tatum, H. Jr. (1986). Maxillary and sinus implant reconstructions. *Dental Clinics of North America,* Vol.30, No.2, (April 1986), pp.207-229, ISSN 0011-8532

Taylor, K.H., Middlefell, L.S., & Mizen, K.D. (2010). Osteonecrosis of the jaws induced by anti-RANK ligand therapy. *British Journal of Oral and Maxillofacial Surgery,* Vol.48, No.3, (April 2010) pp. 221-223, ISSN 0266-4356

van Bezooijen, R.L., Svensson, J.P., Eefting, D., Visser, A., van der Horst, G., Karperien, M., Quax, P.H., Vrieling, H., Papapoulos, S.E., ten Dijke, P., & Löwik, C.W. (2007). Wnt but not BMP signaling is involved in the inhibitory action of sclerostin on BMP-stimulated bone formation. *Journal of Bone and Mineral Research,* Vol.22, No.1, (January 2007), pp.19–28, ISSN 0884-0431

Vitkov, L., Gellrich, N.C., & Hannig, M. (2005). Sinus floor elevation via hydraulic detachment and elevation of the Schneiderian membrane. *Clinical Oral Implants Research,* Vol.16, No.5, (October 2005), pp.615-621, ISSN 0905-7161

10

Clinical Complications of Dental Implants

Su-Gwan Kim
Dept. of Oral and Maxillofacial Surgery, School of Dentistry, Chosun University
Republic of Korea

1. Introduction

Dental implant surgery has become routine treatment in dentistry and is generally considered to be a safe surgical procedure with a high success rate. However, complications should be taken into consideration because they can follow dental implant surgery as with any other surgical procedure. Many of the complications can be resolved without severe problems; however, in some cases, they can cause dental implant failure or even life-threatening circumstances. Avoiding complications begins with careful treatment planning based on accurate preoperative anatomic evaluations and an understanding of all potential problems. This chapter contains surgical complications associated with dental implant surgery and management.

2. Complications associated with implant surgery

2.1 Hemorrhage

The submental artery (2mm in average diameter) (Greenstein et al., 2008 as cited in Hofschneider et al., 1999) is a branch of the facial artery. The sublingual artery (2 mm in average diameter) arises from the lingual artery and is found coronal to the mylohyoid muscle (Greenstein et al., 2008 as cited in Martin et al., 1993). The arterial blood supply of the floor of the mouth is formed by an anastomosis of the sublingual and submental arteries. In the canine area, the vessels are located closer to the lingual plate and alveolar crest than they are in more posterior areas (Dubois et al., 2010). Intraosseous hemorrhage is not a serious event, and control of the hemorrhage can be ensured by compressing the area with a directional indicator, an abutment, or the implant (Annibali et al., 2009). However, severe bleeding and the formation of massive hematomas in the floor of the mouth are the result of an arterial trauma. A vascular wound may occur after detrimental surgical manipulations or tearing of the lingual periosteum, but in most cases, it is attributed to perforations of the lingual cortical plate. Mechanical pressure exerted by the expanding hematomas displaces the tongue and floor of the mouth both superiorly and posteriorly (Kalpidis & Setayesh, 2004). This occurrence may lead to extensive bleeding into the submandibular space, resulting in a life-threatening acute airway obstruction within the first few hours after surgery (Goodacre et al., 1999). The hemorrhage can easily spread in the loose tissues of the floor of the mouth (Fig. 1.), the sublingual area, and the space between the lingual muscles, which may require intubation or an emergency tracheostomy (Dubois et al., 2010). The surgeons also should consider other sources of potential hemorrhage and subsequent hematoma formation, including injuries to muscles or other soft tissues (Isaacson, 2004) (Fig.

2.). The escalating symptomatology of massive bleeding and progressive respiratory distress strongly resemble the clinical development of Ludwig's angina. Most important is the immediate bimanual compression at the suspected site of perforation and transport of the patient to the nearest hospital to secure the airway without delay (Dubois et al., 2010).

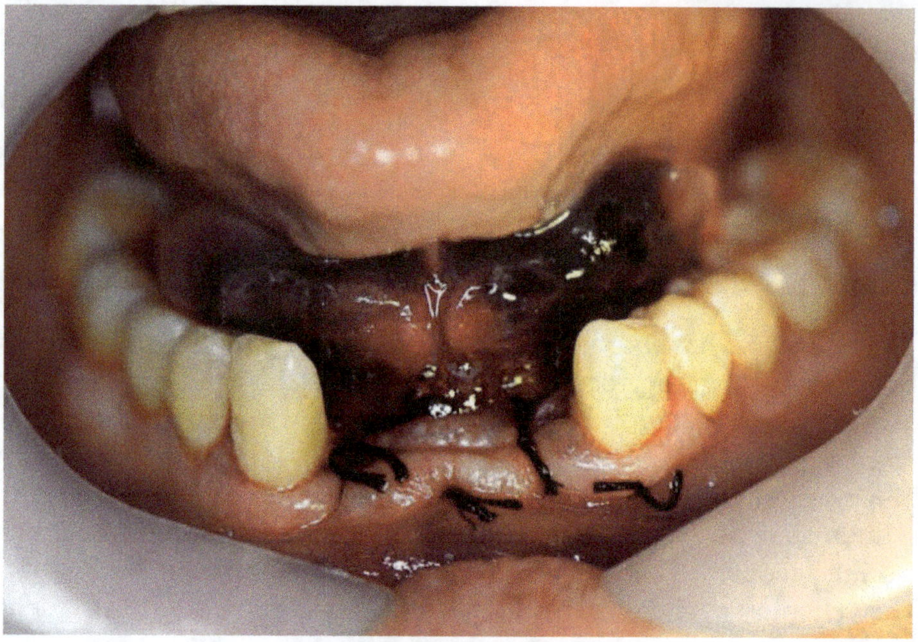

Fig. 1. A severe hematoma on the anterior floor of the mouth after implant placement in the anterior mandible.

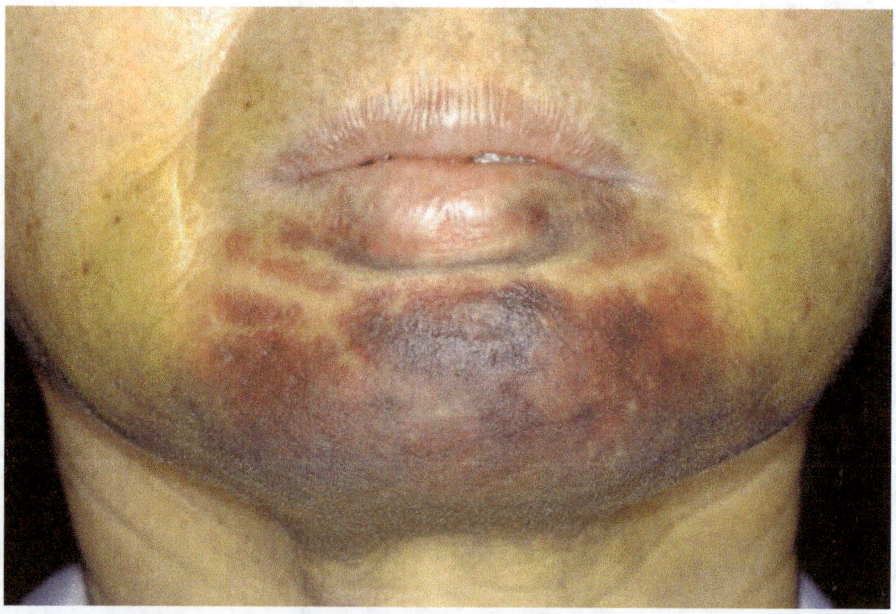

Fig. 2. Ecchymosis on the chin after implant placement in the anterior mandible.

Once the airway is controlled, efforts are undertaken for the definitive resolution of the hemorrhage (Kalpidis & Setayesh, 2004 as cited in Givol, 2000). Hemorrhages can be controlled by gauze tamponage, application of hemostatic agents, cauterization, or digital compression. If a hemorrhage cannot be controlled by these methods, ligation of the bleeding vessel should be performed. An endovascular angiography is an alternative diagnostic tool that can overcome unsuccessful attempts to define and isolate the bleeding source (Fig. 3.) (Kalpidis & Setayesh, 2004). Incisions in the mucosa to relieve the hematoma should be avoided because they may promote further bleeding. The removal of an already inserted implant would also be ineffective (Fig. 4.) (Kalpidis & Setayesh, 2004) (Table 1).

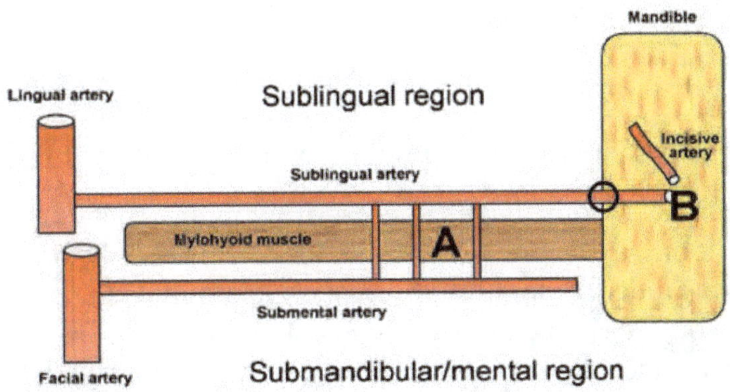

Fig. 3. A schematic representation of the arterial anatomy in the floor of the mouth (Kalpidis & Setayesh, 2004).

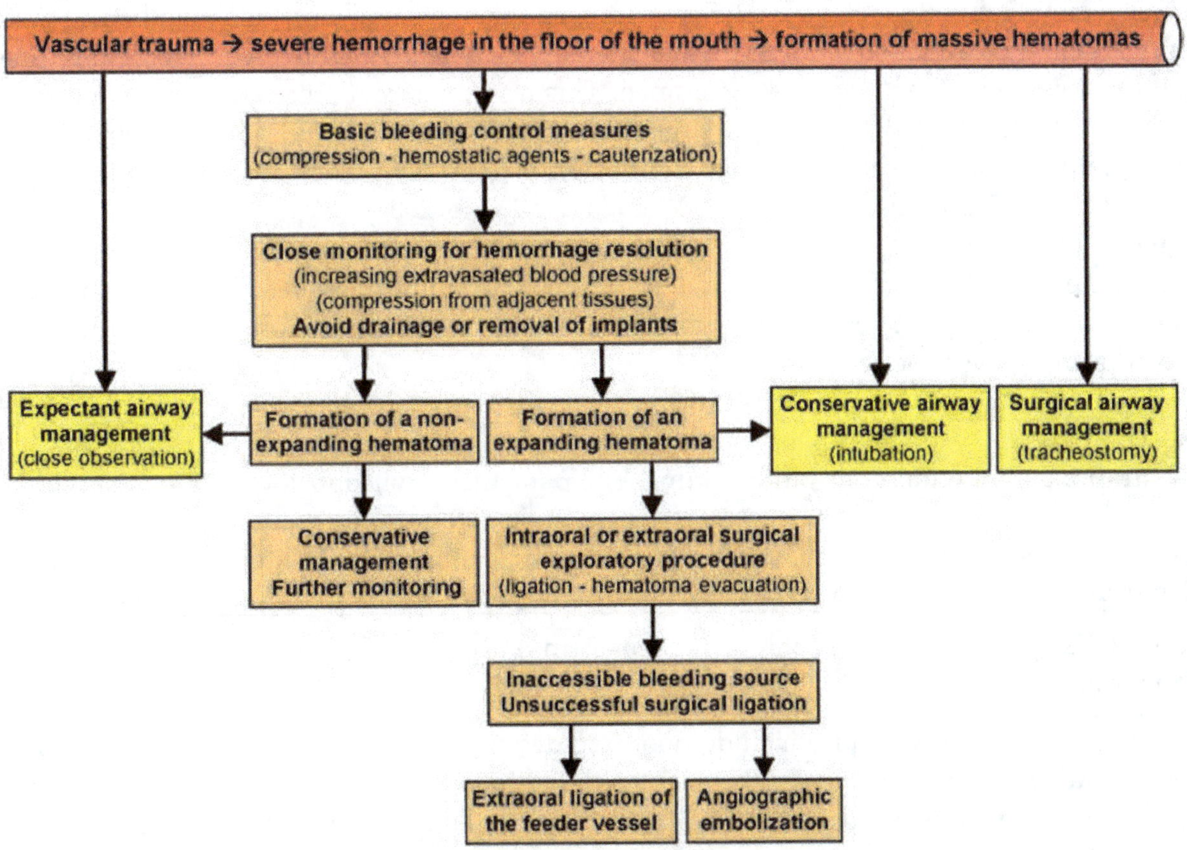

Fig. 4. A flow diagram of airway management and control of massive hemorrhage in the floor of mouth associated with implant placement in the anterior mandibular region (Kalpidis & Setayesh, 2004).

Bleeding site during implant osteotomy	Arteries	Treatments
Posterior mandible	Mylohyoid	Finger pressure at the site
Middle lingual of mandible	Submental	Surgical ligation of facial and lingual arteries
Anterior lingual of mandible	Terminal branch of sublingual or submental	Compression, vasoconstriction, cauterization, or ligation
Invading the mandibular canal	Inferior alveolar artery	Bone graft

Table 1. Treatment of a hemorrhage at an implant osteotomy site (Park & Wang, 2005)

To prevent unintentional hemorrhages in cases involving the immediate placement of implants or recent tooth extractions, the practitioner should be careful not to use the extraction socket as a guide for angulation because this may lead to the perforation of the lingual cortex (Isaacson, 2004 as cited in Givol, 2000). Soft-tissue management during the procedure is essential, and clinicians should make every attempt to avoid subperiosteal tears (Isaacson, 2004).

2.2 Neurosensory disturbances

The inferior alveolar nerve is midway between the buccal and lingual cortical plates in the first molar region (Tammisalo et al., 1992). In about 1% of patients, however, the mandibular canal bifurcates in the inferior superior or medial lateral planes. Thus, a bifurcated mandibular canal will manifest more than one mental foramen. This may or may not be seen on panoramic or periapical films. Accordingly, Dario suggested that clinicians should consider obtaining a preoperative tomogram to avoid nerve injuries prior to implant placement above the inferior alveolar canal (Greenstein & Tarnow, 2006 as cited in Dario, 2002).

A mean incidence of neurosensory disturbance incidence after implant surgery was 6.1% (Goodacre et al., 1999) to 7% (Goodacre et al., 2003), with a range between 0.6% and 39%. Nerve damage can have results ranging from mild paresthesia to complete anesthesia or even disabling dysesthesia (Table 2).

Neurapraxia	There is no loss of continuity of the nerve; it has been stretched or has undergone blunt trauma. The parasthesia will subside, and feeling will return in days to weeks.
Axonotmesis	Nerve is damaged but not severed; feeling returns within 2 to 6 months.
Neurotmesis	Severed nerve; poor prognosis for resolution of parasthesia.

Table 2. Classification of nerve injuries (Greenstein & Tarnow, 2006 as cited in Jalbout & Tabourian, 2004)

Possible causes of nerve injury include poor flap design, traumatic flap reflection, accidental intraneural injection, traction on the mental nerve in an elevated flap, penetration of the osteotomy preparation and compression of the implant body into the canal (Fig. 5.)(Misch & Wang, 2008). Nerve injuries may be caused indirectly by postsurgical intra-alveolar edema or hematomas that produce a temporary pressure increase, especially inside the mandibular canal. Direct traumas are the most frequent causes of nerve injury, and they may occur through five mechanisms: compression, stretch, cut, overheating, and accidental puncture

(Annibali et al., 2009). Finally, prolonged pressure from neuritis may lead to the permanent degeneration of the affected nerve (Park & Wang, 2005).

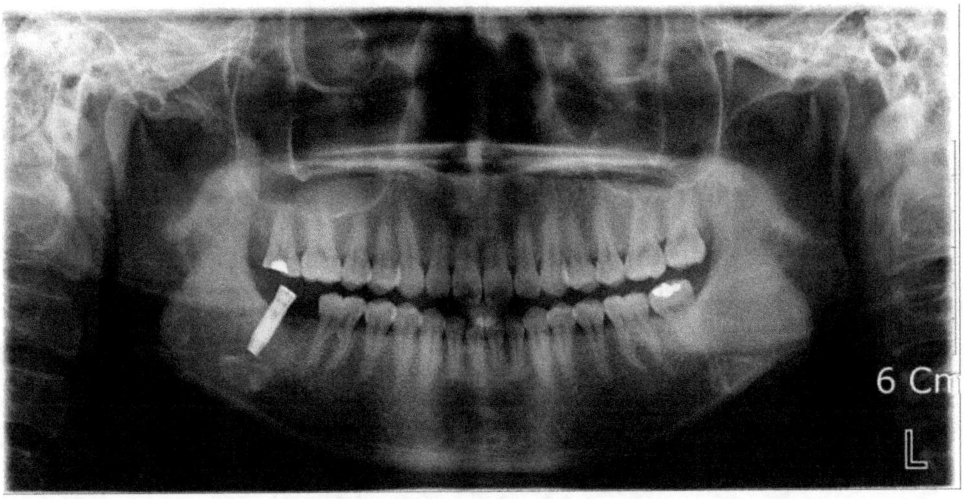

Fig. 5. An inferior alveolar nerve injury after implant placement of #47.

The mental nerve is at particular risk of iatrogenic injury because it arises from asymmetric foramina and forms a concave loop anteriorly. In edentulous patients, it may be very close to the bone surface or the top of the crest.

The nerve injury may cause one of the following conditions: parasthesia (numb feeling), hypoesthesia (reduced feeling), hyperesthesia (increased sensitivity), dysthesia (painful sensation), or anesthesia (complete loss of feeling) of the teeth, the lower lip, or the surrounding skin and mucosa (Greenstein & Tarnow, 2006 as cited in Sharawy & Misch, 1999).

Overpenetration occurs when the cortical portion of the alveolar crest places resistance on the drill. However, as it enters the marrow spaces, a drill may drop into the neurovascular bundle unless the surgeon has excellent control (Misch & Wang, 2008).

For implants placed in the atrophic posterior mandible, the routine use of intraoperative periapical radiographs during the drilling sequence can help avoid the risk of injury to the inferior alveolar nerve. Periapical radiographs used intraoperatively to obtain working length measurements are similar in concept to techniques used in root canal therapy. This method can reliably determine safe distances between the implant and the inferior alveolar canal, thus avoiding the risk of injury to the nerve altogether (Burstein et al., 2008).

The appropriate magnification correction factor should be used, and drill guards can be placed on burs to avoid the unintentional overpenetration of the drill. A safety margin of 2 mm between the entire implant body and any nerve canal should be maintained (Greenstein et al., 2008, as cited in Greenstein & Tarnow, 2006; Worthington, 2004). Additionally, surgical placements of implants should be at least 3 mm in front of the mental foramen (Greenstein & Tarnow, 2006). When placing implants in proximity to the mental foramen, the clinician must take into consideration the anterior loop of the nerve and the available bone above the mental foramen, because the inferior alveolar nerve often rises as it approaches the mental foramen (Kraut & Chahal, 2002). Finally, although the depths of the implant bur are variable, the drill bur may be longer than the implant according to the manufacturers (Table 3).

Be sure to include nerve injury as an item in the informed consent document. Measure the radiograph with care. Apply the correct magnification factor. Consider the bony crestal anatomy: If the ridge is thin buccolingually, is this useless bone or should an augmentation procedure be done? Is the buccolingual position of the crestal peak of bone influencing the measurement of available bone? Consider the buccolingual position of the nerve canal.	Use coronal true-size tomograms where needed. Allow a 1 to 2 mm safety zone. Use a drill guard. Take care with countersinking not to lose support of the crestal cortical bone. Use the aforementioned formula to calculate implant length. Keep the radiograph and the calculation in the patient's chart as powerful evidence of meticulous patient care.

Table 3. Recommendations to avoid nerve injuries during implant placement (Worthington, 2004)

The mental foramen may be located at or near the crest of an atrophic mandible. To avoid damage to the mental nerve in patients with atrophic mandibles, the clinician may need to make incisions in the area of the mental foramen that are lingual to the crest of the mandible (Kraut & Chahal, 2002).

If an implant is in danger of violating the canal, its depth should be decreased in the bone (i.e., by unscrewing it a few turns) and left short of the canal or removed. Because the altered sensation may be due to an inflammatory reaction, a course of steroid treatment or a high dose of nonsteroidal anti-inflammatory medication (e.g., ibuprofen [800 milligrams] three times per day) should be prescribed for three weeks (Kraut & Chahal, 2002). Adjunct drugs such as clonazepam, carbamazepine, or vitamin B-complex might alleviate neuritis via their known neuronal anti-inflammatory actions.

If improvement is noted at three weeks on the basis of a repeated neurosensory examination, the clinician can prescribe an additional three weeks of anti-inflammatory drug treatment. If the improvement is seen, however, the patient should be referred to a microneurosurgeon (Kraut & Chahal, 2002).

The patient should be referred for microsurgery if total anesthesia persists, or if after 16 weeks, dysesthesia is ongoing (Misch & Wang, 2008, as cited in Day, 1994; Nazarian et al., 2003).

Many studies have reported favorable patient responses to inferior alveolar nerve repairs. All have emphasized the need for repair before Wallerian degeneration of the distal portion of the inferior alveolar nerve has occurred; because this degeneration is a slow process, repair is possible four to six months after the injury has occurred (Kraut & Chahal, 2002).

2.3 Injury to adjacent teeth

Damage to teeth adjacent to the implant site may occur subsequent to the insertion of implants along an improper axis or after placement of excessively large implants (Figs. 6, 7.). This problem arises more frequently with single implants (Annibali et al., 2009). Adjacent teeth should be evaluated before implant placement. Pulpal and periradicular conditions such as small periapical radiolucencies, root resorption and large restorations in/near the vital pulp are often misdiagnosed. Dilacerated roots and excessive tilting in the mesiodistal direction that invades the implant space often prevent ideal placement (Misch & Wang, 2008). The tilt of adjacent teeth should be assessed before drilling. The damage of an adjacent tooth by implant placement may cause the tooth to become non-vital, and the tooth may require subsequent endodontic treatment. This will not only result in damage to an adjacent tooth but also implant failure (Sussman, 1998). Use of a surgical guide, radiographic analysis and CT scan can help locate the implant placement, thereby avoiding damage to adjacent teeth. The angulation of adjacent teeth and dilacerations of roots must be radiographically assessed prior to implant placement. Ideally, 1.5 to 2 mm of bone should be present between an implant and the adjacent tooth. Furthermore, inspection of a radiograph with a guide pin at a depth of 5 mm will facilitate osteotomy angulation corrections (Greenstein et al., 2008). To prevent a latent infection of the implant from the potential endodontic lesion, endodontic treatment should be performed (Sussman, 1998). Discrepancies between the apical and crestal interdental spaces as a result of mesial or distal tipping of the roots can be corrected orthodontically (Annibali et al., 2009).

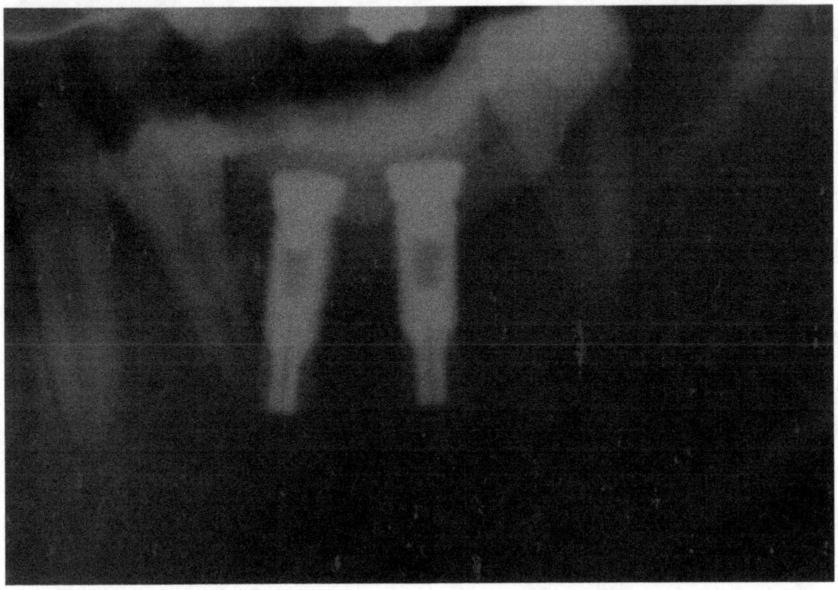

Fig. 6. Injury of an adjacent tooth by a malpositioned implant.

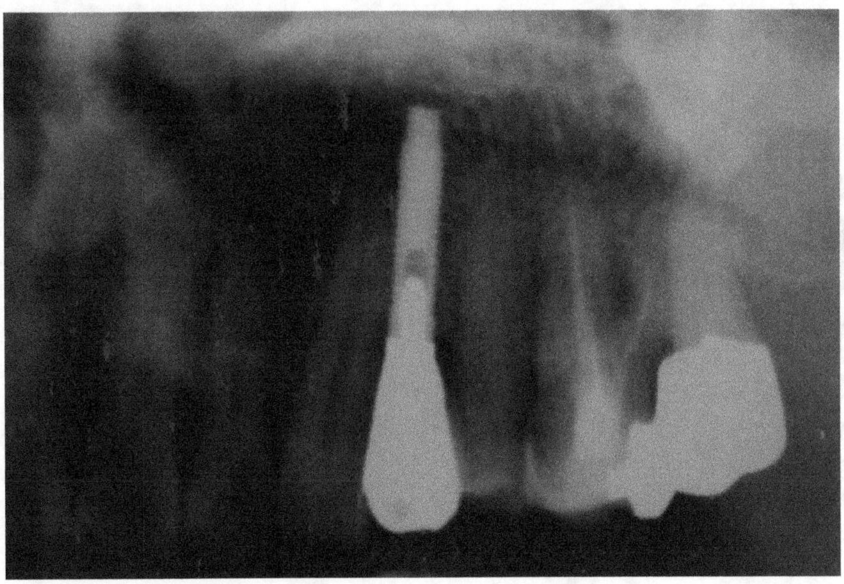

Fig. 7. A malpositioned implant hitting an adjacent tooth.

2.4 Flap dehiscence and exposure of graft material or barrier membrane

The most common postoperative complication is wound dehiscence, which sometimes occurs during the first 10 days (Greenstein et al., 2008). Contributing factors of dehiscence and exposure of the graft material or barrier membrane include flap tension, continuous mechanical trauma or irritation associated with the loosening of the cover screw, incorrect incisions and formation of sequestration of bone debris (Park & Wang, 2005). Premature exposure of barrier membranes may also cause contamination of the graft and its eventual loss (Figs. 8, 9.).

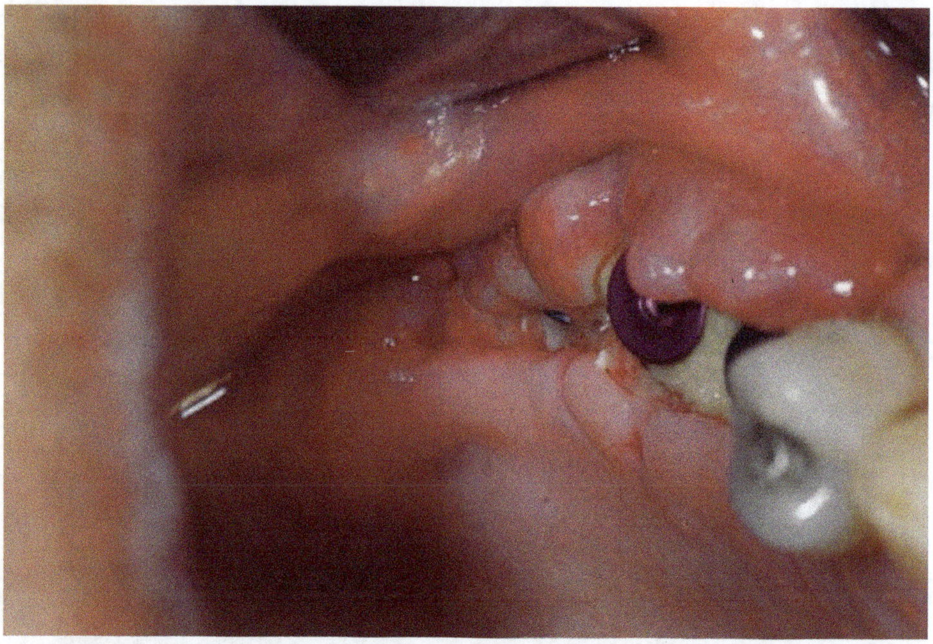

Fig. 8. A dehiscence after guided bone regeneration and implant placement using a non-resorbable membrane.

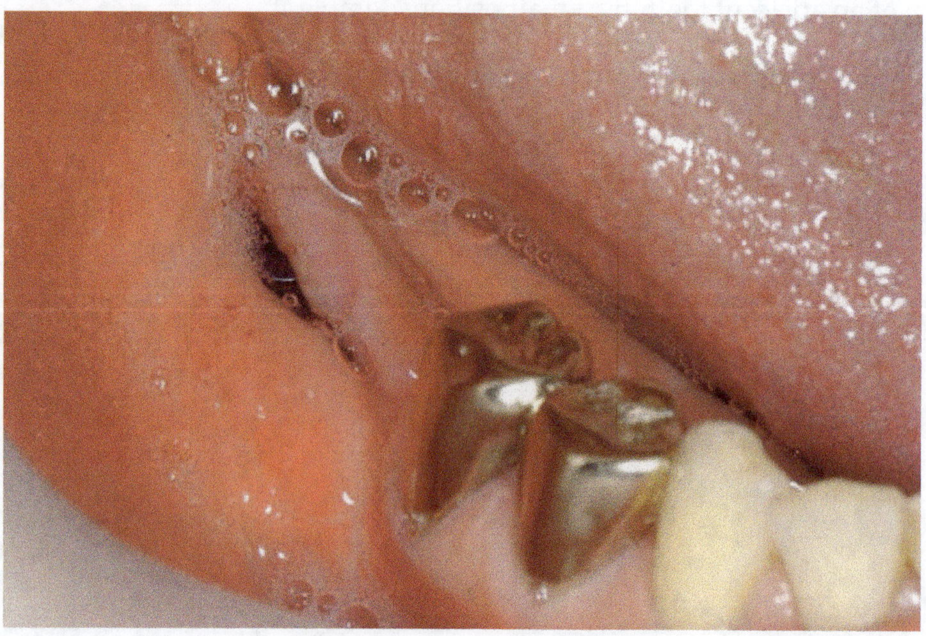

Fig. 9. A dehiscence after implant placement.

To avoid wound dehiscence, tension-free closure using a buccal releasing incision is most important. Dentures should be relieved with a tissue conditioner. Mattress sutures combined with interrupted sutures are also useful. When the dehiscence is small and occurs within 24 to 48 hours, the clinician can immediately resuture the dehiscence. Once the diameter of the wound is large (2 to 3 cm) or the time elapsed is > 2 days, it is suggested that the margins of the wound be excised and resutured (Fig. 10.) (Greenstein et al., 2008 as cited in Sadig & Almas, 2004). If the suture is not possible, chlorhexidine rinses twice a day and/or systemic antibiotics should be considered.

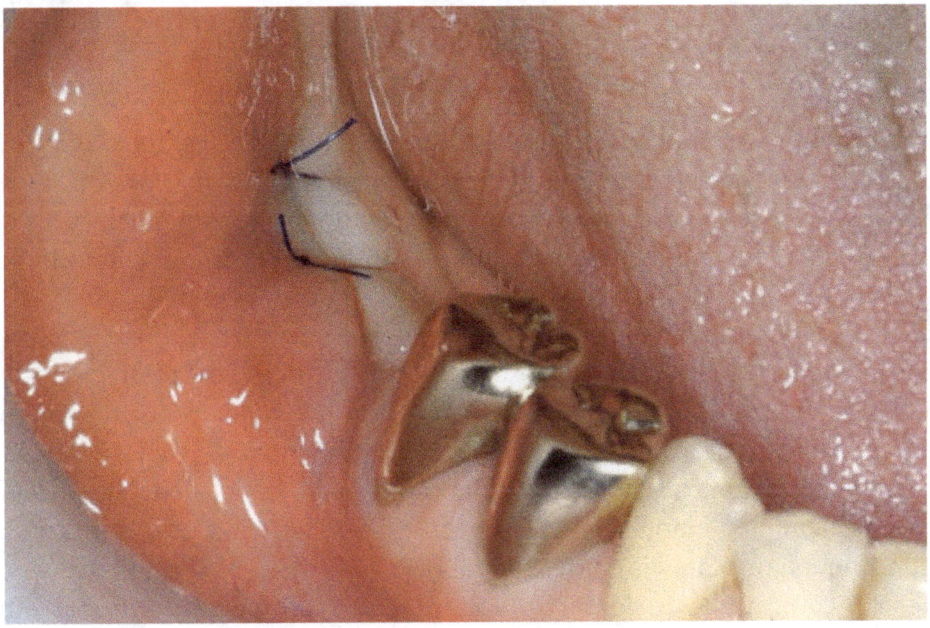

Fig. 10. Resuturing was performed to achieve closure of the dehiscence.

2.5 Bisphosphonate-related osteonecrosis

Bisphosphonates are drugs that inhibit bone resorption; they are widely used for the treatment of osteoporosis, multiple myeloma and skeletal complications of bone metastases (Table 4). The American Association of Oral and Maxillofacial Surgeons (AAOMS) states that patients are considered to have bisphosphonate-related osteonecrosis of the jaw (BRONJ) if they have the following three characteristics: current or previous treatment with a bisphosphonate, exposed or necrotic bone in the maxillofacial regin that has persisted for more than 8 weeks, and no history of localized radiotherapy to the jaws (Advisory Task Force on Bisphosphonate-Related Ostenonecrosis of the Jaws, 2007). The risk of BRONJ associated with oral bisphosphonates appears to increase when the duration of therapy more than 3 years. This time may be shortened in the presence of certain comorbidities. Type 2 diabetes mellitus (Abu-Id et al., 2008), prolonged steroid therapy (Advisory Task Force on Bisphosphonate-Related Ostenonecrosis of the Jaws, 2007), and health-threatening habits such as smoking (Wessel et al., 2008; Yarom et al., 2007) were suggested as predisposing conditions for the development of BRONJ.

If systemic conditions permit, discontinuation of oral bisphosphonates for a period of 3 months prior to and 3 months after elective invasive dental surgery may lower the risk of BRONJ. The risk reduction may vary depending on the duration of bisphosphonate exposure (Advisory Task Force on Bisphosphonate-Related Ostenonecrosis of the Jaws, 2007).

Active ingredient	Trade name	Administered
Alendronate	Fosamax®,Fosavance®	Orally
Etidronate	Osteum®, Difosfen®	Orally
Resedronate	Actonel®, Acrel®	Orally
Tiludronate	Skelid®	Orally
Zoledronate	Zometa®, Aclasta®	Intravenously
Pamidronate	Aredia®, Linoten®, Pamifos®, Xinsidona®	Intravenously
Ibandronate	Bondronat®	Orally, Intravenously
Clodronate	Bonefos®	Orally, Intravenously

Table 4. Different types of bisphosphonates in current usage (Montoya-Carralero et al., 2010)

Currently, there are no reliable or widely available tests for the risk of BRONJ. Marx et al. recommend a blood test, specifically involving a serum C-terminal telopeptide test (CTX) to assess a surrogate marker of bone turnover in patients taking oral bisphosphonates. Categorization of <100 pg/mL as high risk, 100 pg/mL to 150 pg/mL as moderate risk, and >150 pg/mL as minimal risk provides the clinician (Marx et al., 2007).

Many articles have confirmed that implant surgery in patients receiving oral bisphosphonate therapy does not result in BRONJ. (Bell &Bell, 2008; Fugazzotto et al., 2007; Grant et al.,2008; Jeffcoat, 2006) Nevertheless, patients taking bisphosphonates who either had implants that failed to integrate or had integrated implants that subsequently failed have been reported (Goss & Backhous, 2007; Stark & Epker, 1995; Wang et al., 2007).

The prognosis of dental implants that have been placed remains uncertain, and the use of osseointegrated dental implants is controversial.

AAOMS does not contraindicate dental implant placement in patients who have been taking bisphosphonates orally for less than three years prior to surgery, provided that they do not present other risk factors such as medications with corticosteroids or advanced age (e.g., older than seventy years). It has been reported that oral bisphosphonates had a lower risk because they took longer to develop bisphosphonate-induced osteonecrosis given their slower accumulation rates in bone (Ruggiero et al., 2004). Moreover, a drug holiday is recommended 3 to 6 months in duration before dental implant placement in patients with a history of oral bisphosphonate use for longer than 3 years (Ruggiero et al., 2009). Finally, current guidelines contraindicate the placement of dental implants in cancer patients treated with intravenous bisphosphonates (Ruggiero et al., 2009; Khan et al., 2008).

Although bisphosphonates tend to accumulate in sites of active bone remodeling like the jaws, surgical trauma to the alveolar bone during implant surgery could further stimulate the postoperative accumulation of the drug in the implanted site. The localized interference of bisphosphonates on areas of bone turnover may reduce the peri-implant bone resistance to oral bacteria in the long term, thus increasing the risk of peri-implantitis. The potential role of infection on implant failure and BRONJ occurrence is still debated. However, at least one study has reported a reduced incidence of BRONJ in patients who were given prophylactic antibiotics (Montefusco et al., 2008). In addition, the use of perioperative antibiotics and a chlorhexidene mouth wash have been suggested. Great attention should be paid to the oral hygiene and plaque control of implant-prosthetic restorations (Bedogni et al., 2010). Patients treated with bisphosphonates who receive implants should be followed for long periods of time. All patients treated with

oral bisphosphonates must be informed of the potential complications of implant failure and BRONJ development in both the short and long term before the placement of dental implants (Bedogni et al., 2010).
AAOMS has proposed the use of the following staging categories and treatment guidelines regarding BRONJ (Table 5).

BRONJ Staging	Treatment Strategies
At risk category: No apparent exposed/ necrotic bone in patients who have been treated with either oral or IV bisphosphonates	No treatment indicated Patient education
Stage 1: Exposed/necrotic bone in patients who are asymptomatic and have no evidence of infection	Antibacterial mouth rinse Clinical follow-up on a quarterly basis Patient education and review of indications for continued bisphosphonate therapy
Stage 2: Exposed/necrotic bone associated with infection as evidenced by pain and erythema in the region of the exposed bone with or without purulent drainage	Symptomatic treatment with broad-spectrum oral antibiotics, e.g., penicillin, cephalexin, clindamycin, or first generation fluoroquinolone Oral antibacterial mouth rinse Pain control Only superficial debridements to relieve soft tissue irritation
Stage 3: Exposed/necrotic bone in patients with pain, infection, and one or more of the following: pathologic fracture, extraoral fistula, or osteolysis extending to the inferior border	Antibacterial mouth rinse Antibiotic therapy and pain control Surgical debridement/resection for longer term palliation of infection and pain

Table 5. Staging and treatment strategies (Advisory Task Force on Bisphosphonate-Related Ostenonecrosis of the Jaws, 2007)

3. Complications associated with maxillary sinus lift

3.1 Schneiderian membrane perforation

The Schneiderian membrane, which is characterized by periosteum overlaid with a thin layer of pseudociliated stratified respiratory epithelium, constitutes an important barrier for the protection and defense of the sinus cavity. The integrity of the sinus membrane is essential in maintaining the healthy and normal function of the maxillary sinus (Ardekian et al., 2006).
The mucociliary apparatus protects the sinus against infection while the membrane also acts as a biologic barrier. If a perforation occurs, the membrane perforation could represent a window for bacterial penetration and invasion into the grafted area (Zijderveld et al., 2008). Failure to atraumatically elevate the Schneiderian membrane may result in graft migration or loss, exposure of the graft or the implant to the sinus, and postoperative site infection. In addition to contaminating the recipient site, disruption of the mucosa may alter the normal

mucociliary flow patterns, causing retention of secretions and infections around the foreign body (Ward et al., 2008).

The most common intraoperative complication seems to be Schneiderian membrane perforation, which occurs in 10% to 60% of all procedures (Ardekian et al., 2006; Pikos, 1999; Proussaefs et al., 2004). The risk of membrane perforation increases when anatomical variations such as a maxillary sinus septum, spine, or sharp edge are present (Chanavaz, 1990; van den Bergh et al., 2000). Very thin or thick maxillary sinus walls create higher risks of perforating the Schneiderian membrane. The angulation between the medial and lateral walls of the maxillary sinus seemed to exert an especially large influence on the incidence of membrane perforation. For example, sharper angles observed at the inner walls of the sinus in the vicinity of the second upper bicuspid presents a higher risk of perforation (Zijderveld et al., 2008).

The occurrence of iatrogenic sinus membrane perforations during surgery does not seem to be related to sinusitis in healthy people (Ardekian et al., 2006). However, large tears can cause sinusitis, graft infection, or graft displacement into the sinus, which could compromise new bone formation and implant survival (Reiser et al., 2001).

To minimize Schneiderian membrane perforations, surgeons must evaluate the maxillary sinus anatomy while considering the lateral thickness of the lateral wall, slope of the sinus wall, location of septa, membrane thickness through the radiography and CT analysis before maxillary sinus augmentation. Piezoelectric surgery is usually more time-consuming than other techniques, though the frequency and number of Schneiderian membrane perforations or lacerations are generally lower. If the bony lateral wall is thick, a reduction of the thickness of the wall before formation of the lateral window is recommended. In cases involving a very thin maxillary sinus wall, careful reflection of the mucoperiosteum is recommended while the Schneiderian membrane already shines a dark grayish-bluish color through the sinus wall. It is advised that clinicians not begin the lateral door preparation with a round stainless-steel burr; they should use a round diamond bur directly, thereby reducing the risk of a membrane perforation (Zijderveld et al., 2008). To prevent a perforation, some additional small holes in the suction device are recommended to diminish the suction power and to avoid the direct contact of the suction device with the Schneiderian membrane (Zijderveld et al., 2008).

If a tear in the membrane occurs along the periphery of the osteotomy and it is difficult to reengage the membrane, this situation can be managed by extending the outline of the osteotomy several millimeters past the original window and reestablishing contact with the membrane (Greenstein et al., 2008). In general, small tears (<5 to 8 mm) are mitigated simply by folding the membrane up against itself as the membrane is elevated (Chanavaz, 1990). Larger tears do not lend themselves to closure by infolding, and they would need additional methods to contain the graft in its desired position. It has been reported that large sinus membrane perforations should be repaired with collagen or a fibrin adhesive. In severe perforations, some investigators have even suggested abandoning the procedure for 6 to 9 months while the membrane regenerates (Karabuda et al., 2006).

3.2 Hemorrhage

The blood supply of the maxillary sinus is derived from the infraorbital artery, the greater palatine artery and the posterior superior alveolar artery (Chanavaz, 1990; Uchida et al., 1998a). Bleeding during sinus augmentation is rare because the main arteries are not within the surgical area. Although accidental laceration of the vessel is not life-threatening because of the small size of the artery, an impaired visualisation may compromise the elevation of the Schneiderian membrane and interfere with the placement of the graft material (Elian et al., 2005; Testori et al., 2010).

The blood supply to the buccal antral portions relevant to sinus floor elevation surgery occurs via two arteries: the posterior superior alveolar artery and the infraorbital artery, as well as their intraosseous branches and anastomoses (Solar et al., 1999). Anatomically, anastamosis between the posterior superior alveolar artery and infraorbital artery is always found at the lateral antral wall (Traxler et al, 1999); bleeding via damage to these arteries may occur during the formation of the lateral window. The average distance from the artery to the alveolar crest was 16.4 mm (Elian N et al., 2005) to 18.9 mm (± 2.82 mm) (Solar et al., 1999).

The height of the residual bony ridge appears to play a significant role in the location of the vessel. In classes A, B and C (Lekholm & Zarb classification (Lekholm & Zarb, 1985)), the vessel was found >15 mm from the alveolar crest, but in classes D and E, the value was >7 mm (mean 10.4 mm). It is recommended, therefore, to place the superior border of the osteotomy up to 15 mm from the alveolar crest in classes A, B and C, which is sufficient for sinus exposure and placement of long dental implants. In severely atrophic ridges, or classes D and E, where the surgeon has a tendency to place the osteotomy of the sinus wall too far cranially, there is a high probability of transecting the vessel (Mardinger et al., 2007b). Such bleeding can usually be controlled by pressure with a moist gauze pad (Fig. 11.)(Elian et al., 2005).

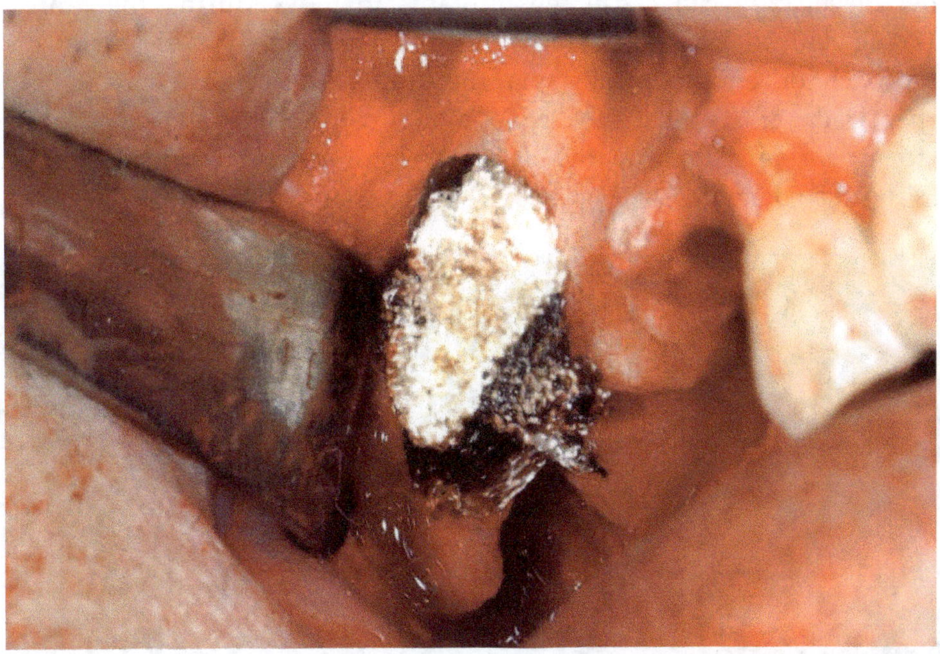

Fig. 11. Hemostasis was achieved using Surgicel during maxillary sinus augmentation.

A preoperative CT examination is essential to detect the location of the intraosseous anastomoses. In addition, piezoelectric surgical inserts may be beneficial in minimizing lacerations of vessels and membrane (Testori et al., 2010). A vestibular extraosseous anastomosis runs below the zygomatic process (Solar et al., 1999). This anastaomosis is located in the area of the periosteum overlying the lateral wall at a higher level than the intraosseous anastamosis. The vascular compromise would be the result of an inappropriate anterior releasing incision or vertical incision (Elian et al., 2005). To avoid damage to the extraosseous anastomosis, vertical mucosal incisions should extend superiorly as little as possible, and the periosteum should be prepared carefully (Solar et al., 1999).

3.3 Loss of the implant or graft materials into the maxillary sinus

The displacement of implants or graft materials into the maxillary sinus can result in a foreign-body reaction and cause serious complications. Migration of a dental implant into the maxillary sinus may present a risk for the development of maxillary sinusitis. Immediate implant insertion should be performed only if the residual bone is stable and high enough to ascertain high primary stability (Becker et al., 2008).
An implant can easily migrate into the sinus without apparent force in the posterior maxilla, clearly showing a lack of osseointegration (Fig. 12.). Various mechanisms have been proposed to explain the migration of an implant into the maxillary sinus, which fall under three main categories: changes in intrasinal and nasal pressures; autoimmune reaction to the implant, causing peri-implant bone destruction and compromising osseointegration; and resorption produced by an incorrect distribution of occlusal forces (Galindo et al., 2005). The changes in intrasinal and nasal air pressures produce a suction effect because of the negative pressure exerted by these cavities. A portion of the bone grafting material can become dislodged in the maxillary sinus at either the initial ridge augmentation or during the implant placement surgery. The natural ciliary movement in the maxillary sinus will transport foreign material toward the ostium (Hunter et al., 2009). In cases with less than 5 mm of bone, mastication can cause the implants to move during the graft maturation timeframe (Peleg et al., 2006). The implants must be immediately retrieved surgically via an intraoral approach or endoscopically via the transnasal route to avoid inflammatory complications (Ueda & Kaneda, 1992). To avoid complications when bone volume is inadequate to support an implant with sufficient length, a bone reconstruction procedure of the maxilla should be performed.

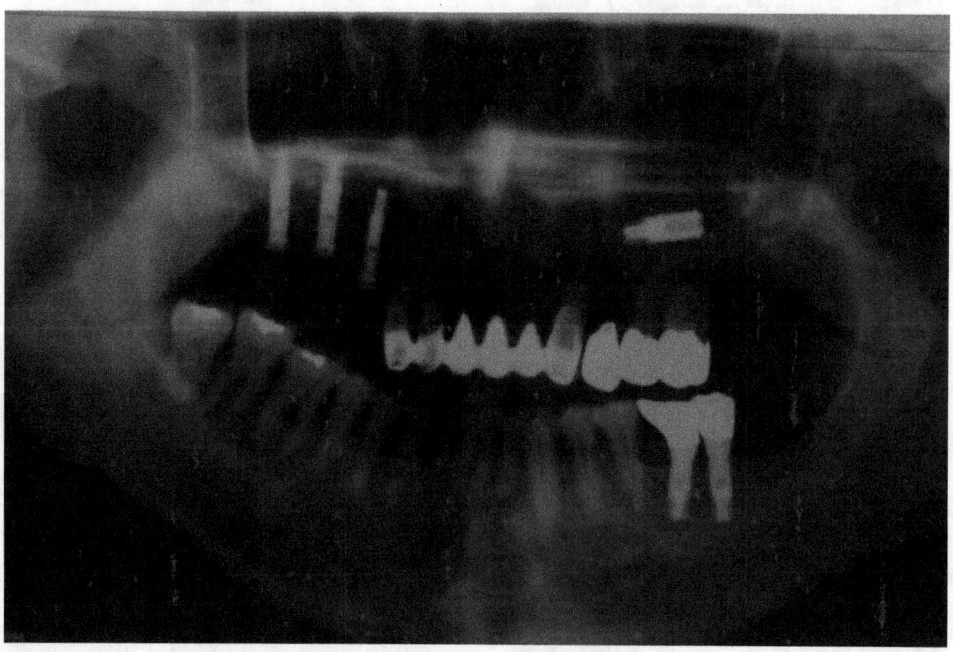

Fig. 12. Displacement of an implant into the maxillary sinus.

3.4 Postoperative maxillary sinusitis

The mean height of the maxillary sinus is 36 to 45 mm, the mean width mesiodistally is 25 to 35 mm, and the mean depth is 38 to 45 mm (laterally–medially). The average total maxillary sinus volume is 13.6±6.4 cc. The minimum maxillary sinus volume is 3.5 cc, while the maximum is 31.8 cc (Uchida, 1998b). The ostium is located on the superior aspect of the medial wall of the maxillary sinus above the first molar (van den Bergh et al., 2000). The normal drainage pattern of the maxillary sinus is into the middle nasal meatus by way of a naturally occurring ostium.

The ostium is usually 35 mm superior to the floor of the maxillary sinus (Zinner et al., 2008). This information can be used to prevent maxillary sinus complications such as sinusitis by the obstruction of the ostium. Radiographic imaging of the osteo-meatal complex is crucial in fully evaluating the physiologic health of the maxillary sinus and the likelihood of avoiding infections following maxillary bone grafting (Zinner et al., 2008).

Maxillary sinusitis can occur as a result of contamination of the maxillary sinus with oral or nasal pathogens or via ostial obstruction caused by postoperative swelling of the maxillary mucosa, hematoma and seroma. Mucosal swelling may lead to the reduction of the patency of the ostio-meatal unit (Figs. 13, 14.). This unit plays a key role in the development of sinusitis, through impairment of the mucociliar cleansing system (Bertrand & Eloy, 1992). Maxillary sinusitis can also occur because of non-vital bony fragments floating freely in the maxillary sinus. Another cause is the lack of asepsis during sinus augmentation (Timmenga et al., 2001). Maintenance of normal maxillary sinus physiology should be a major goal while ostium patency must be preserved. Therefore, the use of a systemic decongestant, such as pseudoephedrine, and a nasal spray containing a vasoconstrictor, such as phenylephrine, is recommended after implant surgery (Regev et al., 1995).

The development of sinusitis following sinus augmentation can be directly related to drainage disturbances, mainly as a result of septal deviation and allergies combined with oversized inferior and middle turbinates (Mardinger, 2007a). In the event of an inadvertent laceration or puncture of the Schneiderian membrane and inoculation of the maxillary sinus

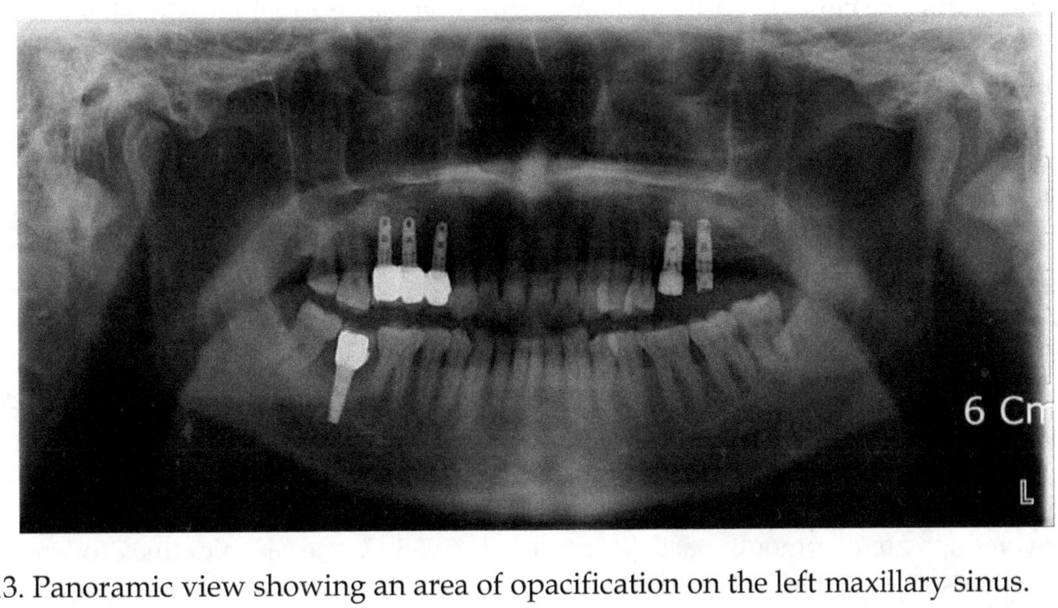

Fig. 13. Panoramic view showing an area of opacification on the left maxillary sinus.

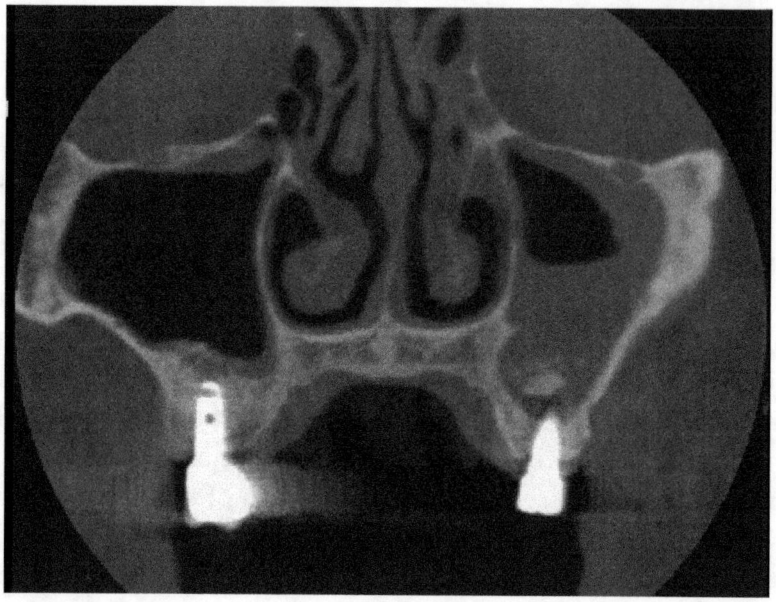

Fig. 14. Computed tomography scan clearly shows significant mucosal thickening along the entire lining of the sinus.

with oral bacteria, a healthy sinus with a patent osteo-meatal complex will usually remove the offending bacteria and remain healthy (Zinner et al., 2008). With no patent drainage pathway, the maxillary sinus quickly became obstructed, inflamed, and then infected (Hunter et al., 2009).

Timmenga et al. reported that the occurrence of postoperative sinusitis after bone grafting of the sinus floor is limited to patients with a predisposition for sinusitis (Timmenga et al., 1997). To minimize the occurrence of a postoperative infection, possible causes should be removed prior to sinus augmentation.

A history of excessive yellow or green nasal discharge, particularly with worsening nasal obstruction, is a relatively strong predictor of possible chronic bacterial sinusitis and may warrant further assessment for chronic sinusitis (Ward et al., 2008). A nasoendoscopic evaluation should be considered for patients with a history of frequent sinusitis to rule out the presence of an obstructive phenomenon as a risk factor before undergoing sinus augmentation (Manor et al., 2010).

Most implant failures occur 3 to 6 months after surgery, and they are usually not associated with an infection of the maxillary sinus (Becker et al., 2008). The clinical diagnosis of sinusitis is characterized by a triad of symptoms: nasal congestion, secretion or obstruction, and headache (Manor et al., 2010). If an infection develops (e.g., pain, redness, and tenderness) without fluctuance, antibiotics are administered. Once there is fluctuance, incision and drainage are performed in conjunction with systemic antibiotics (Barone et al., 2006; Regev et al., 1995).

Pathogens found have included *β-hemolytic* Strepococcus, *Enterococcus*, *Peptostreptococcus*, *Pneumococcus*, *Staphylococcus* (Doud Galli et al., 2001) and *Actinomycosis* (Roth & Montone, 1996). The antibiotics most effective in alleviating sinus infections are amoxicillin, trimethoprim sulfamethoxazole, and cefaclor. Amoxicillin with clavulanic acid and clindamycin also are commonly used (Regev et al., 1995). General guidelines for treatment of sinusitis was represented in Tables 6, 7.

Transient sinusitis	Chronic sinusitis
1. Use of decongestants and antibiotics 2. Follow-up after 2 weeks 3. If no recovery, transient sinusitis has possibly evolved into subacute sinusitis needing further treatment: a. Continuation of decongestants and antibiotics b. Maxillary drains for sinus irrigation c. CT scanning and consideration of functional endoscopic sinus surgery if no recovery within 3 weeks	1. Use of decongestants and antibiotics 2. CT scanning and functional endoscopic sinus surgery

Table 6. General guidelines for the treatment of transient and chronic maxillary sinusitis after maxillary sinus augmentation (Timmenga et al., 2001)

1. Preoperative evaluation of sinus clearance-related factors 2. Postsurgery: a nasal decongestant (xylomethazoline 0.05%) and topical corticosteroid (dexamethasone 0.01%) to prevent postsurgery obstruction of the ostium 3. Perioperative antibiotic prophylaxis (cephradine 1 g 3 times daily, starting 1 hour before surgery and continued for 48 hours after surgery)

Table 7. General guidelines for the prevention of transient and chronic maxillary sinusitis after maxillary sinus augmentation (Timmenga et al., 2001)

4. Conclusions

Although serious complications are uncommon, dental implant placement is not free of complications, as complications may occur at any stage (Table 8). Therefore, careful analysis via imaging, precise surgical techniques and an understanding of the anatomy of the surgical area are essential in preventing complications. One should be aware of the possible complications related to implant placement so that the patient can be properly informed. Prompt recognition of a developing problem and proper management are needed to minimize postoperative complications.

Problems	Possible causes	Solutions
Nerve injury	Mechanical injury by stretching, compression, and partial or total trans-section	Remove implant Wait for a period Rivotril®, Tegretol®, Vitamin B6
Hemorrhage during drilling	Injury of an artery	Extraoral pressure from the submental against the body of mandible Implant placement will stop bleeding

Fracture of mandible	Atrophic mandible	Immediate implant retrieval Bone graft Monocortical miniplates
Penetration of nasal/sinus floor	Type IV bone	Primary closure Antibiotic, decongestant, chlorhexidine
Lack of primary stability	Type IV bone, grafted bone, imprecise preparation, excessive countersinking	Remove implant, replace with larger diameter or longer implant
Maxillary sinus lift	Preexisting condition, surgical handling	Seal by folding the excess membrane, collagen membrane, bone graft, primary closure Antibiotics, decongestant, chlorhexidine
Significant bleeding	Subclinical bleeding diathesis, surgical handling	Atraumatic surgical technique, compression for >10min
Devitalization of adjacent teeth	Not enough space in between implant and adjacent tooth	Endodontic treatment

Table 8. Intraoperative surgical-related complications (Park & Wang, 2005)

5. References

Abu-Id, MH.; Warnke, PH. & Gottschalk J. (2008). "Bis-phossy jaws"- High and low risk factors for bisphosphonate-induced osteonecrosis of the jaw. *J Craniomaxillofac Surg,* Vol. 36, No. 2, (January 2008), pp. 95-103, ISSN 1010-5182, Edinburgh, Scotland

American Association of Oral and Maxillofacial Surgeons. (2007). Advisory Task Force on Bisphosphonate-Related Osteonecrosis of the Jaws, American Association of Oral and Maxillofacial Surgeons position paper on bisphosphonate-related osteonecrosis of the jaws. *J Oral Maxillofac Surg,* Vol. 65, No. 3, (March 2007), pp. 369-76, ISSN 0278-2391, Philadelphia, Pennsylvania, USA

Annibali, S.; Ripari, M., La Monaca, G., Tonoli, F. & Cristalli MP. (2009). Local accidents in dental implant surgery: prevention and treatment. *Int J Periodontics Restorative Dent* Vol. 29, No. 3, (June 2009), pp. 325-31, ISSN 0278-2391, Philadelphia, Pennsylvania, USA

Ardekian, L.; Oved-Peleg, E., Mactei, E. & Peled, M. (2006). The clinical significance of sinus membrane perforation during augmentation of the maxillary sinus. *J Oral Maxillofac Surg,* Vol. 64, No. 2, (February 2006), pp. 277-82, ISSN 0278-2391, Philadelphia, Pennsylvania, USA

Barone, A.; Santini, S., Sbordone, L., Crespi, R. & Covani, U. (2006). A clinical study of the outcomes and complications associated with maxillary sinus augmentation. *Int J*

Oral Maxillofac Implants, Vol. 21, No. 1, (Jan-Fab 2006), pp. 81-5, ISSN 0882-2786, Illinois, USA

Becker , ST.; Terheyden, H., Steinriede, A., Behrens, E., Springer, I. & Wiltfang, J. (2008). Prospective observation of 41 perforations of the Schneiderian membrane during sinus floor elevation. *Clin Oral Implants Res*, Vol. 19, No. 12, pp. 1285-9, ISSN 0905-7161, Oxford, England

Bedogni, A.; Bettini, G., Totola, A., Saia, G. & Nocini, PF. (2010). Oral bisphosphonate-associated osteonecrosis of the jaw after implant surgery: a case report and literature review. *J Oral Maxillofac Surg*, Vol. 68, No. 7, pp. 1662-6, ISSN 0278-2391, Philadelphia, Pennsylvania, USA

Bell, BM.; Bell R. (2008). Oral bisphosphonates and dental implants: A retrospective study. *J Oral Maxillofac Surg*, Vol. 66, Vol. 5, pp. 1022-4, ISSN 0278-2391, Philadelphia, Pennsylvania, USA

Bertrand, B.; Eloy, P. (1992). Relationship of chronic ethmoidal sinusitis, maxillary sinusitis, and ostial permeability controlled by sinusomanometry: statistical study. *Laryngoscope*, Vol. 102, No. 11, (Nov 1992), pp. 1281-4, ISSN 0023-852X, Philadelphia, Pennsylvania, USA

Burstein, J.; Mastin, C. & Le, B. (2008). Avoiding injury to the inferior alveolar nerve by routine use of intraoperative radiographs during implant placement. *J Oral Implantol*, Vol. 34, No. 1, pp. 34-8, ISSN 0160-6972, Kansas, USA

Chanavaz, M. (1990). Maxillary sinus: Anatomy, physiology, surgery, and bone grafting related to implantology—Eleven years of surgical experience. *J Oral Implantol*, Vol. 16, No. 3, pp. 199-209, ISSN 0160-6972, Kansas, USA

Dario, LJ. (2002). Implant placement above a bifurcated mandibular canal: a case report. *Implant Dent*, Vol. 11, No. 3, pp. 258-61, ISSN 1056-6163, Philadelphia, Pennsylvania, USA

Day, RH. (1994). Microneurosurgery of the injured trigeminal nerve. *Oral Maxillofac Surg Knowledge Update*, Vol. 1, pp. 91-116

Doud Galli, SK.; Lebowitz, RA., Giacchi, RJ., Glickman, R. & Jacobs, JB. (2001). Chronic sinusitis complicating sinus lift surgery. *Am J Rhinol*, Vol. 15, No. 3, (May-Jun 2001), pp. 181-6, ISSN 1050-6586, Rhode Island, USA

Dubois, L.; de Lange, J., Baas. E. & Van Ingen, J. (2010). Excessive bleeding in the floor of the mouth after endosseus implant placement: a report of two cases. *Int J Oral Maxillofac Surg*, Vol. 39, No. 4, (Apr 2010), pp. 412-5, ISSN 0901-5027, Edinburgh, Scotland

Elian, N.; Wallace, S., Cho, SC., Jalbout, ZN. & Froum, S. (2005). Distribution of the maxillary artery as it relates to sinus floor augmentation. *Int J Oral Maxillofac Implants*, Vol. 20, No. 5, (Sep-Oct), pp. 784-7, ISSN 0882-2786, Illinois, USA

Fugazzotto, PA.; Lightfoot, WS., Jaffin, R. & Kumar, A. (2007). Implant placement with or without simultaneous tooth extraction in patients taking oral bisphosphonates: Postoperative healing, early follow-up, and the incidence of complications in two private practices. *J Periodontol*, Vol. 78, No. 9, (Sep 2007), pp. 1664-9, ISSN 0022-3492, Chicago, Illinois, USA

Galindo, P.; Sánchez-Fernández, E., Avila, G., Cutando, A. & Fernandez, JE. (2005). Migration of implants into the maxillary sinus: two clinical cases. *Int J Oral Maxillofac Implants*, Vol.20, No. 2, (Mar-Apr 2005), pp. 291-5, ISSN 0882-2786 Illinois, USA

Givol, N.; Chaushu, G., Halamish-Shani, T. & Taicher, S. (2000). Emergency tracheostomy following life-threatening hemorrhage in the floor of the mouth during immediate implant placement in the mandibular canine region. *J Periodontol*, Vol. 71, No. 12, (Dec 2000), pp. 1893-5, ISSN 0022-3492, Chicago, Illinois, USA

Goodacre, CJ.; Kan, JY. & Rungcharassaeng, K. (1999). Clinical complications of osseointegrated implants. *J Prosthet Dent*, Vol. 81, No. 5, (May 1999), pp. 537-52, ISSN 0022-3913, New York, USA

Goodacre, CJ.; Bernal, G., Rungcharassaeng, K. & Kan, JY. (2003). Clinical complications with implants and implant prostheses. *J Prosthet Dent*, Vol. 90, No. 2, (Aug 2003), pp. 121-32, ISSN 0022-3913, New York, USA

Goss, AN.; Backhouse, P. (2007). Bisphosphonates and osteonecrosis of the jaws. *Aust Prescriber*, Vol. 30, pp. 96-7, ISSN 0312-8008, Deakin, Australia

Grant, BT.; Amenedo, C., Freeman, K. & Kraut, RA. (2008). Outcomes of placing dental implants in patients taking oral bisphosphonates: A review of 115 cases. *J Oral Maxillofac Surg*, Vol. 66, No. 2, (Feb 2008), pp. 223-30, ISSN 0278-2391, Philadelphia, Pennsylvania, USA

Greenstein, G.; Tarnow, D. (2006). The mental foramen and nerve: clinical and anatomical factors related to dental implant placement: a literature review. *J Periodontol*, Vol. 77, No. 12, (Dec 2006), pp. 1933-43, ISSN 0022-3492, Chicago, Illinois, USA

Greenstein, G.; Cavallaro, J., Romanos, G. & Tarnow, D. (2008). Clinical recommendations for avoiding and managing surgical complications associated with implant dentistry: a review. *J Periodontol*, Vol. 79, No. 8, pp.1317-29, ISSN 0022-3492, Chicago, Illinois, USA

Hofschneider, U.; Tepper, G., Gahleitner, A. & Ulm, C. (1999). Assessment of the blood supply to the mental region for reduction of bleeding complications during implant surgery in the interforaminal region. *Int J Oral Maxillofac Implants*, Vol. 14, No. 3, (May-Jun 1999), pp. 379-83, ISSN 0882-2786, Illinois, USA

Hunter, WL 4th.; Bradrick, JP., Houser, SM., Patel, JB. & Sawady, J. (2009). Maxillary sinusitis resulting from ostium plugging by dislodged bone graft: case report. *J Oral Maxillofac Surg*, Vol. 67, No. 7, pp. 1495-8, ISSN 0278-2391, Philadelphia, Pennsylvania, USA

Isaacson, TJ. (2004). Sublingual hematoma formation during immediate placement of mandibular endosseous implants. *J Am Dent Assoc*, Vol. 135, No. 2, (Feb 2004), pp. 168-72, ISSN 0002-8177, Chicago, Illinois, USA

Jalbout, Z.; Tabourian, G. (2004). Glossary of Implant Dentistry, *Proceedings of International Congress of Oral Implantologists*, Upper Montclair, New Jerjey 2004

Jeffcoat, MK. (2006). Safety of oral bisphosphonates: Controlled studies on alveolar bone. *Int J Oral Maxillofac Implants*, Vol. 21, No. 3, (May-Jun 2006), pp. 349-53, ISSN 0882-2786, Illinois, USA

Kalpidis, CD.; Setayesh, RM. (2004). Hemorrhaging associated with endosseous implant placement in the anterior mandible: a review of the literature. *J Periodontol* , Vol. 75, No. 5, (May 2004), pp. 631-45, ISSN 0022-3492, Chicago, Illinois, USA

Karabuda, C.; Arisan, V. & Ozyuvaci, H. (2006). Effects of sinus membrane perforations on the success of dental implants placed in the augmented sinus. *J Periodontol* , Vol. 77, No. 12, (Dec 2006), pp. 1991-7, ISSN 0022-3492, Chicago, Illinois, USA

Khan, AA.; Sándor, GK., Dore, E., Morrison, AD., Alsahli, M., Amin, F., Peters, E., Hanley, DA., Chaudry, SR., Dempster, DW., Glorieux, FH., Neville, AJ., Talwar, RM., Clokie, CM., Al Mardini, M., Paul, T., Khosla, S., Josse, RG., Sutherland, S., Lam, DK., Carmichael, RP., Blanas, N., Kendler, D., Petak, S., St-Marie, LG., Brown, J., Evans, AW., Rios, L. & Compston, JE. (2008). Canadian consensus practice guidelines for bisphosphonate associated osteonecrosis of the jaw. *J Rheumatol* Vol. 35, No. 7, pp. 1391-7, ISSN 0315-162X, Toronto, Ontario, Canada

Kraut, RA.; Chahal, O. (2002). Management of patients with trigeminal nerve injuries after mandibular implant placement. *J Am Dent Assoc*, Vol. 133, No. 10, (Oct 2002), pp. 1351-4, ISSN 0002-8177, Chicago, Illinois, USA

Lekholm, U.; Zarb, GA. (1985). Patient selection and preparation, In: *Tissue- Integrated Prostheses: Osseointegration in Clinical Dentistry*, Bra°nemark, PI., Zarb, GA. & Albrektsson, T., pp. 199-209, Quintessence, ISBN: 0-86715-129-3, Illinois, USA

Manor, Y.; Mardinger, O., Bietlitum, I., Nashef, A., Nissan, J. & Chaushu, G. (2010). Late signs and symptoms of maxillary sinusitis after sinus augmentation. *Oral Surg Oral Med Oral Pathol Oral Radiol Endod*, Vol. 110, No. 1, (Jul 2010), pp. e1-4, ISSN 1079-2104, New York, USA

Mardinger, O.; Manor, I., Mijiritsky, E. & Hirshberg, A. (2007). Maxillary sinus augmentation in the presence of antral pseudocyst: a clinical approach. *Oral Surg Oral Med Oral Pathol Oral Radiol Endod*, Vol. 103, No. 2, (Feb 2007), pp. 180-4, ISSN 1079-2104, New York, USA

Mardinger, O.; Abba, M., Hirshberg, A. & Schwartz-Arad, D. (2007). Prevalence, diameter and course of the maxillary intraosseous vascular canal with relation to sinus augmentation procedure: a radiographic study. *Int J Oral Maxillofac Surg*, Vol. 36, No. 8, (Aug 2007), pp. 735-8, ISSN 0901-5027, Edinburgh, Scotland

Martin, D.; Pascal, JF., Baudet, J., Mondie, JM., Farhat, JB., Athoum, A., Le Gaillard, P. & Peri, G. (1993). The submental island flap: a new donor site. Anatomy and clinical applications as a free or pedicled flap. *Plast Reconstr Surg*, Vol. 92, No. 5, (Oct 1993), pp. 867-73, ISSN 0032-1052, Philadelphia, Pennsylvania, USA

Marx, RE. ; Cillo, JE. Jr. & Ulloa, JJ. (2007). Oral bisphosphonate-induced osteonecrosis: risk factors, prediction of risk using serum CTX testing, prevention, and treatment. *J Oral Maxillofac Surg*, Vol. 65, No. 12, (Dec 2007), pp. 2397-410, ISSN 0278-2391, Philadelphia, Pennsylvania, USA

Misch, K.; Wang, HL. (2008). Implant surgery complications: etiology and treatment. *Implant Dent*, Vol. 17, No. 2, (Jun 2008), pp. 159-68, ISSN 1056-6163, Philadelphia, Pennsylvania, USA

Montefusco, V.; Gay, F., Spina, F., Miceli, R., Maniezzo, M., Teresa Ambrosini, M., Farina, L., Piva, S., Palumbo, A., Boccadoro, M. & Corradini, P. (2008). Antibiotic prophylaxis before dental procedures may reduce the incidence of osteonecrosis of the jaw in patients with multiple myeloma treated with bisphosphonates. *Leuk Lymphoma* Vol. 49, No. 11, (Nov 2008), pp. 2156-62, ISSN 1042-8194, Ebingdon, England

Montoya-Carralero, JM.; Parra-Mino, P., Ramírez-Fernández, P., Morata-Murcia, IM., Mompeán-Gambín Mdel, C. & Calvo-Guirado, JL. (2010). Dental implants in patients treated with oral bisphosphonates: a bibliographic review. *Med Oral Patol Oral Cir Bucal*, Vol. 15, No. 1, (Jan 2010), pp. e65-9, ISSN 1698-4447, Valencia, Spain

Nazarian, Y.; Eliav, E. & Nahlieli, O. (2003). Nerve injury following implant placement: Prevention, diagnosis and treatment modalities. *Refuat Hapeh Vehashinayim*, Vol. 20, No. 3, (Jul 2003), pp. 44-50, ISSN 0792-9935, Israel

Park, SH.; Wang, HL. (2005). Implant reversible complications: classification and treatments. *Implant Dent*, Vol. 14, No. 3, pp. 211-20, ISSN 1056-6163, Philadelphia, Pennsylvania, USA

Peleg, M.; Garg, AK. & Mazor, Z. (2006). Predictability of simultaneous implant placement in the severely atrophic posterior maxilla: A 9-year longitudinal experience study of 2132 implants placed into 731 human sinus grafts. *Int J Oral Maxillofac Implants*, Vol. 21, No. 1, pp. 94-102, ISSN 0882-2786, Illinois, USA

Pikos, M. (1999). Maxillary sinus membrane repair. Report of a technique for large perforations. *Implant Dent*, Vol. 8, No. 1, pp. 29- 34, ISSN 1056-6163, Philadelphia, Pennsylvania, USA

Proussaefs, P. ; Lozada, J., Kim, J. & Rohrer, MD. (2004). Repair of the perforated sinus membrane with a resorbable collagen membrane: A human study. *Int J Oral Maxillofac Impl*, Vol. 19, No. 3, (May-Jun 2004) pp. 413-420, ISSN 0882-2786, Illinois, USA

Regev, E.; Smith, RA., Perrott, DH. & Pogrel, MA. (1995). Maxillary sinus complications related to endosseous implants. *Int J Oral Maxillofac Implants*, Vol. 10, No. 4, (Jul-Aug 1995), pp. 451-61, ISSN 0882-2786, Illinois, USA

Reiser, GM.; Rabinovitz, Z., Bruno, J., Damoulis, PD. & Griffin, TJ. (2001). Evaluation of maxillary sinus membrane response following elevation with the crestal osteotome technique in human cadavers. *Int J Oral Maxillofac Implants*, Vol. 16, No. 6, (Nov-Dec 2001), pp. 833-40, ISSN 0882-2786, Illinois, USA

Roth, M.; Montone, KT. (1996). Actinomycosis of the paranasal sinuses: a case report and review. *Otolaryngol Head Neck Surg*, Vol. 114, No. 6, pp. 818-21, ISSN 0194-5998, New York, USA

Ruggiero, SL.; Mehrotra, B., Rosenberg, TJ. & Engroff, SL. (2004). Osteonecrosis of the jaws associated with the use of bisphosphonates: a review of 63 cases. *J Oral Maxillofac Surg*, Vol. 62, No. 5, (May 2004), pp. 527-34, ISSN 0278-2391, Philadelphia, Pennsylvania, USA

Ruggiero, SL.; Dodson, TB., Assael, LA., Landesberg, R., Marx, RE. & Mehrotra, B. (2009). American Association of Oral and Maxillofacial Surgeons: Position paper on bisphosphonate-related osteonecrosis of the jaws—2009 update. *J Oral Maxillofac Surg*, Vol. 67, No. 5 suppl, pp. 2-12, ISSN 0278-2391, Philadelphia, Pennsylvania, USA

Sadig, W.; Almas, K. (2004). Risk factors and management of dehiscent wounds in implant dentistry. *Implant Dent*, Vol. 13, No. 2, pp. 140-147, ISSN 1056-6163, Philadelphia, Pennsylvania, USA

Schwartz-Arad, D.; Herzberg, R. & Dolev, E. (2004). The prevalence of surgical complications of the sinus graft procedure and their impact on implant survival. *Journal of Periodontology*, Vol. 75, No. 4, (Apr 2004), pp. 511-516, ISSN 0022-3492, Chicago, Illinois, USA

Sharawy, M.; Misch, CE. (1999). Anatomy for dental implants. In: *Contemporary Implant Dentistry, 2nd ed,* Misch, CE. pp. 217-224, The CV Mosby Company, ISBN 0815170599, St. Louis, USA

Shlomi, B.; Horowiz, I., Kahn, A., Dobriyan, A. & Chaushu, G. (2004). The effect of sinus membrane perforation and repair with Lambone sheet on the outcome of maxillary sinus floor augmentation: A radiographic assessment. *Int J Oral Maxillofac Implants,* Vol. 19, No. 4, (Jul-Aug 2004), pp. 559-62, ISSN 0882-2786, Illinois, USA

Solar, P.; Geyerhofer, U., Traxler, H., Windisch, A., Ulm, C. & Watzek, G. (1999). Blood supply to the maxillary sinus relevant to sinus floor elevation procedures. *Clin Oral Implants Res*, Vol. 10, No. 1, (Feb 1999), pp. 34-44, ISSN 0905-7161, Oxford, England

Stark, WJ.; Epker, BN. (1995). Failure of osseointegrated dental implants after bisphosphonate therapy for osteoporosis. A case report. *Int J Oral Maxillofac Implants,* Vol. 10, No. 1, (Jan-Feb), pp. 74-8, ISSN 0882-2786, Illinois, USA

Sussman, HI. (1998). Tooth devitalization via implant placement: a case report. *Periodontal Clin Investig*, Vol. 20, No. 1, pp. 22-4, ISSN 1065-2418, USA

Tammisalo, T.; Happonen, RP. & Tammisalo, EH. (1992). Stereographic assessment of mandibular canal in relation to the roots of impacted lower third molar using multiprojection narrow beam radiography. *Int J Oral Maxillofac Surg*. Vol. 21, No. 2, (Apr 1992), pp. 85-9, ISSN 0901-5027, Edinburgh, Scotland

Testori, T.; Rosano, G., Taschieri, S. & Del Fabbro, M. (2010). Ligation of an unusually large vessel during maxillary sinus floor augmentation. A case report. *Eur J Oral Implantol*, Vol. 3, No. 3, (Autumn 2010), pp. 255-8, ISSN 1756-2406

Timmenga, NM.; Raghoebar, GM., Boering, G. & Weissenbruch, R. (1997). Maxillary sinus function after sinus lifts for the insertion of dental implants. *J Oral Maxillofac Surg,* Vol. 55, No. 9, pp. 936-9, ISSN 0278-2391, Philadelphia, Pennsylvania, USA

Timmenga, NM.; Raghoebar, GM., van Weissenbruch, R. & Vissink, A. (2001). Maxillary sinusitis after augmentation of the maxillary sinus floor: a report of 2 cases. *J Oral Maxillofac Surg*, Vol. 59, No. 2, Feb 2001), pp. 200-4, ISSN 0278-2391, Philadelphia, Pennsylvania, USA

Traxler, H.; Windisch, A., Geyerhofer, U., Surd, R., Solar, P. & Firbas, W. (1999). Arterial blood supply of the maxillary sinus. *Clin Anat*, Vol. 12, No. 6, pp. 417-421, ISSN 0897-3806, New Jersey, USA

Uchida, Y.; Goto, M., Katsuki, T. & Akiyoshi, T. (1998) A cadaveric study of maxillary sinus size and aid in bone grafting of the maxillary sinus floor. *Journal of Oral and Maxilofacial Surgery*, Vol. 56, No. 10, (Oct 1998), pp. 1158-1163, ISSN 0278-2391, Philadelphia, Pennsylvania, USA

Uchida, Y.; Goto, M., Katsuki, T. & Soejima, Y. (1998). Measurement of maxillary sinus volume using computerized tomographic images. *Int J Oral Maxillofac Implants*, Vol. 13, No. 6, (Nov-Dec 1998), pp. 811-8, ISSN 0882-2786, Illinois, USA

Ueda, M.; Kaneda, T. (1992). Maxillary sinusitis caused by dental implants: report of two cases. *J Oral Maxillofac Surg*, Vol. 50, No. 3, (Mar 1992), pp. 285-7, ISSN 0278-2391, Philadelphia, Pennsylvania, USA

van den Bergh, JP.; ten Bruggenkate, CM., Disch, FJ. & Tuinzing, DB. (2000). Anatomical aspects of sinus floor elevations. *Clin Oral Implants Res*, Vol. 11, No. 3, (Jun 2000), pp. 256-265, ISSN 0905-7161, Oxford, England

Wang, HL.; Weber, D. & McCauley, LK. (2007). Effect of long-term oral bisphosphonates on implant wound healing: Literature review and a case report. *J Periodontol*, Vol. 78, No. 3, (Mar 2007), pp. 584-94, ISSN 0022-3492, Chicago, Illinois, USA

Ward, BB.; Terrell, JE. & Collins, JK. (2008). Methicillin-resistant Staphylococcus aureus sinusitis associated with sinus lift bone grafting and dental implants: a case report. *J Oral Maxillofac Surg*, Vol. 66, No. 2, (Feb 2008), pp. 231-4, ISSN 0278-2391, Philadelphia, Pennsylvania, USA

Wessel, JH.; Dodson, TB. & Zavras, AI. (2008). Zoledronate, smoking, and obesity are strong risk factors for osteonecrosis of the jaw: A case-control study. *J Oral Maxillofac Surg*, Vol. 66, No. 4, pp. 625-31, ISSN 0278-2391, Philadelphia, Pennsylvania, USA

Worthington, P. (2004). Injury to the inferior alveolar nerve during implant placement: a formula for protection of the patient and clinician. *Int J Oral Maxillofac Implants*, Vol. 19, No. 5, (Sep-Oct 2004), pp. 731-4, ISSN 0882-2786, Illinois, USA

Yarom, N.; Yahalom, R., Shoshani, Y., Hamed, W., Regev, E. & Elad, S. (2007). Osteonecrosis of the jaw induced by orally administered bisphosphonates: Incidence, clinical features, predisposing factors and treatment outcome. *Osteoporos Int*, Vol. 18, No. 10, (Oct 2007), pp. 1363-70, ISSN 0937-941X, Godalming, England

Zijderveld, SA.; van den Bergh, JP., Schulten, EA. & ten Bruggenkate, CM. (2008). Anatomical and surgical findings and complications in 100 consecutive maxillary sinus floor elevation procedures. *J Oral Maxillofac Surg*, Vol. 66, No. 7, (Jul 2008), pp. 1426-38, ISSN 0278-2391, Philadelphia, Pennsylvania, USA

Zinner, ID.; Shapiro, HJ., Gold, SD. (2008). Sinus graft complications. Problem solving. *N Y State Dent J*, Vol. 74, No. 4, (Jun-Jul 2008), pp. 40-3, ISSN 0028-7571, New York, USA

11

Factors Affecting the Success of Dental Implants

Carlos Nelson Elias
Instituto Militar de Engenharia, Biomaterials Laboratory Rio de Janeiro, RJ, Brazil

1. Introduction

Dental implants are fully placed in the bone in order to replace the natural root of the tooth and allow the installation of a dental prosthesis. The implant has gained importance with the work of Professor Per Ingvar Brånemark, who studied the microcirculation in bone tissue. Brånemark used stainless steel optical chambers to investigate the anatomy and physiology of tissue injury. The chamber was inserted in rabbit and dog legs. In some experiments the chamber structure of stainless steel was replaced by titanium. At the end of the experiments, Prof Brånemark observed that the titanium chamber was firmly attached to the bone (Brånemark et al., 1964). In fact, the titanium chamber could not remove from the surrounding bone once it had healed. Histological studies showed complete integration of titanium with the bone. After this chance observation, Brånemark developed a new concept of osseointegration which led to dental implants. The use of titanium-based dental implants in humans begun in 1965.

Dental implant technology was improved in recent years, providing patients with unparalleled levels of effectiveness, convenience, and affordability. This is one of the main reasons why so many dentists recommend dental implants as their preferred method to replace missing teeth. Titanium dental implants can offer many benefits. Because they present osseointegration with the jawbone, they are more stable than dentures. Patients with dental implants may be able to talk and eat more easily because they do not face the risk of their dentures dislodging. Dentures require replacement when the gum tissue shrinks and changes the fit; implants are not affected by this problem. The maintenance and hygiene of dental implants are easier than with dentures. Another reason for continued growth of the global market for dental implants is that dental implants offer an effective treatment for edentulism and because of the rising demand for cosmetic dentistry worldwide across all age groups.

The conventional clinical protocol proposed by Brånemark (Brånemark, 1990) for placement of dental implants involves two phases. The first is the placement of the implant in a surgical cavity prepared in the bone. The protocol recommends a healing period for tissue reorganization. The waiting time for healing to occur depends on bone quality and the region in which the implant was performed and was estimated by Brånemark as between 3 months to 6 months. The second phase of treatment is the prosthesis placement. With this technique, all natural teeth can be replaced, restoring function and aesthetics to the patient.

The conventional protocol can be changed so that insertion of the implant and prosthesis placement can be made in a single step. In this case, the protocol is called immediately loading. The dentistry has an interest in reducing the healing time after surgery and loading the implants with oral forces safely. To meet this expectation one must consider that the body has a minimum time to perform the reactions that lead to osseointegration. In order to shorten the healing time, the strategy is to alter the biocompatibility of titanium implant surfaces, modifying the surgical technique and changing the implant design.

Despite the influence of the implant shape on the primary stability and the distribution of oral loads, there is no standardization of implant design. As shown in figure 1, there are dental implants on the market with different shapes. The cylindrical screw threaded implants are the most commonly used. Based on biomechanics and clinical observations, it was found that tapered implants have a higher compression capacity than cylindrical ones. During insertion the tapered implant induces compression stresses on the bone and increases the implant primary stability. However, the tapered implant is not suitable for all applications.

In an attempt to increase the success rate of implants, some researchers used the control of surface properties to select the type of cell that interact with the implant. It is known that osteoblastic cells adhere more quickly to rough surfaces of titanium than to smooth surfaces (Zhu et al., 2004; Puleo & Bizios, 1992). Despite the advances in prosthodontic, the explanation of the influence of the implant surface on osseointegration remains incomplete. The new surfaces improve the success of implants in patients with low bone quality and quantity. However, there is still an unexplained loss of implants.

Several papers in the literature (Wennerberg, 1998; Tete et al., 2008; Suzuki et al. 2009; Stadlinger et al. 2008; Richards, 1996) describe the importance of titanium surface properties in implant osseointegration. These works studied the morphology, topography, roughness, chemical composition, surface energy, surface energy, surface composition, chemical potential, residual stress, the existence of impurities, thickness of titanium oxide film and the presence of metallic and nonmetallic compounds on the surface. The mentioned factors influence the concentration of cells involved in osseointegration. The importance of this work is the fact that by controlling the surface one can reduce the healing time of the implant and the bone-implant interface has enough mechanical strength to withstand the forces in the oral environment (Schucker et al., 2006).

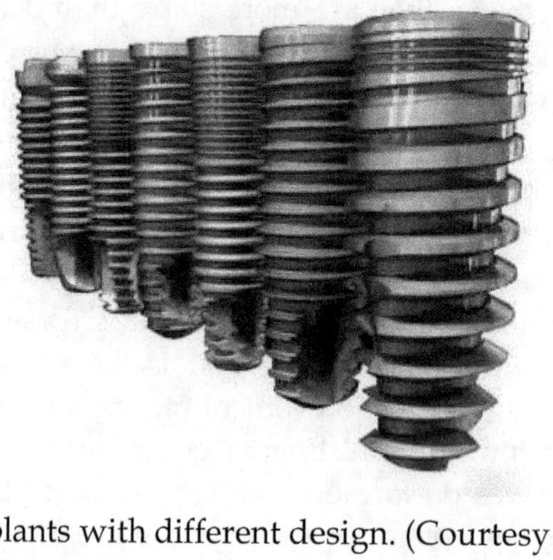

Fig. 1. Available dental implants with different design. (Courtesy of Conexão Sistemas e Prótese Company, Brazil).

As discussed below in detail, besides biomechanics, the shape and dimensions of the implant, the quality and quantity of the bone, the surgical technique and the loading conditions (load intensity, direction of the forces involved) influence the stability of the implants and the maintenance of osseointegration.

2. Biocompatibility

The modern concept of biocompatibility involves, not only compatibility of the material with the tissue but its ability to perform a specific function. The response to specific individual materials could vary from one application site to another. Therefore, biocompatibility is defined only for a determined application. For example, the biomaterial used in intraocular lenses is not adequate for dental implants, although both show biological compatibility. In practice, there is no material that is biocompatible for all applications. Thus biocompatibility could not solely be dependent on the material properties (physical, chemical, mechanical) but also had to be defined by the situation in which the material is used (Williams, 2008).

The requirement for biocompatibility in a medical device intended for long term contact with the tissues of the human body is that the material does no harm to the tissues, and this presupposes chemical and biological inertness. However, in the case of dental implants, there is a need for osseointegration, which implies in a need for specific and direct interactions between biomaterials and tissue components.

The main factors influencing the biocompatibility of biomaterials are chemical composition, mechanical properties, electrical charge and surface features. The biocompatibility of materials used in dental implants is evaluated by studying the reaction between the implant and the bone. The reaction between the implant and the soft tissue is also important. The region where the implant is in contact with the soft tissue is responsible establishing a kind of seal that isolates implant and the bone from the mouth environment.

The analysis of the biocompatibility of biomaterials is accomplished by testing *in vitro* and complemented with tests *in vivo*. Tests *in vitro* involve cell culture, characterization of the chemical composition of surfaces, identification of the types of oxides and crystalline structures, determination of the thickness of the oxide layer, and quantification of resistance in mechanical loading conditions and dynamic resistance corrosion. The implant stability, surface roughness and surface wettability are also important.

The implant tests *in vivo* are done in animals, especially mice, rabbits, dogs, sheep and pigs. The last testing stage involves analysis of human clinical trials. In tests *in vivo*, after implant removal from the animal, the samples are analyzed by microscopy to determine the tissue quality around the implant. In such tests certain types of tissue reaction have been repeatedly observed. Another important test is the interface implant-bone mechanical resistance after osseointegration of the implant. This measurement is indirectly determined by measuring the minimum torque required to remove the implant.

Tests *in vivo* are done to evaluate the corrosion resistance and the breakdown between toxicity, hijacking (non-vascular tissue and thick in contact with the implant, the absence of pathological cells) and inertia (vascularized tissue and loose connective tissue). It is known that a relationship exists between the material toxic reaction and a high corrosion rate. Co, Cu, Ni and V give rise to increased degradation in this order, and the degree of toxicity is increased in the same order. Metals that have corrosion passivation, i.e., high resistance to corrosion, do not trigger a negative response of tissues. This behavior is observed with Pt,

Ta, Nb, Zr and Ti. It is possible to identify a correlation between biocompatibility, chemical stability and biological performance.

Corrosion resistance, degradation and the corrosion products released are important parameters for materials selection. Morais et al. (Morais et al., 2009) evaluated the concentration of Ti, Al, and V in rabbit tissues (kidney, liver, and lung) after 1 week, 4 weeks, and 12 weeks of placement in the tibiae of Ti-6Al-4V orthodontic mini-implants. Various amounts of Ti, Al, and V were detectable (figure 2), confirming diffusion of Ti, Al and V from orthodontic mini-implants, with accumulation in remote organs (kidney, liver, and lung). Each metallic element had a different release behavior as a function of time. However, it is not enough to know which chemical elements are released; it is also important to analyze their influence on biocompatibility. Despite the tendency of metallic ion release with the Ti alloy, the measurable amounts of metals (Ti, Al, and V) released from Ti-6Al-4V orthodontic mini-implants in rabbits' tissues were significantly below the average dietary intake of these elements through food and drink and did not reach toxic concentrations.

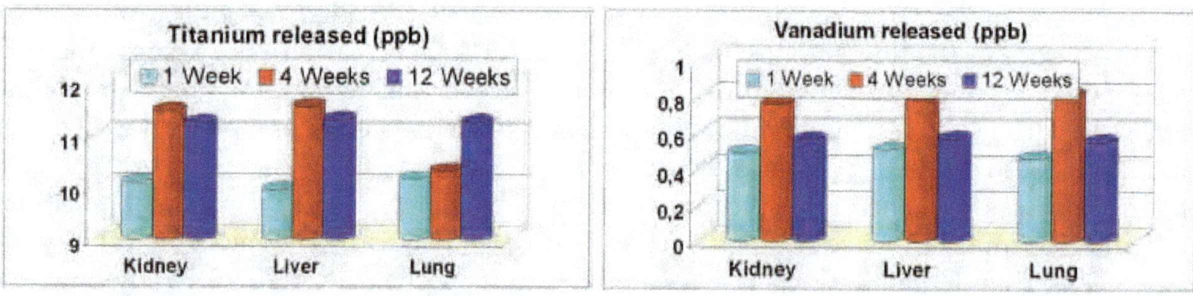

Fig. 2. Levels of metallic ions released from orthodontic Ti-6Al-4V mini-implants inserted in rabbits. (A) Ti (ppb). (B) V (ppb). Adapted from Morais et al. (Morais et al., 2009)

The analysis of biocompatibility becomes more complex when one considers that a low corrosion rate is not sufficient to ensure compatibility between the implant and the host tissue. Despite the fact that the corrosion resistance of stainless steel is about 300 times greater than that of Mg, many steel alloys release nickel, that, depending on the patient, can be highly toxic. A similar behavior problem is observed in Cr-Co alloys (Williams, 2008). The amount of some chemicals that are released in the body is a determinant factor of material biocompatibility. There is evidence that there is correlation between the intrinsic toxicity of the ions and their ability to bind macromolecules. It is thus necessary to study the ability of the products of corrosion of metals to react with host proteins to form a potentially toxic metal-protein, and to analyze the stability of compounds formed during the release of corrosion products. A high corrosion resistance does not ensure biocompatibility; the tissue reaction depends on the concentration and toxicity of the corrosion products.

The materials that ensure osseointegration are cp titanium, tantalum and niobium. Most companies employ cp titanium. Implants made of Ti-6%Al-4%V must be submitted to a surface treatment to exhibit osseointegration.

3. Tissue and dental implant interactions

Dental implants withstand oral loading because they have mechanical interlocking, fibro-osseous retention and osseointegration. The mechanical retention is not dependent on the implant material. Dental implants are primarily anchored in bone by means of mechanical interlocking. For dental implants with a screw shape, axial loading is transmitted to the bone via threads. The factors that affect mechanical interlocking are associated to the implant shape, surface irregularities and roughness, holes and grooves, screw thread type and the number of threads.

The term "fibro-osseous retention" or "fibrointegration" is applied to cases where the implant is attached to the bone by connective tissue. The "fibrointegration" concept is that there is a soft tissue interface surrounding an implant or a dense collagen tissue between implant and bone, whereas the term osseointegration in optical microscopy analysis refers to the physical contact between new bone and the implant, without the interposition of connective tissue.

Osseointegration was defined as a phenomenon where intimate contact between bone and biomaterials occurs at the optical microscopy level, enabling surgical implants to replace load-bearing organs restoring their form and function (Albrektsson et al., 1981). In the case of osseointegrated implants, when there is no fibrous capsule, high resolution microscopic results shows an afibrillar interfacial zone at the bone-implant interface; mineralized tissue generally does not directly touch the biomaterial. The interfacial layer is rich in noncollagenous proteins as well as certain plasma proteins. Titanium-newbone interface presents a thin layer with proteoglycans and glycoproteins. Some researchers have suggested that this interfacial zone provides a mechanism for bonding between hard tissue and cp Ti (Dee, 2002a).

The cellular interactions at the surface of cp Ti implants occur through the weak forces of van der Waals and hydrogen bonds. The first exhibit a binding energy of only 10 kcal/mol, due to molecular electric dipoles. The hydrogen bonds have energy of 1.10 kcal/mol. The strong binding forces, both covalent and ionic, with a binding energy of 10-100 kcal/mol, depend on the microstructural characteristics of the surface at atomic scale. These connections occur at defects such as cations, anions and impurity atoms. The placement of dental implant results in blood leakage, homeostasis, and fibrin blood cot formation at the tissue-bone interface (Cooper, 2003). The first cells to appear on a biomaterial surface during blood contact (adsorption), coagulation, and fibrinolytic phases are blood cells, i.e., platelets, monocytes, and polymorphonuclear granulocytes followed by erythrocytes. Immediately after insertion of dental implants in the surgical alveolus, reactions occur with the host tissues.

Bioactive materials (glass ceramics and hydroxyapatite) induce specific biological reactions on the surface, resulting in the formation of a union between implant and host. These biomaterials form strong bonds with the adjacent tissue. They promote a connection with the bone tissue through bridges of calcium and phosphorus. Titanium does not fit into this classification because it has a titanium oxide layer, which is inert when in contact with the tissue. The micromechanism responsible for connection with the bone depends on specific surface chemical properties.

As Albrektsson et al. (Albrektsson et al., 1982) commercially pure (cp) titanium implants were shown to establish very close contacts with bone, without any interposed cellular layers. There was only a thin (20-40 nm) interfacial collagen-free layer of ground substance, i.e. macromolecules consisting of proteoglycans and glucose aminoglycans attached to a backbone of hyaluronic acid. Such observations, supported by other morphological and functional studies, indicated that cp. titanium was excellently tolerated by the tissues. Johansson et al. (Johansson, 1990) examined the interface between bone and cp Ti implants and found a layer of proteoglycans about 20 nm thick and then, at a distance of about 100 nm, heavily mineralized collagen fibers. Between the two layers, were identified fibrin and no organized mineral deposits.

The oxidized surface of metals on an aqueous environment has a hydroxyl layer. Free metal ions can dissociate the water molecules and saturate or camouflage their positive charge with negatively charged hydroxyl ions. In the case of titanium oxide, for each dissociation of a molecule of water are produced two hydroxyl groups, which are differently positioned on the surface and produce an acid and a base in the neighboring area. These forms act as bipolar or amphoteric that can attract and bind with other molecules. An important feature of the amphoteric materials is the value of their point of zero charge measured by the pH. At point zero, the positive and negative charges on the surface are balanced. The equilibrium point for the titanium oxide is a pH around 6.2. Some amino acids are bipolar and can react as acids (because of the carboxyl groups) or as bases (because of amino groups). These hybrids are ideal for chemical absorption and form a double bond with amphoteric hydroxylated titanium oxide.

Results of a study by Suzuki et al. (Suzuki et al., 2009) supports the suggestion that the implant surface treatment positively influenced the early bone healing, resulting in the presence of lamellar bone morphology due to primary remodeling in the woven bone/vascular rich network observed at the bone surrounding.

4. Osseointegration

It is well known that success in implant dentistry depends on several parameters that may improve considering both biologic and mechanical criteria. To explain the micromechanisms involved in osseointegration is necessary to know concepts of biology, physiology, anatomy, surgery and tissue regeneration. Osseointegration is observed in several areas, including not only dental implants, but also maxillofacial implants, replacement of damaged joints and placement of artificial limbs.

Osseointegration was defined by Brånemark as the direct connection of living bone with the surface of an implant subjected to a functional load. This definition has been modified over the years. Among the important requirements for osseointegration are the existence of a biocompatible surface, the presence of alveolar bone in the potential recipient sites and no traumatic surgery.

To Brånemark et al, the phenomenon of osseointegration is due to new bone formation in close contact with the implant. To achieve this end, protocols were developed, since several parameters have to be defined, from the choice of the metal to the placement and preservation of the prosthesis. Thus, osseointegration depends on the material used in the implant, the machining conditions, the surface finish, the type of bone that receives the implant, the surgical technique, design of the prosthesis and the patient care.

Among the surgical factors that influence osseointegration, implant bed preparation is of critical importance. Drilling the implant bed not only causes mechanical damage to the bone but also increases the temperature of the bone directly adjacent to the implant surface. Mechanical and thermal damage to the tissue surrounding the implant during drilling can have a destructive effect on the initial state of the cavity housing the implant (Anitua et al., 2007).

Necrosis occurs when the temperature exceeds 47 °C for 1 min. Therefore, care must be taken to avoid thermal bone injury during the procedure. External irrigation at room temperature can provide sufficient cooling during drilling and keep the temperature below the critical value of 47 °C. Lower temperature saline was shown to be more effective in cooling the bone, and irrigation of the site should be continued between the drilling steps

(Sener et al., 2009). Other factors affect heat generation during drilling, such as the drilling speed and force.

Bioactive materials bond to bone tissue through bridges of calcium and phosphorus. On the other hand, the chemical bond between non-coated titanium implants and living tissue occurs through weak van der Waals and hydrogen bonds.

The van der Waals forces (polarization and molecular electric dipoles) have bond energy of about 10 kcal/mol. The hydrogen bonds have energy of 1.10 kcal/mol. Covalent and ionic bonds have energy of the order of 10-100 kcal/mol. The types of connections between the implant and the body depend on the microstructural characteristics of the surface on atomic scale. These connections occur at defects such as cations, anions and impurity atoms. The chemical composition of oxide, density and grain boundary impurities exert great influence on the occurrence of strong bonds.

Osseointegration is a biological concept which involves the incorporation of a foreign body to the living bone (host) with fixation and stability when subjected to functional loads. In order for dental implant osseointegration to occur, there must be an adherence of the cells to the surface of the biomaterial. The implant surface characteristics can modulate the adsorption of proteins, lipids, sugar, and ions present in the tissue fluids. Attachment to a surface is a critical first step in cell response because it determine which cells will populate the surface and how many (Boyan et al., 2001). In vitro tests with osteoblastic cells showed that when cell adhesion occurs, the cells change shape and spread. In this phase, reorganization of cytoskeletal proteins occurs. At points of contact between cells and biomaterials there is an exchange of information between cells and the extracellular matrix, leading to activation of specific genes and remodeling. As the chemical composition of biomaterial induces different reactions of the cells, the surface properties of biomaterials induce different reaction mechanisms (Anselme & Bigerelle, 2005). Both the morphology and the surface roughness of biomaterials influence proliferation, differentiation, extracellular matrix synthesis, production of local factors and even cell shape (Jayaraman et al., 2004)

The tests for implant removal by torsion indicate that there is a strong bond between the titanium implant and the bone. In the analysis of implants removed from animals it can be observed that there is a considerable amount of bone attached to the surface of the implant. This is an indication that osseointegration occurred.

Histologically, the identification of osseointegration is by the presence of regenerated bone at the implant-bone interface. The structure of the contact region can be analyzed in detail by means of electron microscopy and microanalysis. Histological preparations are suitable for this purpose. Several studies have found that there is a contact zone between implant and bone after placement. In these works it was possible to identify the presence of titanium atoms in the tissues surrounding the site of the alveoli. There was also the presence of lamellar bone with lacunae characteristics. Microanalysis and mapping of chemical elements in the region around the implant with microprobe indicated the presence of titanium, calcium and phosphorus. By this technique it is possible to verify that the relative intensities of Ca and P are constant, indicating that the bone is completely mineralized. Semiquantitative analysis in the region of the implant-bone interface shows the presence of chemical elements constituting the bone at a distance of 0.5 μm. These results show that the micromechanics of osseointegration is at the molecular level.

The tissue contact with the osseointegrated implant is the result of a process of new bone growth that involves continuous modeling and remodeling. Thus, it is important to understand that integration of bone with the implant is a dynamic process. The formation and stability of new bone about the implant is a combination of resorption and bone apposition. The balance between these processes is affected by various types of stimuli, including biomechanical forces in the dental prosthesis and the potential presence of inflammation (mucositis and peri-implantitis).

5. Influence of movement on the osseointegration

Despite the results obtained in studies to elucidate various aspects of osseointegration, there are doubts as to the actual micromechanisms involved in the formation of the union between bone and titanium, especially regarding the necessity of mechanical stimulation to induce bone connection.

After installation, the dental implants should provide initial mechanical stability to prevent movement. Movement between an implant surface and hard tissue causes fibrous capsule formation around the implant. Clinically, encapsulation is prevalent with stainless steel, alumina, zirconia and rarely seen with cp Ti implants without movement.

In fact, previous studies in animals reported a threshold of micromotion between 50 and 100 mm, above which micromotion induces bone resorption at the interface, thus producing fibrosis around endosseous implants (Soballe et al., 1993; Szmukler-Moncler et al. 2000).

Implant stability depends on direct mechanical connection between implant surface and the surrounding bone and can be divided into primary, secondary and tertiary stability. The stability obtained immediately after insertion of a dental implant is called primary stability. The stability obtained after osseointegration is named secondary stability. The tertiary stability is the maintenance of osseointegration. Primary implant stability is considered to play an essential role in successful osseointegration. It depends on bone quality and quantity, implant geometry and the site preparation technique.

Primary implant stability can be remarkably decreased in "low quality bone" (Beer et al., 2003). There are no conclusive studies of the minimum primary stability that ensures osseointegration. Clinical results indicate that when the dental implant insertion torque is higher than 40 N.cm, the success rate increases. Implant insertion and prosthesis installation in the same surgery procedure is called immediate/early function of dental implants. Immediate loading is today a commonly used term in the dental field and indicates the possibility of applying an occlusal load to dental implants earlier than the traditional healing period of 3 to 6 months. However, the applied load is often reduced or even absent; therefore, it is more correct to use the term "immediate/early function" rather than "immediate/early loading." Moreover, the subdivision between "immediate function" (when the prosthesis is applied within hours from the implant insertion) and "early function" (when the prosthesis is applied earlier than the traditional period of 3 to 6 months) has been accepted (Bogaerde et al., 2010).

6. Importance of titanium oxide layer in osseointegration

Although titanium is used extensively in the manufacture of dental implants since the early 1970's, there are still doubts about the mechanisms involved in its biological response.

Titanium spontaneously forms a very thin oxide film on its surface. This passive film protects titanium against corrosion attack or degradation in a wide range of harsh or aggressive environmental conditions. The biocompatibility of titanium as an implant material is attributed to surface oxides spontaneously formed in air and/or physiological fluids (Williams, 1981).

During machining of titanium, absorption of O_2 molecules occurs. After about 10 nanoseconds, the molecules dissociate and a monolayer of atomic oxygen is deposited. This oxygen reacts with titanium to form a titanium oxide film with a thickness between 50 and 100 Å (5 a 10 nm). This film, which forms spontaneously at ambient temperature and pressure, is called native oxide. Titanium oxide films can also be artificially grown by heating, acid etching and electrolytic oxidation also known as anodizing.

Titanium oxide films with thicknesses up to 800 nm can be formed by anodizing. At the body pH, the stable form of titanium oxide is TiO_2. After the implant has remained in place for some time, its surface becomes covered with plasma protein, especially fibronectin and vitronectin.

Some researchers studied the titanium oxide films on dental implant surfaces, measuring properties such as the crystalline structure, composition and thickness of the film. These studies showed that healing around titanium implants occurs through a gradual process of mineralization, i.e., osseointegration involves mechanisms that do not start at the implant surface (Larsson et al., 1996). Moreover, during healing, which occurs in a few days and remodeling, which requires weeks or even years, the biological processes that occur at the interface affect the properties of the initial oxide layer. The thickness of the oxide layer increases with time and incorporates ions of Ca, P and S from the physiological environment.

The surface properties of implants, such as morphology, roughness, thickness of the oxide layer, impurity level and types of oxide depend on the treatment to which the material was submitted. These surface properties have a significant effect on new bone formation.

After machining and cleaning, commercial dental implants are submitted to a surface treatment in order to attain the desired roughness and an adequate thickness of the titanium oxide film. It is important to remember that contact between the implant and the body established through a titanium oxide film; there is no contact between metallic titanium and the body.

The main difficulty for studying the influence of titanium oxide on osseointegration lies in isolating the variables that characterize the surface and analyze then one at a time. For instance, in a specific study it is necessary to change only the type of oxide layer (crystalline structure) while maintaining the same roughness and thickness; in a second study, it is necessary to change only the roughness and so on.

Larsson et al. (Larsson et al., 1996) investigated the bone formation around titanium implants with varied surface morphologies (machined, electropolished and electropolished followed by anodizing). The results showed that after one week a thin layer of bone covered with osteoid from the endosteum has been observed around the implants. After seven weeks the amount of bone around electropolished implant surfaces is lower than for anodized and machined machined implants with grooves between 1 and 10 μm. Anodic oxidation of the electropolished surfaces, which produced areas of increased roughness and a thicker surface oxide, had an enhancing effect on the rate of bone formation. Electropolished implants have less bone formation around the implant due to a lower surface roughness and the presence of a thin oxide layer. This behavior can be attributed to the fact that osteoblast cells adhere and spread more easily on rough surfaces than on smooth ones. They concluded that both surface topography on the submicrometer scale and oxide thickness influence the bone response to titanium.

Since host cells interact with adsorbed proteins and not with the material itself, the types and states of adsorbed proteins are critical determinants of cells responses to implanted

biomaterials. Albumin, fibrinogen and immunoglobulin predominate on many blood and tissue contact biomaterial (Tang & Hu, 2005). But blood has over 150 proteins. On the basis of mass transport considerations, more abundant proteins and proteins with the highest diffusion coefficient will be first to arrive at the surface. The most abundant proteins are albumin (40 mg/mL), IgG (15 (mg/mL), α_1–Antitrypsin (3 mg/mL), fibrinonogen (3 mg/mL). Because of its highest concentration and diffusion coefficient (6.1×10^{-7} cm^2/s), albumin dominates initial interaction with surface. Fibrinogen can dominate the surface because of greater affinity, even though its rate of arrival is more than 100 times less than that of albumin (Dee et al., 2002b).
In the past, implants coated with hydroxyapatite (HA) were widely used. They are no longer used due to the huge number of periimplantitis observed. However, HA-coated implants had a larger amount of bone overlying the surface compared to uncoated implants. In these implants the number of gaps between the HA coating and bone was lower and the formation of mineralized nodules was more pronounced.

7. Interaction of cells with the biomaterial surface

Any material placed in the body will cause a biological response, and the implants interact with the body environment through their surface. Consequently, the study of the properties of the outmost layer of a dental implant is critically important in the analysis of both the biological response to the implant and the titanium responses to the physiological environment.
With insertion of the biomaterial in the human body and contact with the material with the body fluids (BF), multiple events are triggered. In the past, it was believed that identification of a foreign body by the cells led to defensive strategies and inflammatory reactions that resulted in encapsulation of the biomaterial to isolate it from the body. Currently, it is known that through material selection, processing and surface coating, it is possible to obtain the desired cell response. One can favor the adsorption and absorption of a specific type of cell or even prevent the adhesion of organic material. For example, the surface of coronary stents must have properties that prevent cell adhesion. Moreover, the surface of dental implants must allow the adsorption of specific proteins to trigger the mechanisms involved in osseointegration.
As soon as an implant is inserted, adsorption of cells on the surface of the foreign body begins. The cells activate mechanisms to identify the chemical composition of the material and induce different reactions. Cell react differently to bioinert, bioactive and bioreactive materials (Wolner et al., 2006). In the case of bioinert materials (stainless steel, Co-Cr alloy, zirconia, alumina, nylon, etc.) the body induces the formation of a capsule of fibrous tissue surrounding the biomaterial. Bioactive materials (titanium, niobium and tantalum), on the other hand, induce mechanisms that lead to osseointegration. For bioreative biomaterials (hydroxyapatite, calcium phosphate, bioglass), ionic changes occur in the body and the biomaterial is resorbed.
When a bioactive implant is inserted into bone, its surface is modified by ions and proteins. The increased surface energy may alter plasma proteins adsorbed to the surface and activate cell membrane receptors. The process of coagulation is triggered and platelet activation initiates an inflammatory response by recruiting neutrophils and monocytes to the wound area. Platelet-derived cytokines such as IGF, TGF-ß and PDGF enhance the osteogenic response and bone formation by stimulating the migration and proliferation of osteogenic

cells, which differentiate into osteoblasts and eventually produce bone matrix. Thus, the cascade of events induced by the activation of platelets, including the release of chemotactic and mitogenic factors, increased production of thrombin and the recruitment and activation of neutrophils and monocytes may explain the faster bone repair around surfaces of different chemical composition (Togashi et al., 2007; Kikuchia, 2005).

New technologies and new materials have emerged based on these concepts (Kashiwagi et al., 2009; Li et al., 2008). The new biomaterials are developed with the aim of presenting biocompatibility for a specific application. Unfortunately, sometimes the foreign material inserted into the human body does not induce the desire response. In some cases, the physiological reactions are deleterious. Better understanding and control of material properties can eliminate or minimize the critical reactions and allow the advancement of technology of biomaterials. One of the critical responses to foreign materials is directly related to the interaction between the material surface and adsorption proteins (Le Duc & Wang, 2006).

In the body fluid (BF) there are ions in solution as well as lipids, carbohydrates and proteins that can be adsorbed on the biomaterial surface. The biomaterials are selected to obtain a specific response necessary for certain applications (Niinomi, 2002). In this process, proteins play an important role to induce the desired response.

After the initial reaction of proteins with the foreign body a physiological response occur, following by a sequence of events leading to acceptance or rejection of the material. These responses involve the recruitment of several cell types that are present at the interface of the material and perform activities such as extracelular matrix remodeling (Thull, 2002). In the case of dental implants, recruitment of cells, that leads to implant encapsulation, is not desirable. Proper implant surface preparation, adequate loading conditions and control of micromovements are essential and decisive to avoid formation of fibrous tissue in the bone-implant interface. The use of commercially pure titanium is no guarantee of osseointegration.

Based on the concepts presented, it is concluded that the surface properties of implants are extremely important for controlling the reactions that lead to improved performance and osseointegration of the implant. Among the properties of the implant surface that influence the attraction, repulsion, adsorption and absorption of proteins and cells as well as on osseointegration are roughness, wettability, electrical charge, chemical composition, surface energy, residual stresses and morphology.

The wettability of a liquid is defined as the contact angle between droplets of the liquid in thermal equilibrium on a horizontal surface. Depending on the type of surface and liquid the droplet may take a variety of shapes as illustrated in figure 3. The wetting angle θ is given by the angle between the interface of the droplet and the horizontal surface. The liquid is seemed wetting when $90 < \theta < 180$ degrees and non-wetting when $0 < \theta < 90$. When $\theta = 180$ degrees corresponds to perfect wetting and the drop spreads forming a film on the surface. Figure 4 shows hydrophilic dental implant surface.

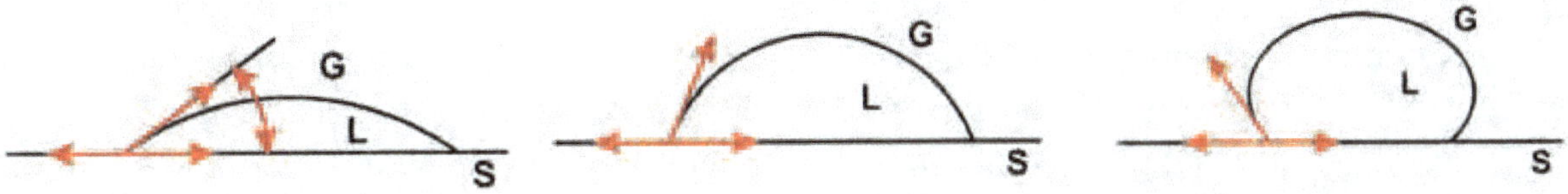

Fig. 3. Wetting ability of material surface. Hydrophilic surface (left), normal hydrophilic surface (middle) and hydrophobic surface (right).

Cell adhesion involves short term events such as physicochemical linkages between cells and substrates and long term events leading to the regulation of cell expression involving extracellular proteins, cell membrane proteins and cytoskeleton proteins (Anselme, 2000). The chemical composition and microstructure of a surface can regulate the adsorption of components present in the extracellular fluid. It is known that rough and chemically activated surfaces provide the ideal conditions for direct protein adsorption and alter the adsorption of fibronectin and albumin due to modifications in their ionic state. These mechanisms are important for implant osseointegration.

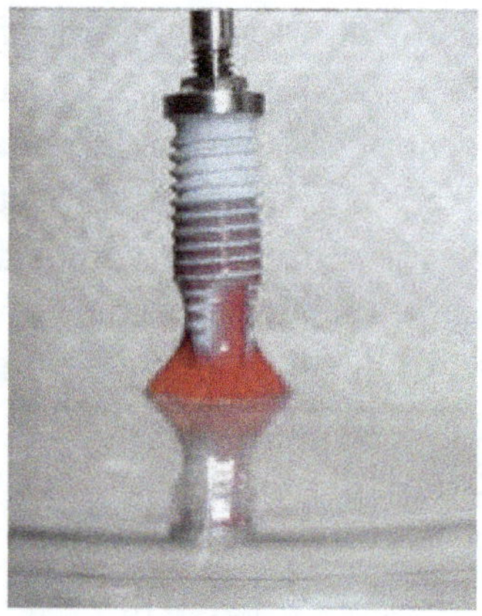

Fig. 4. Vulcano Actives™ dental implant showing its high hydrophilic surface.

Adhesion is a basic cellular process that directly influences cell growth, differentiation and migration, as well as morphogenesis and healing. The extracellular matrix (ECM) elaborated by cells constitutes a regulator of cell adhesion and differentiation and contributes to the mechanical properties of the tissue. These regulatory effects of ECM are mediated through transmembrane proteins specialized in cell substrate adhesion. These cell surface receptors are called integrins, which are αβ heterodimeric proteins. The αβ association is essential for integrins to bind to their ligand and determines the specific ligand binding (a ligand is an ion or molecule that binds to a central metal atom to form a coordination complex. The bonding between metal and ligand generally involves formal donation of one or more of the ligand electron pairs. The nature of metal-ligand bonding can range from covalent to ionic). Some integrins are able to bind several ligands, $\alpha 3\beta 1$ is a laminin, collagen, fibronectin, and, enctatin receptor (Verrier et al., 2002). All these mechanisms depend on the surface properties of the biomaterial.

The arrangement of atoms in the surface of metals is different from the atomic arrangement in the bulk and makes is more receptive to adsorption of atoms and molecules from the environment. The reactions between the environment and the biomaterial surface increases when the energy per unit area at the metal surface increases.

Titanium, having a high energy surface, will easily adsorb O_2 molecules, which dissociate and form titanium oxide in a few milliseconds. Therefore, even in the implants without surface treatment, there is no body contact with metallic titanium, but only with a layer of titanium oxide. Therefore, for the biocompatibility of commercially pure Ti implants, the properties of the oxide layer are more important than those of the metal.

The thickness of the protein coating on the surface of the implants depends on the surface energy of the material. Histological observations made on implants with high surface energy indicated that they have layers of proteins with greater thickness than those with low energy, revealing that cellular activity varies with the surface energy. When implants with low surface energy were mechanically separated from the capsule tissue and inspected under a microscope, it was found that most of the surface did not have tissue. In implants with low surface energy, the cells remain with an almost spherical shape, lose their attachment and can easily be separated from one another. The globular appearance of these cells allowed identifying them histological as fibroblasts. The globular appearance of the cells is associated with poor cell growth, but is not related to the normal activity of fibroblasts in the healing process.

In order to study the biocompatibility of materials and the extent of osseointegration, one needs quantitative and qualitative information on the surface energy of the implants, since it affects the interactions between biomaterial surfaces with proteins, cells and bacteria. Different cell types use different mechanisms when attaching to different surfaces and, as a rule, cells do not interact with the surface directly, but via proteins secreted by the cells and adsorbed by the surface, forming a distinct layer. Adhesive compounds such as fibronectin and vitronectin are present in the serum adsorbed on the substrate and adhesion is in fact an interaction with these compounds. This interaction is of the type ligand-receptor because the cells have specialized receptors (integrins) through which they identify the adsorbed adhesive proteins-ligands. Guided by the substrate surface properties, conformational alterations of the adsorbed proteins possibly change their biological behavior. In this context, the initial cellular interactions depend on surface physicochemical properties such as wettability, charge, heterogeneity, topography, roughness and the presence of functional groups (Vladkova, 2010)

The direct biochemical interactions between the surface of titanium implants and tissue molecules are short range; the predominant type of chemical bonds is the weak forces of van der Waals and hydrogen bonds such as polarization and molecular electric dipoles. The surface energy is directly proportional to the tendency to adsorb molecules. The general rule is that materials with a surface tension between 20 and 30 dynes/cm^2 exhibit a low adsorption. Materials with surface tension values above this range are more adsorptive.

The sessile drop technique is a method used for the characterization of solid surface energies, and in some cases, aspects of liquid surface energies. The main premise of the method is that by placing a droplet of liquid with a known surface energy, the shape of the drop, specifically the contact angle (figure 3), and the known surface energy of the liquid are the parameters which can be used to calculate the surface energy of the solid sample.

The Owens/Wendt theory (Owens et al., 1969) divides the surface energy into two components: surface energy due to dispersive interactions and surface energy due to polar interactions. The no dispersive or polar component arises from electrostatic interactions, metallic bonding forces, hydrogen bonding and dipole interactions. The dispersive or no polar component has its origin in interactions between molecules and covalent bonds. These two components can be calculated as t he ratio of the contact angles with surfaces with known properties and the contact angles with the surface under investigation.

There is a relationship between critical surface tension and biocompatibility. The surface energy model includes contributions from the solid phase (implant) and the liquid phase (blood) to the physiological results. The basic premise is that the driving force for protein adsorption is the surface free energy. Thus, proteins are not strongly absorbed in a surface with low interfacial free energy and remain in solution. In the case of dental implants, the properties of the liquid phase can be changed by drugs to activate tissue mechanisms that facilitate adherence. The use of drugs and an adequate preparation of the implant surface are seen as complementary methods to improve osseointegration.

Materials with a high surface energy adsorb macromolecules more easily, have a higher number of favorable sites for cell adhesion, and facilitate the growth of layers that stimulate cell binding. In order to improve osseointegration, it is desirable that the strength of the non-dispersive component of the surface tension be as low as possible, while the dispersive component remains high.

8. Types of dental implants

There is not a consensus among researchers as to the best surface roughness and even the shape of the implants. As shown in figure 1, there are a number of types of dental implants available. The same manufacturer produces implants with different shapes and surfaces. It is common knowledge that the geometric shape of the implant should be chosen in such a way to provide the largest bone-implant contact area in order to improve osseointegration decrease the stress concentration close to cervical area.

Commercial dental implants can be divided into groups according to shape, type of connection to the prosthetic component, surface treatment and roughness.

a. Shape (figure 5): cylindrical, conical, hybrid;
b. Type of connection (figure 6): external hexagon, internal hexagon, Morse taper, dodecagon;
c. Surface treatment (figure 7): acid etching, sandblasting, anodizing, coated by plasma sprays, nanoparticles deposition, laser treatment,
d. Surface roughness: macroroughness (figure 7D and 6E), microroughness (figure 7A), nanoroughness

In an attempt to improve the interaction between bone and implant, increase the surface area, improve the distribution of forces to the bone and achieve a better primary stability, various implants shapes were developed. Screw-shaped dental implants dominate the dentistry market. The screw shape provides a large contact area between implant and bone, increases primary stability, reduces the shear stress in the bone-implant interface, reduces the stress concentration in the cervical region and relieves stress concentration. The thread profile is characterized by the depth, pitch, flank angle, the top radius of curvature, and the straight part at the bottom of the thread. The rounded thread top relieves stress concentration and reduces the stress on the bone. However, there is no recommendation or standardization for the screw of dental implants. During bone repair, it is important that implant micromotions do not submit the tissues to any kind of trauma. Destabilization of the bone-implant interface leads to the interposition of fibrous tissue on its surface and prevents osseointegration.

Implants with large thread steps increase bone-implant interface shear stresses which should be avoided because bones have a lower strength to shear than to tension and compression.

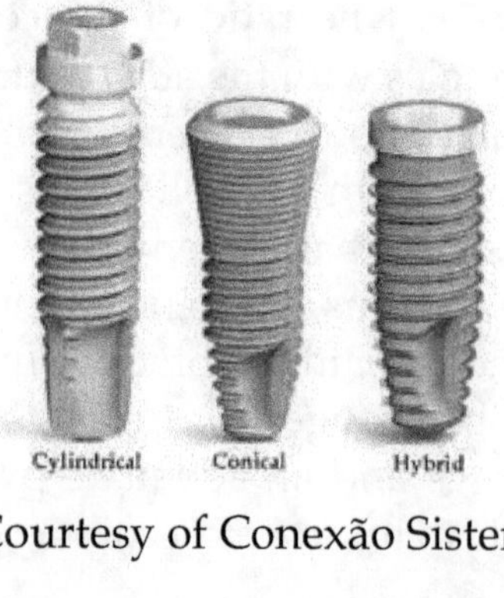

Fig. 5. Dental implants design. (Courtesy of Conexão Sistemas e Prótese, Brazil).

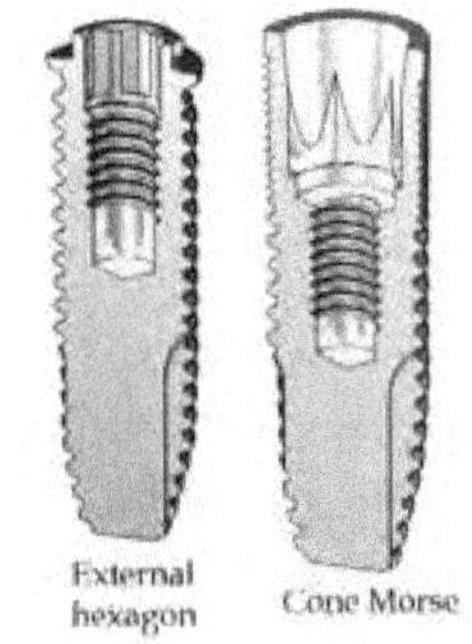

Fig. 6. Dental implant with external hexagon and internal Morse taper. (Courtesy of Conexão Sistemas e Prótese)

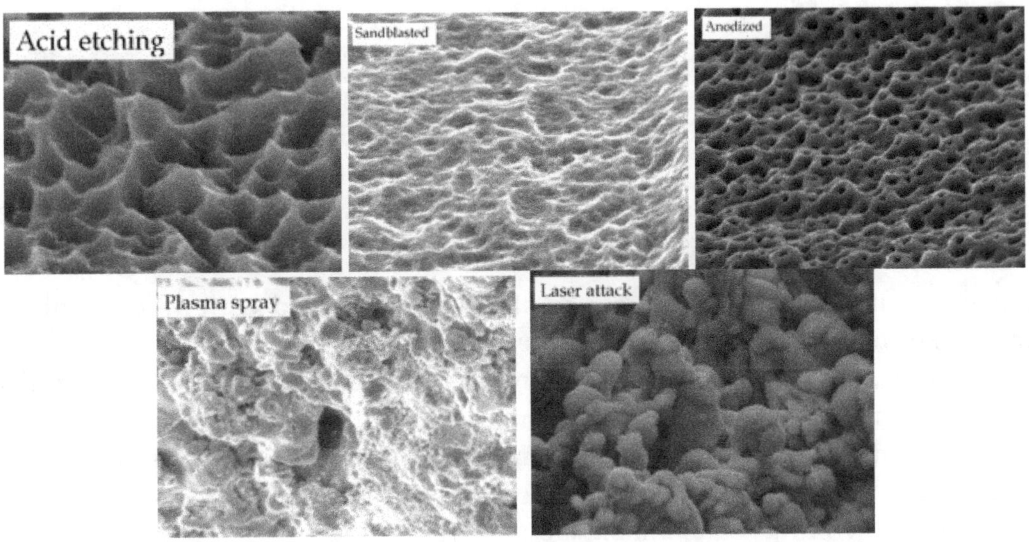

Fig. 7. Surface morphologies of available titanium dental implant. (A) Acid etching. (B) Sandblasting. (C) Anodizing. (D) Coated with TiO_2 by plasma spray. (E) Laser treatment.

By varying the profile of fillets of tapered threads is possible to increase the surface area of the conical implant relative to cylindrical implants with the same diameter and length (table 1). Implant thread fillets are not standardized. The fillet can be triangular, square, V-shaped, rounded or trapezoidal (figure 8).

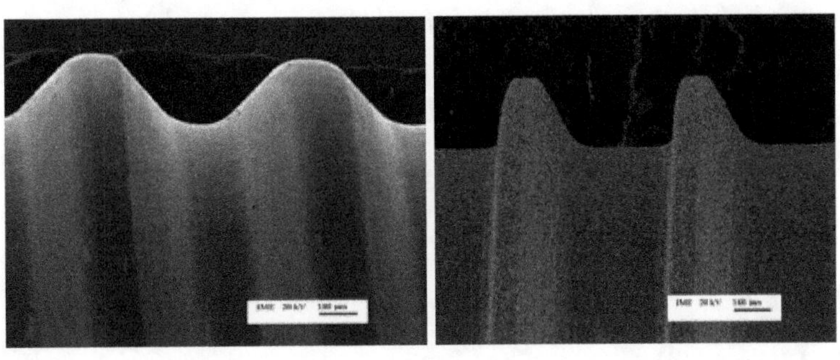

Fig. 8. Profiles of fillets. Cylindrical implant (left) and conical implant (right).

Initially, prostheses were composed of seven parts: implant, intermediate, intermediate screw, abutment, abutment screw, bolt retainer and prosthesis. However, clinical experience has shown that the larger the number of components, the greater the possibility of failure.

Currently, cemented prostheses are composed of four elements: implant, abutment, abutment screw fixation and prosthetic crown. Screwed prostheses are made of implant, abutment, abutment screw, crown and screw crown. These sets require a strict control of manufacturing and design to ensure that the chewing forces are properly transferred to the host. There is an apparent lack of consensus as to the implant shape that provides the best performance. For some, the choice of a threaded cylindrical implant takes into account the prevalence of compressive stresses in relation to shear; the choice of a cylindrical implant maximizes the importance of maximum resistance to shear stress.

Length (mm)	Cylindrical	Conical
8.5	217.57	-
10.0	252.55	283.69
11.5	283.52	311.76
13.0	316.92	343.44
15	360.18	383.51

Table 1. Influence of dental implant design on the surface area. Implant diameter equal to 5.0 mm.

With respect to length and diameter, the implants are marketed with different dimensions, in order to take into account different clinical treatment. Dental implants with cylindrical threads are commercially available with diameters between 3.25 and 6.0 mm and lengths between 5 and 18 mm. For implants with similar surface treatments, the larger the size, the greater the resistance to removal of the implant after osseointegration. The choice of implant size is determined by the available space, bone quality and implant bed. Based on the characteristics and volume of available bone in the region of surgery, the professional defines the type, shape and size of the implant to be used.

Among the different parts of the implants, the dimensions of the cervical region deserve the most attention. About 12% of connections show loosening of the abutment screw during the first year of use due to lack of stability. To minimize this problem, many implants are designed with an external or internal hexagon. However, only changes in the design of implants are not sufficient to eliminate the problem; one must examine the dimensional tolerances of the implants, the interchangeability of parts and the couplings between parts. Binon (Binon, 1998) found that the lack of fit between implant and prosthesis causes instability of the joints connecting the system. In other words, a difference between the dimensions of the implant hexagon and hexagon connection impairs the system stability Therefore, one should take special attention to dimensional tolerances of the implants and connections, which depend on factors related to part manufacturing, surgery planning and execution and the implant quality.

9. Roughness

The importance of implant surface topography for successful osseointegration was first pointed out by Albrektsson et al. (Albrektsson et al., 1981). More recent studies have confirmed that the surface roughness of implants affects osseointegration and the mechanical stability of dental implants (Werner et al., 2009; Zhu et al., 2004; Puleo, 1992;

Wennerberg et al., 1998a) . Several mechanisms involved in osseointegration depend on surface morphology, since the cells react differently in contact with smooth surfaces and rough surfaces. Fibroblasts and epithelial cells adhere more strongly to smooth surfaces and the ability of osteoblast proliferation and collagen synthesis is greater in surface with moderate roughness (Wennerberg et al., 1998b; Cochran et al., 1998). Despite the importance of roughness in osseointegration, there is no standard for the roughness of dental implants.

The surface of dental implants is greatly influenced by the action of the cutting tool. Elements such as tool shape, speed, feed, and cutting fluid can be varied to affect the surface topography. Other factors affecting the surface are the instability of the cutting tool due to chatter or imbalance in the grinding wheel, and errors in the machine tool guideway (Morton, 1994).

Machined dental implants have a pattern of grooves from the manufacturing process that can be detrimental for osseointegration (figure 9). To improve osseointegration it is important that the surface treatment creates the right kind of defects. Depending on size, surface topography can be defined in terms of surface roughness, waviness and form (Figure 10). For dental implants, roughness is the most important feature.

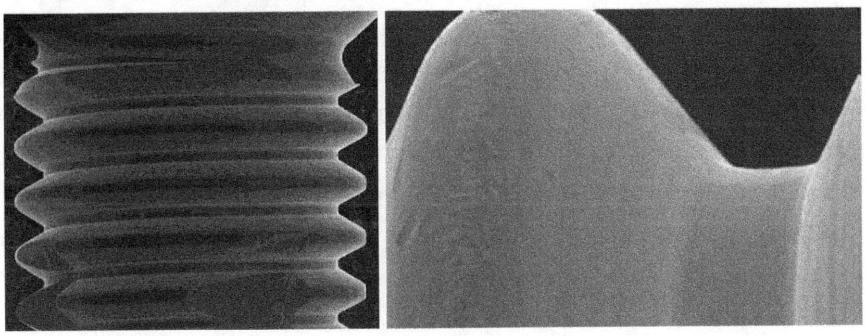

Fig. 9. Surface morphology of machined dental implant, showing the grooves left by the manufacturing tools.

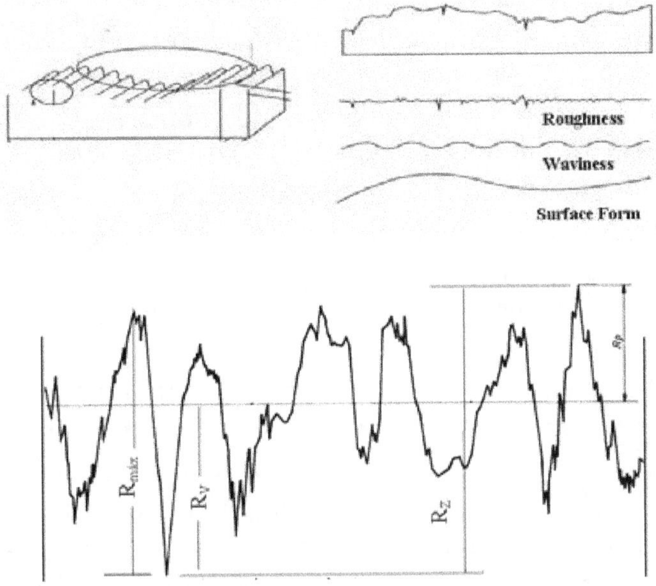

Fig. 10. Sketch representing the surface topography and roughness parameters.

Surface roughness is the primary component of texture and refers to high frequency irregularities. In the case of dental implants, surface roughness consists of fine imperfections on the order of micrometer (μm) due to the cutting process (figure 9) or due to a surface treatment (figure 7). In machined implants, roughness is closely related to the cutting tool and consists of a regular pattern of shallow grooves.

Surface waviness refers to the secondary component of texture upon which roughness is superimposed. It is as a series of regular deviations of approximately sinusoidal shape and a size on the order of millimeters. It is attributed to the deformations and vibrations of the machine and the part during manufacturing.

Surface form is some irregularity the general shape of the surface, neglecting roughness and waviness, which is frequently caused by errors in the machine tool guideway and deformations due to stress patterns in the component.

Since the basic types of surface geometry are caused by different factors and tend to have different relationships to the performance of the component, it is usual to consider them separately during analysis. In general, if control of dental implant performance related to surface topography is required, roughness is main parameter to be analyzed.

For effective analysis of surface roughness, the profile is evaluated according to internationally recognized mathematical formulas called parameters (ISO 468: Surface roughness parameters. ISO 4287: Surface texture: Profile method, terms, definitions and surface texture parameters. ISO 4288: Surface texture: Profile method, rules and procedures for the assessment of surface texture. ISO 8785: Surface imperfections, terms, definitions and parameters. BS 1134-1: Assessment of surface texture, methods and instrumentation. BS EN ISO 3274: Geometric product specifications (GPS). Surface texture and profile method. ASME B46.1: Surface texture: surface roughness, waviness, and lay). The purpose of using a parameter is to resort to a number that can characterize a certain aspect of the surface and hence eliminate the need for subjective operator assessment. Since it is not possible to characterize a surface completely with a single parameter, a combination of parameters is normally used.

Despite the importance of surface roughness on osseointegration of dental implants, there are no standards to measure the roughness of the implants. The procedure adopted has been to adopt the same parameters used in engineering. Moreover, previous studies of the subject (Wennerberg 1996; Elias et al., 2008) analyze only a few parameters and offer no conclusive explanation of the influence of each roughness parameter on osseointegration.

Roughness measurements are performed using mechanical or electronic devices, such as a style instrument called profiler. The use of a contact roughness meter (mechanical) has several limitations, including the fact that the values of peak heights and depths of valleys are limited by the tip shape. The most common non-contact technique uses a laser beam. It is also possible to evaluate the surface roughness by atomic force microscopy; however, this technique is limited to a small region of the specimen.

Surface roughness is characterized by small protrusions (peaks) and holes (valleys) on the surface in relation to a reference plane. The parameters used to quantify this roughness are determined in two dimensions (2D) or three-dimensional (3D). The letter "R" is used for parameters related to roughness and the letter "S" for parameters related to the surface profile. The measured parameters can be divided into three groups:

a. Spaciousness parameters are measures of the height of the irregularities or vertical deviations on the surface. They are determined by the peak heights and depths of valleys, or both, regardless of the spacing between the irregularities along the surface (R_a, R_q, R_z, R_{sk}, R_{ku}, R_t, S_a, S_q, S_z, S_{sk}, S_{ku}, S_t, R_p, R_v, R_c, R_m).

b. Spacing parameters are determined by the distance between irregularities along the surface (Sm and Scx)

c. Hybrid parameters describe a combination of the amplitude and spacing of surface irregularities (S_{qd} and S_{dr}).

Roughness average (R_a), the most common1y used roughness parameter, is defined as the mean height of the roughness profile. Its main drawback is the fact that different profiles may have the same Ra and differ significantly in performance. Another averaging parameter, R_q, defined as the root mean square of the roughness profile, is more sensitive to surface variations. After a surface treatment of the implant, it may be more adequate to specify the maximum roughness height, R_{max}, or the peak-to-valley height, R_z, rather than use the mean height given by R_a. The R_{max} parameter measures the highest and lowest points of the profile. There are doubts as to whether the variations in the heights of surface irregularities are more important than the distance between them, or what the best combination of these factors for osseointegration is.

The definitions of the main roughness parameter are:

- R_a (average roughness): R_a is average value of the amplitudes in relation to a reference line. This parameter quantifies the average vertical distance between the five highest peaks and five major valleys.
- R_q or R_{ms} (root mean square roughness): R_q is the square root of the squares of the amplitudes in relation to the midline. The squaring of the values of irregularity increases the effect of the irregularities that deviate markedly from the average.
- R_z (average partial roughness): R_z is the arithmetic mean of five values of the partial roughness Z_i. The partial roughness Z_i is defined as the sum of the absolute values of the ordinates of the points of greatest deviations (above and below the midline) existing within a sampling length. Graphically, this represents the height between the maximum and minimum points of the profile within the sampling length.
- R_{max} (maximum roughness). R_{max} is the largest value of partial roughness Z_i along the measurement path. Another parameter similar to R_{max} for measuring surface roughness is R_y, defined as the maximum distance between the highest peak and the largest valley within the sampling length.
- R_t (total depth). R_t is the vertical distance between highest peak and the deepest valley.
- R_{3z} (average roughness of the third peak). In each module are plotted the distances between the third highest peak and the third deepest valley. R_{3z} is the height of this peak plus the depth of the valley.

Other amplitude parameters are:

- R_{sk}: asymmetry factor (skewness);
- R_{ku}: flattening profile (kurtosis);
- R_p or Z_p: maximum height of the highest peak of surface roughness, situated above the midline.
- R_v or Z_v: depth profile of the largest valley
- R_c: average height of the profile elements
- R_{om}: depth of the deepest valley
- S_m: mean distance between furrows or average distance between peaks
- R_{Sm}: average width of the profile elements

- PC: number of peaks per unit length

The mean values of some roughness parameters for a titanium surface are displayed in Table 1. After surface treatment, significant changes are observed in the roughness parameters that affect the cell-surface interaction, as measured by implant removal torque. Multiple comparisons Tukey's HSD tests have shown a statistically significant difference in R_a after surface treatment. The machined surface has grooves, which increase roughness. The surface area (A_1 and A_2 in Table 2) was larger after sandblasting and anodizing; statistically significant differences were found between these groups and the others (Elias et al., 2008).

Group	R_a (μm)	R_q (μm)	R_z (μm)	R_{max} (μm)	R_{pkx} (μm)	A_1 (μm²)	A_2 (μm²)
Machined	0.65±0.11	0.81±0.17	6.09±0.37	7.76 ± 1.37	21.6±0.41	24.71 ± 5.42	70.66±16.20
Acid	0.51±0.10	0.71±0.07	5.09±0.46	6.78 ± 1.33	1.77±0.37	34.76 ± 7.35	103.86±14.80
Blasted	0.75±0.05	0.98±0.04	5.55±0,21	12.44 ± 9.7	6.75±0.76	99.75± 6.76	190.13± 4.90
Anodized	0.87±0.14	1.12±0.18	5.14±0.69	19.84±2.13	16.71±2.47	97.67±11.43	215.37± 1.67

Table 2. Mean value ± SD of titanium cylinder surface roughness parameters.

A previous study (Links et al., 1998) pointed out the importance of the surface topography of implants on the regulation of the osteoblast physiology. For instance, on smooth surfaces osteoblasts seem to have decreased adhesion, but proliferate at a high extent. On rougher surfaces they seem to adhere further, proliferate at a low extent and show an increased protein secretion, resembling a more differentiated phenotype. However, if the peaks of the surface topography are too high or the distance between them is too great, the cells may be essentially dealing with smooth surfaces.

Also important is the osteoblast attachment, which is affected by surface treatment. Menezes et al. (Menezes et al., 2003) analyzed osteoblast adhesion onto titanium implant acid etched (HNO3) for 20 seconds (Group 1), 60 seconds (Group 2) and 90 seconds (Group 3). They observed a tendency of increase in cell attachment as the surface becomes rougher. Figure 11 shows the influence of osteoblast attachment onto surface acid etched during different time.

Data concerning cell attachment reveal a tendency of smooth surfaces to be a poorer substrate for osteoblast attachment when compared to rougher ones. (Eriksson et al., 2001) demonstrated that leukocyte adhesion on rough titanium surfaces is higher as well as its expression of adhesion receptors when compared to smooth counterparts. This could also occur with osteoblasts onto titanium surfaces.

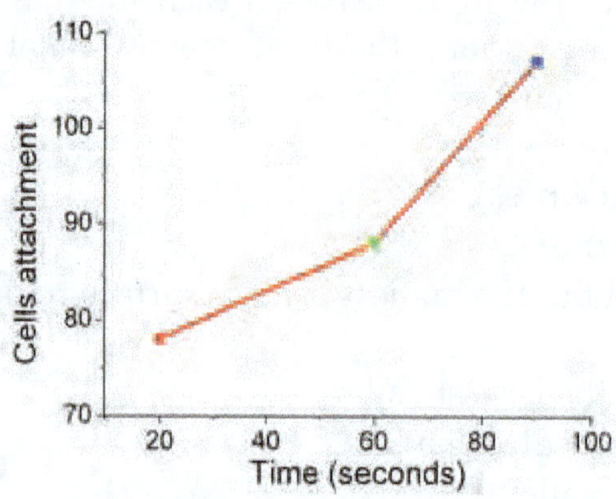

Fig. 11. Osteoblast cell attachment on titanium surfaces acid etched after 20, 40 and 60 seconds. (Adapted from Menezes et al., 2003)

The fact that osteoblasts on smoother surfaces exhibited a lengthened shape may be reflecting the grooves on the surface formed by the machining tolls (figure 12) Cells tend to grow along the grooves where those are seen. In consequence, if the grooves of the surface are arranged parallel to each other, cells become arranged in the same way. Osteoblasts also tend to spread over large areas in smooth surfaces. Thus, a rectangular shape and an arrangement in a continuous monolayer are expected to occur. Menezes et al. (Menezes, 2003) conclude in their work that smooth implant surfaces are poorer substrates for osteoblast attachment. Also, differentiation of the cells surrounding the implant should be the primary concern as long as a calcified bone around the implant is wanted.

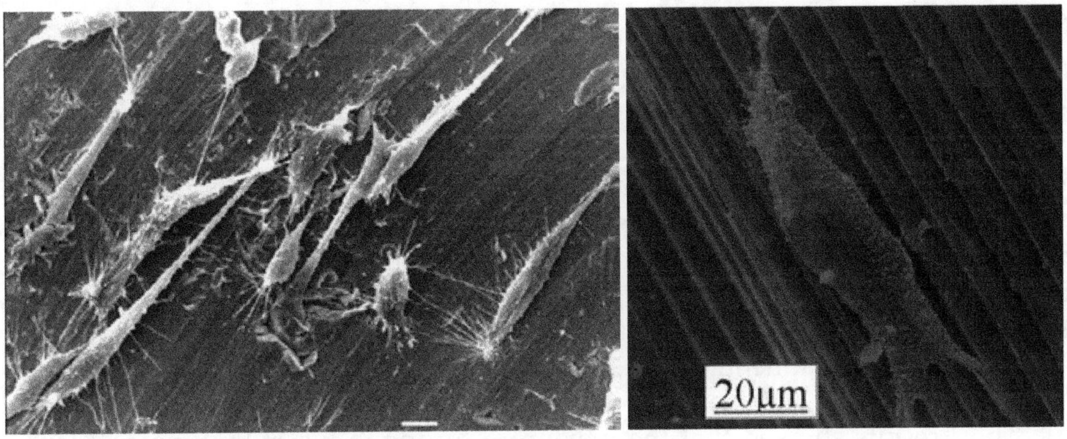

Fig. 12. Osteoblast cells growing along the grooves. (Menezes et al. 2003)

10. Influence of the implant surface on primary stability

Javed and Romanos (Javed & Romanos, 2010) evaluated the role of primary stability for successful of immediate loading (IL) of dental implants. This analysis is important because a fundamental prerequisite for implant success is substantial primary stability at the time of insertion and following loading of the implant. It may be considered as the unifying principle behind the need for adequate bone volume and density, longer or wider implants, and the 3–6-month delay recommended before implants are placed in function. A poor primary stability is one of the major causes of implant failure.

Although establishment of a good primary stability has been the primary focus during implant placement, there are numerous other factors that may contribute to the initial retention of the implant. Therefore, it is critical to maintain the integrity of the peri-implant tissues since bone resorption takes place with or without implant placement in the fresh extraction site. Specifically, for immediately loaded implants, the role of the primary implant stability with the surrounding, mature bone seems to be crucial for long term success.

Studies have shown that surface topography and roughness positively influence the healing process by promoting favorable cellular responses and cell surface interactions. Implant surface characteristics have also been shown to influence primary stability (Santos et al., 2009). Rough surfaces are considered to enhance primary stability as they present a larger surface area and allow a firmer mechanical link to the surrounding tissues (Romanos et al., 2002). Figure 13 shows the influence of surface finishing on dental implant primary stability.

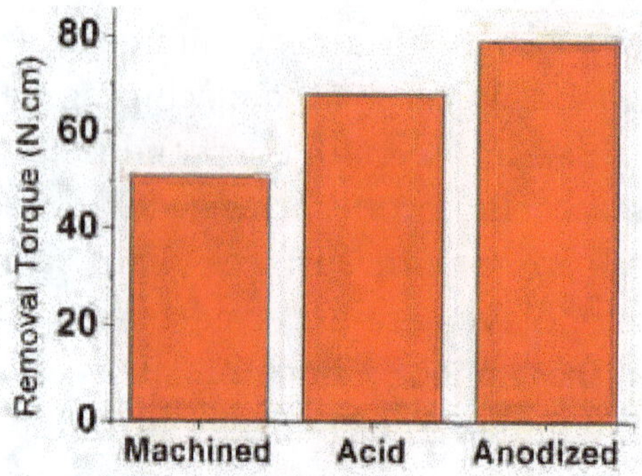

Fig. 13. Effect of the implant surface treatment on the insertion torque (N.cm). (adapted from Santos et al., 2009)

The primary stability of an implant fixture at the time of placement is often estimated by judging the presence of any mobility. In clinical work, primary stability can be evaluated either by the mobility from percussing an implant with a blunt instrument such as a mirror handle. The follow up of the implants can be estimated by devices such as Periotest, Periometer, resonance frequency analysis (RFA) and placement torque. Some factors affect the implant's primary stability, including the bone density, the implant design, the surgical technique, the insertion torque, and the instrumentation protocol. Among these parameters, the insertion torque has not yet been sufficiently analyzed. The insertion torque is a function of the implant surface treatment, design, and screw-thread geometry.

Santos et al. (Santos et al., 2009) analyzed the influence of dental implant surface on primary stability. Their results showed that the maximum torque to insert the implant depends on the friction coefficient between the implant surface and the placement wall, implant design, implant thread geometry and surface treatment.

For the same finishing surface, the differences in insertion torques reflect different implant geometries. The torque to install a conical implant is larger than the torque to install a cylindrical implant (figure 14). This difference can be attributed to the different thread geometry. Figure 8 and 15 show the cylindrical and the conical implants threads geometries. The screw threads are different in cylindrical and conical implants. The thread geometry of the conical implant increases the implant surface area in contact with the host tissue. The reduction in pitch of the conical implant thread increases its contact area as compared to the cylindrical implant. The conical implant has a larger area than the cylindrical implant (table 1). As surface area increases, the friction surface between the implant and the site wall increases, demanding a larger insertion torque.

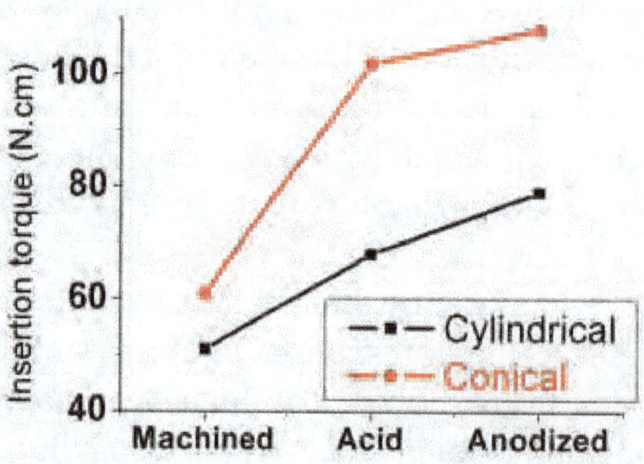

Fig. 14. Effect of the dental implant design and surface treatment on the insertion torque (N.cm). (adapted from Santos et al., 2009).

The implants submitted to a surface treatment presented a higher roughness and higher friction coefficient than the machined one. The implant that required the smaller insertion torque was the machined one, which possesses a smooth surface compared to the acid-etched or anodized samples. The insertion torque for the acid-etched implant was significantly different from the anodized implant.

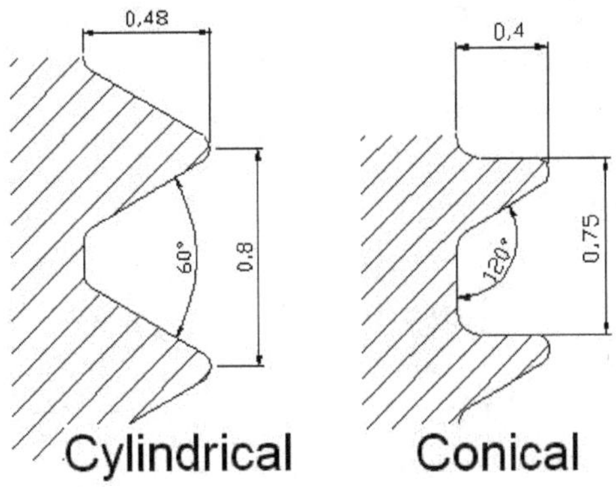

Fig. 15. Thread geometries of implants with cylindrical and conical design.

Javed et al. (Javed et al., 2011) reviewed the influence of surface morphology on the primary stability of dental implants. They conclude that rough-surfaced implants have significantly higher success rates compared with dental implants with smooth surfaces. Although the results in the literature show a direct relationship between surface roughness and overall implant stability, the influence of surface roughness on primary stability remained undetermined. Therefore, it is important to differentiate the initial implant stability gained from surface topographical features from that gained by the BIC.

11. Wettability

Dental implant surface wettability influences the degree of contact with the physiological environment. Highly hydrophilic surfaces seem more desirable than hydrophobic ones in view of their interactions with biological fluids, cells and tissues. Complete moistening and distribution of a liquid on a surface indicates high surface energy, biocompatibility and hydrophilicity of a material. Measurement of the contact angle of a liquid is one way to quantify the surface free energy of solids or the ability of the liquid to wet the solid. When the contact angle is greater than 90 degrees the surface is hydrophobic, as opposed to less than 90 degrees, when the surface is hydrophilic.

When a drop is placed in contact with the surface of a solid, there is interaction between the atoms of the liquid, the solid and the surrounding air. This interaction is observed in form of an attractive force between the atoms of the three materials. The greater the interaction between the surface and the liquid, the greater is the flattening of the drop (figure 3).

Baier and Meyer (Baier & Meier, 1988) related the critical surface tension between implants and biocompatibility. According to these authors, materials with high surface free energy adsorb more easily and have a higher number of favorable sites to allow connections to the cells. The general rule is that materials with a surface tension between 20 and 30 dynes/cm ^{2} exhibit low adhesion and materials with surface tension above this range have better results for osseointegration.

Baier (Baier & Meier, 1988) observed the effect of surface energy of titanium in bioactivity and found that the thickness of the protein that forms on the surface of the implants after 10 days of deployment depends on the surface energy. Histological observations made on implants with high surface energy indicated that they have layers of proteins with greater thickness than those with low energy. The cellular activity varies with the surface energy of the sample. When implants with low surface energy were mechanically separated from the capsule tissue and analyzed under a microscope, it was found that soft tissues occurred in most of the surface. It was observed that the host tissue in contact with implant with low surface energy has cells with globular appearance, almost spherical, that can easily be separated. The globular appearance of these cells identified them as fibroblasts and is associated with poor cell growth, but is not related to the normal activity of fibroblasts in the healing process.

Elias et al. (Elias et al., 2008) analyzed the influence of the dental implant surface treatment on contact angle and on removal torque (Table 3). The results showed that the surface treatment changes the surface wettability. The implants with treated surfaces showed greater roughness, higher friction coefficient, lower contact angle and demanded a larger insertion torque than machined implants. The contact angle of NaCl (highest hydrophilic liquid tested) with the anodized surface had the smallest value. No statistically significant difference ($P < 0.05$) in the contact angle between blood and any titanium surface was observed, except between blood and the anodized surface.

	Mean value ± SD contact angle (degree)				**Removal**
Implant Treatment	**Water**	**DMSO**	**NaCl**	**Blood**	**Torque (N.cm)**
Machined	85.20 ± 3.55	72.4 ± 2.3	51.6 ± 1.8	66.4 ± 0.5	57.0 ± 18.6
Acid etched	96.24 ± 9.20	68.7 ± 2.5	44.4 ± 1.6	61.6 ± 0.7	75.45 ± 10.5
Sandblasted	79.86 ± 4.85	52.5 ± 2.6	43.0 ± 0.9	61.8 ± 0.1	72.15 ± 14.9
Anodized	47.25 ± 2.94	38.3 ± 2.1	25.3 ± 1.3	55.5 ± 0.3	83.15 ± 12.7

Table 3. Mean value ± SD contact angle of treated titanium surfaces and dental implant removal torque from rabbit.

12. Influence of bone

Theoretically, for implants with the same dimensions, the choice of surface finishing is based on the type of bone that will receive the implant. Lekholm and Zarb (Lekholm & Zarb, 1985) classified the types of bones based on the quality of cortical bone and trabecular bone density. According to them, the bones can be classified as type D1, D2, D3 and D4.

The D1 bone has dense cortical and trabecular bone. Clinically, the D1 bone has little bleeding during surgery, indicating a slight vascularization. Because it is a harder bone, one should take extra care during the preparation of the implant insertion site to prevent overheating. Localized heating prevents the initial necrosis, which can be prolonged by ischemia caused by compression of the implant on the walls of the bone, keeping the contact area of bone in a state of compression. Implants with a length of 10 mm can be used.

The D2 has satisfactory cortical bone and a less dense and vascularized trabecular bone. In D2 bone there is lots blood in contact with the implant surface and initial stability is good. The implant should be at least 12 mm length and is required that at least 50% of the surface keeps the initial contact with the bone.

The cortical and trabecular in D3 bone is less dense than D2 and lower mechanical strength. Clinically, it is a brittle bone, with cortical and trabecular fragile little dense, which can often lead to poor initial anchor the implant.
The D4 bone has cortical papyracea (slender), slightly mineralized trabecula and has low mechanical strength. This type is very fragile, leading to a delicate surgical procedure to achieve initial implant anchorage.
Normally, the bone is of type D1 and D2 in the region between the mental foramen in the mandible and anterior maxilla. The bone type D3 can be found in the region of upper premolars and lower type D4 and will always be found in the molar region of mandible and maxilla.
For bone D1 and D2 can indicate machined dental implants without surface treatment. For the bone type D3 and D4 must be employed treated implant surface, which has higher contact area than machined and can improve the mechanisms involved in osseointegration. For the D3 and D4 bone type should always choose implants with surface treatment Misch (Misch, 2008) suggested for the D4 bone the use of implants larger than 12 mm and the largest diameter possible. The cavity preparation must be done very carefully, since due to low mechanical strength of bone, small lateral movements can easily move the slope of the planned implant.

13. Influence of surface morphology on implant osseointegration

Although titanium is used extensively as a biomaterial, there are still doubts about the procedure to obtain the best biological response. When analyzing the importance of the surface of the implant osseointegration to occur, one should separate the discussion of the influence of implant shape (design) and surface morphology. In shape analysis consider the dimensions of the implant (length, diameter, thickness), shape (barrel shape, cylindrical, conical and hybrid), type of threads (triangular, square, trapezoidal, rounded, microthread), height of fillets of threads, the thread angle, thread pitch and implant-prosthesis connection type (extern hexagon, internal connection in the form of a hexagon, cone Morse, star grip). These parameters influence the primary stability, the distribution of forces and mechanical properties of the implant. As for surface morphology should be analyzed macro and nanomicroestructure as well as the homogeneity of the surface, the chemical and physical properties.
Several researchers (Wennerberg et al., 1998; Hayakawas et al., 2000; Kokubo et al., 1999) examined the influence of surface properties of titanium implants on bone apposition into surface and the results showed that the biological response depends on the morphology, surface composition and titanium oxides on the implant surface in contact with the physiological environment. These results are important because the dentistry selects the roughness of the implant according to the surgical protocol, site of insertion, quality and quantity of available bone.
The surface properties of implants such as morphology, roughness, thickness of the oxide layer, impurity level and types of oxides depend on the surface treatment process. The difficulty in analyzing the influence of these parameters is the current inability to change only one parameter at a time keeping the others unchanged. For example, it is not feasible to modify only the titanium oxide crystalline structure or chemical composition, without change the oxide thickness.
During insertion of the implants immediately after the surface comes in contact with blood, a protein cover the implant surface. Titanium in contact with the physiological environment

absorbs molecules from the plasma, as so absorb factor I, factor III, Ig G and C1q. A few seconds after inserting the implant can find polymorphonuclear granulocytes and platelets adhered on its surface. Then there is the adhesion of mature granular leukocytes, neutrophils, basophils and acidophilus. The granulocytes polymorphonuclear leukocytes are the first recruited by the titanium surface exposed to contact with blood. Depending on the surface preparation is no difference in the absorption and reaction of cells exposed to titanium by contact with human blood (Werner et al., 2009; Puleo &Bizios, 1992; Kasiwagi et al., 2009; Novak et al., 2009; Eriksson et al., 2001). The adhesion of monocytes (mononuclear leukocytes of intense phagocytic activity, representing 3-7% of circulating blood leukocytes) is sensitive to variations in the thickness of the titanium oxide layer (Eriksson et al., 2001). Polymorphonuclear granulocytes are more dependent on surface roughness of the implant. Macrophages prefer areas with lower roughness.

A few months after insertion, the implants with treated surface have a higher amount of bone overlying the surface than machined implants with lower roughness. Possibly, the success depends on the speed of osteogenesis around the implant, ie, early osteoblast adhesion on implant surface. Despite this finding, it is unclear how the implant surface promotes or inhibits osteogenesis. The behavior of cells is dependent on the interaction of action and triggering activity of the cells and molecules (Henessy et al., 2009).

Cells have mechano-receptor properties that can identify whether or not the surface has features appropriate to begin the process of differentiation and bone matrix. The proteins attached on the surface of the implants induce adsorption and pre-osteoblastic cells. Research results show that the surface treatments affect the interfacial forces, wettability, roughness, energy and adsorption capacity of the molecules that recognize osteoblasts (Eriksson et al., 2001). Biomaterials in contact with the biological environment suffer dynamic changes in their surface properties, involving a cascade of reactions at the interface between the environment and biomaterial, forming a "conditioning film" that modulates the responses cellular (Puleo & Bizios, 1992). The wettability and surface energy influence on the adsorption of proteins and increase focal adhesions of osteoblasts on the surface of implant (Kashiwagi et al., 2009).

14. Surface treatment of implants

Numerous surface modification approaches have been developed for all classes of dental implants to modulate biological responses and improve the osseointegration and primary stability. Study of the surface treatment of dental implants is multidisciplinary, involving researchers from Materials Science, Mechanical Engineering, Mathematics, Computer Science, Dentistry, Surgery, Biophysics and Veterinary Medicine. The involvement of professionals from various fields and diverse knowledge facilitates the work, the analysis of results and development of new shapes and surfaces for the implants. Research results show that despite of the high success (95 to 98%) of titanium dental implants, it is necessary to analyze the surface characteristics of the implant with respect to surface finishing, physical properties, chemical composition, residual stress, morphology, microstructure and type of oxide (Henessy et al., 2009). A finishing deficiency of the implant can jeopardize the success of surgery, especially when there are contaminants from the manufacturing process, presence of burrs and stress concentration that compromises the mechanical performance of the implant during loading.

The success of dental implants will not occur when the implant surface morphology does not present features that allow adhesion and cell growth. The problem is increased by the presence of contaminants, mainly alumina particles used in the blast, which are toxic and lead to apoptosis. The deleterious effect of the existence of machining chips or holes in the surface of the implants refers to the possibility of these defects releases during implant insertion into the cavity and compromise the osseointegration. The process of machining and processing further determine the surface properties of implants, especially the electronic structure, crystalline oxide, chemical composition, mechanical and chemical properties.

The primary stability depends on the shape and surface morphology of implant. The secondary stability depends mainly on the implant surface. The differences among surfaces of available dental implants are the roughness, chemical composition, surface energy, chemical potential, the segregation of hydrides and nitrides, work hardening, the presence of metallic and nonmetallic, existence of impurities resulting from the manufacture or handling, type titanium oxide, crystal structure and oxide thickness of the oxide layer. This is important since the proteins interact with the oxides of the implant surface and the interaction depends on these parameters.

Surface roughness of dental implants can be analyzed in three orders of magnitude: macroscopic, microscopic and nanoroughness. Each size of the roughness provides contacts with different cells and biological molecules and is responsible for the intensity and types of biological bonding. A priori, it is expected that the increased surface area of the implant, increase the number of sites to bind to cells, facilitates tissue growth and increase the mechanical stability. However, this is not a general rule. Fibroblasts avoid rough surfaces and accumulate in the smooth surface. In contrast, macrophages exhibit rugophily behavior, or prefer to attach to rough surfaces. The epithelial cells are more attracted to rough surfaces than for smooth. Osteoblast cells adhere more easily on rough surfaces like those found on commercial implants with treated surfaces than in machined (Jayaraman et al., 2004; Le Duc & Wang, 2006; Thull, 2002; Lim et al., 2004).

The chemical composition of the surface determines the stability and reactivity of the implant, which shall consist solely of titanium oxide. Although there are no conclusive studies of the influence of impurities on the surface of the implants, the surface should contain the lowest possible levels of contamination. The surface energy and the existence of residual stresses after sandblasting modify the reactivity of the surface. Implant with coating has a complete different behavior. The coating modifies the behavior of cells and cascade reactions.

The surface morphology of dental implants is modified by chemical, mechanical and electrochemical treatments. By treating the surface of implants is possible to reduce the healing and loading time after surgery, accelerate growth and bone maturation, to increase the primary stability and to ensure the successful application in bone with less quality and quantity. There are many variables, combinations of parameters related to the implant surface treatment and factors that influence osseointegration (material, implant shape, implant surface, bone quality and quantity, surgical technique and loading condition).

The companies adopt a variety of techniques for surface treatment of commercial implants. By treating the surface of implants, it is possible to increase the stability, the wettability, the contact between implant and bone, the strength of the bone-implant interface and the success of treatment in patients seen as critical. Furthermore, it is possible to improve the retention of tissue, stimulate the healing process and reduce the loading time.

The choice of the methodology to be used in surface treatment is initiated by selecting the desired roughness, since the procedures for macroroughness, microroughness and nanoroughness are different. The current trend is to obtain hybrid surfaces, i.e., a morphology with micro- and nanoroughness. In some cases, the chemical composition of the implant surface is changed with addition of calcium, phosphorus and fluoride (Ellingsen et al. 2004). The precise role of surface chemistry and topography on the early events in dental implant osseointegration remain poorly understood.

For study purposes, the surface modification of dental implants shown in figure 7 and 9 can be divided in the followings classes:

a. machined surface (untreated surface);
b. plasma spray;
c. laser treatment;
d. acid etching;
e. sandblasting and sandblasting followed by acid etching;
f. anodizing;
g. deposition of nanoparticles by physical or chemical methods.

14.1 Implants with untreated surface (as machined)

Implants with untreated surface (machined) were the first to be used, but are seldom employed nowadays After manufacturing, these implants are subjected to cleaning, decontamination, passivation, and sterilization. The implants without surface treatment are inappropriately called "smooth". The term "smooth" is inadequate, since scanning electron microscopy shows that the surface of these implants has tool marks from the machining process (figure 9).

The disadvantage regarding to the morphology of untreated implants is the fact that osteoblastic cells are rugophilic – that is, they are prone to grow along the grooves existing on the surface, as shown in figure 12. This characteristic requires a longer healing time between surgery and implant loading. The use of these implants follows a protocol suggested by Brånemark: 3-6-month healing or waiting time prior to loading. Owing to morphological characteristics and lower resistance to removal torque (Table 1), machined dental implants are becoming commercially unavailable.

14.2 Surface treatment with plasma spray and laser

Two alternative surface treatments are laser ablation and plasma spraying the surface with a ceramic. After both treatments the implant surface has a large roughness (figure 7), which can be characterized as an area under macroroughnesss. The macroroughnesss influence the primary stability and mechanical fixation of bone formation but does not alter the behavior of cells during the period of osseointegration.

Gaggl et al. (Gaggl et al., 2000) cited that (i) surfaces of laser-treated Ti implants showed a high purity with appropriate roughness for good osseointegration, and (ii) the laser-treated Ti had regular patterns of micropores with interval of 10-12 μm, diameter of 25 μm, and depth of 20 μm.

Cho and Jung (Cho & Jung, 2003) evaluated the significance of different surface textures by comparison of the removal forces for laser-treated and machined titanium screw 8 weeks after the installation in rabbit tibia. They observed that laser treatment created a deep and regular honey-comb pattern with small pore, while machined treatment created the typical microscopically grooved and relatively smooth surface characteristic. In the laser surface, the distance between the pore was 10–12 μm. Eight weeks after implant placement, the

average removal torque was 23.58 ± 3.71Ncm for the machined implants, 62.57 ± 10.44Ncm for the laser-treated implants.
The micropores in laser treated implants, evaluated by Gaggl et al. (Gaggl et al., 2000) and by Cho and Jung (Cho & Jung, 2003), do not improve osseointegration. Figure 16 shows the morphology of an implant surface treated with a laser. The surface exhibits macroroughness at low magnification, whereas melting structures can be observed at high magnification. At higher magnification, a laser-treated surface is smoother than acid etching. The best implant surface has microroughness and nanoroughness.

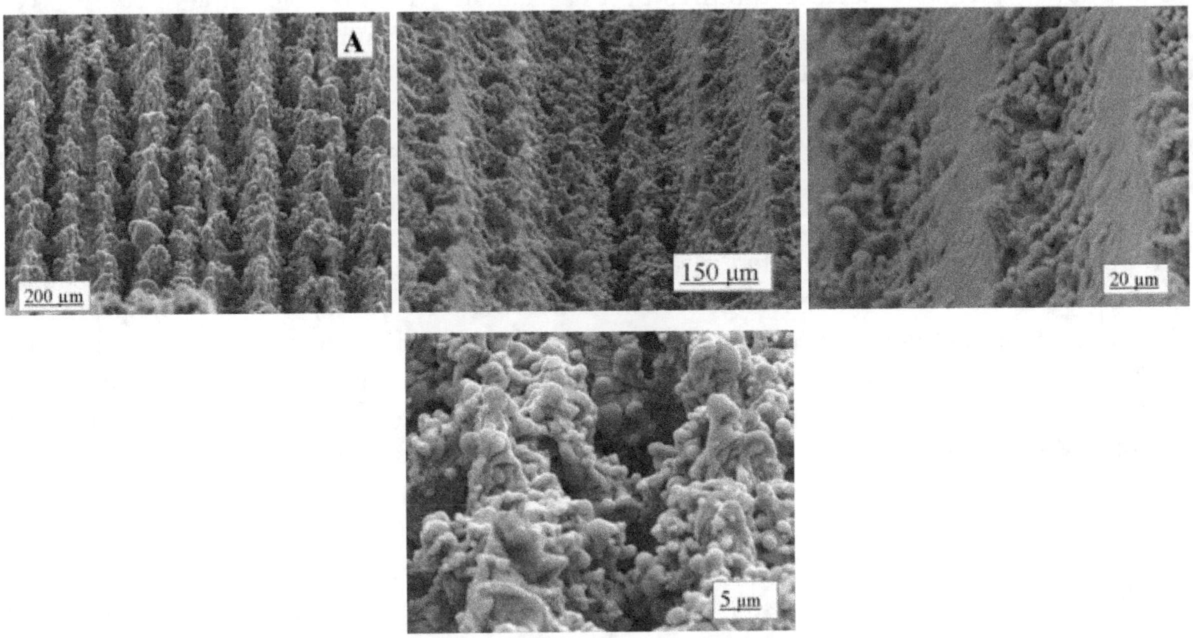

Fig. 16. Surface morphology of titanium after laser treatment. The surface has macroroughness and at high magnification shows melting structure.

Cordioli et al. (Cordioli et al., 2000) reported that average removal torque value was 25.28 N·cm for the machined implants, 26.85 N·cm for the grit-blasted implants, 29.57 N·cm for the plasma-sprayed implants, and 40.85 N·cm for the acid-etched implants under similar conditions. Their results showed that removal torque value of plasma-sprayed implants has approximately the same value of machined or grit-blasted implants.
Plasma spraying and laser treatments are no longer being used, because of the resulting macrorugosities. It is expected that surface characteristics exhibit biological influence during implant installation and interaction with cells by modifying the mechanisms involved in cell adsorption and differentiation.
The osseointegration of dental implants with plasma-sprayed HA is faster than for uncoated implants. However, studies have shown that these coatings may be partially dissolved/resorbed after long periods in use (Sun et al., 2001). [. In addition, the HA coating is chemically unstable and bonds weakly to the implant surface.
Considering the potential of the association between laser ablation and smaller scale HA coatings to create a stable and bioactive surface on titanium dental implants, Faeda *et al.* (Faeda et al., 2009) analyzed the effects of a surface treatment by laser-ablation (neodymium-doped yttrium aluminum garnet [Nd:YAG]) and, later, thin deposition of HA particles by a chemical process. They compared the removal torque of implants treated with

laser followed by acid etching, implants with only laser-ablation and implants with machined surface (MS). After 4, 8 and 12 weeks of healing, the removal torque was measured. Average removal torque in each period was 23.3, 24.0 and 33.9 N·cm for MS, 33.0, 39.9 and 54.6 N·cm for laser modified surface (LMS), and 55.4, 63.7 and 64.0 N·cm for HA (Figure 21). The difference was statistically significant ($p < 0.05$) between the LMS-MS and HA-MS surfaces for all evaluation periods, and between LMS-HA for 4 and 8 weeks of healing. The surface characterization showed a deep, rough and regular topography provided by the laser conditioning that was followed by the HA coating. They conclude that the implants with laser surface modification associated with HA biomimetic coating can shorten the implant healing period by the increase of bone implant interaction during the first 2 months after implant placement.

Although the use of hydroxyapatite-coated endosseous implants in the treatment of dental patients has been established, their clinical predictability remains controversial. A number of clinical and basic studies evaluating the effect of HA coating have been reported. Concerns regarding microbiological susceptibility, resorption, fatigue, and fracture in long-term application have been pointed out. Clinical studies suggest that HA-coated implants have short-term survival rates (ranging from 6 months to 6 years) that are comparable to short-term survival rates of titanium implants (Biesbrock & Edgerton, 1995). In conclusion, the clinician needs to take into consideration the enhanced bacterial susceptibility of HA coatings compared with titanium implants. In addition, the clinician needs to consider the possible failure of HA coatings as a result of coating-substrate interfacial fracture (Ong & Chan, 2000). Dental implants with titanium or hydroxyapatite coating produced by plasma spray are in disuse.

Among commercially available dental implants coated with hydroxyapatite using the plasma spraying technique one can cite the Bonelike® (Biomet 3i, USA) and Calcitek (Sulzer Calcitek Inc., USA)

14.3 Surface treatment with acid

The acid etched dental implant surface presents a superficial morphology that varies with the treatment conditions (acid, chemical composition percentage, etching time and temperature treatment). Through acid etching, it is possible to control the roughness, number, size and porous distribution on micrometer and nanometer scales.

Every manufacturer has its own acid etching method regarding concentration, time and temperature for treating implant surfaces. In general, acid treatment is performed by immersing the implants into solutions of HCl + H2SO4, HF + HNO3 and HNO3. After acid attack, the implant is again immersed into an aqueous solution of HNO3 for passivation of titanium oxide and formation of a stable oxide layer (Elias & Meirelles, 2010). An example of the morphology of an acid-etched surface of a commercially available implant is shown in figure 17.

Acid treatments provide homogeneous roughness, increased active surface area and improve cells adhesion. The morphology of the implant surface shown in figure 16 is isotropic and exhibits micro-cavities with defined edges. This type of surface not only facilitates retention of osteogenic cells, but also allows them to migrate towards the implant surface. Implants having surface morphology similar to that shown in figure 16 induce fibrin retention, favor adsorption of fibronectin and improve the osseointegration (Brunette, 2001; Braceras et al. 2009).

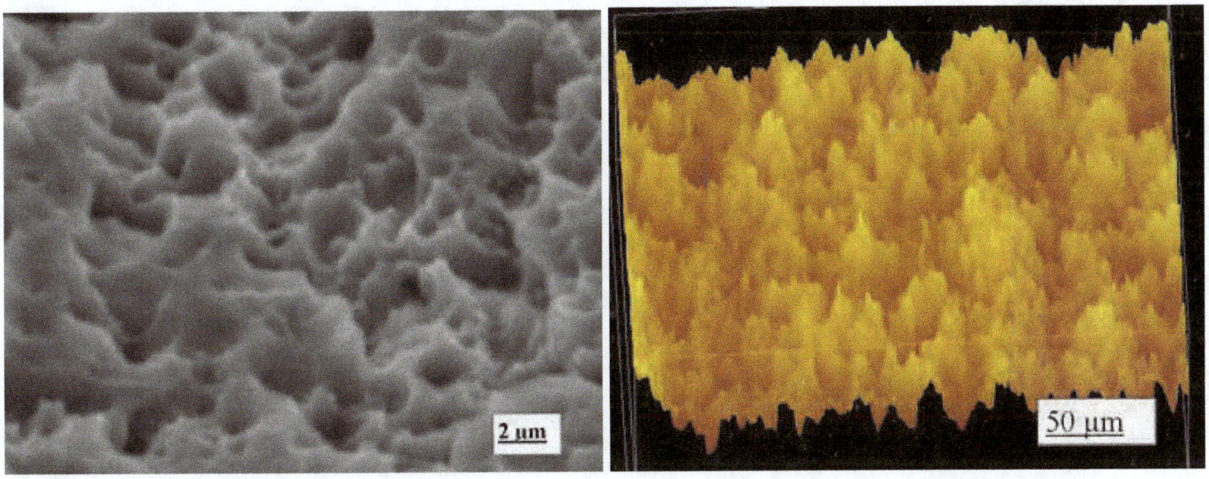

Fig. 17. Surface morphology of dental implant Master Porous™ acid etched, showing microporous.

As Table 3 and figure 14 show, the removal torque of acid etched implants is higher than that of machined implants, which means that the osseointegration mechanisms are faster in acid treated implants than machined implants

Among the commercially available acid-treated implants, one can cite the Master Porous System® (Conexão Sistema de Próteses, Brazil), Osseotite™ (Biomet 3i, USA), Friadenty Plus® (Friadent GmbH, Germany), Defcon TSA® (Impladent SL, Spain) and BlackFix® (TitaniumFix, Brazil).

Wennerberg (Wennerberg et al., 2003) analized some samples of the Osseotite™ implants and measured the roughness surface parameters. They showed that the Tioblast™ has S_a = 0.94 µm, S_{cx} = 11.68 and S_{dr} increased.

14.4 Sandblasting surface treatment

When the implant is blasted with silicon oxide (silica), aluminum oxide (alumina), titanium oxide (rutile), hydroxyapatite and calcium phophate, the implant surface suffers plastic microdeformation. The sandblasting process induces the formation of a fine superficial layer with residual stress. Part of the kinetic energy of the particles is stored in the form of crystal defects, such as dislocations, twins and grain boundaries, and these modifications increase the material surface energy. The superficial layer with residual compressive stress increases the material's fatigue resistance (Askeland, 2006). The residual stress values obtained from blasting procedures depend on both hardness and particles size distribution. The influence of residual stress has not been analyzed in the field of dental implants.

The influence of surface roughness on bone formation on titanium-blasted surfaces was evaluated by Wennerbeg et al. (Wennerbeg et al., 1995). The samples were blasted with Al2O3 particles. After surface preparation, the samples were passivated, washed with distilled water and dried. The results from animal experiments showed higher values for removal torque and bone-to-implant contact for samples blasted with 25 µm and 75 µm sized particles compared with those machined or blasted with 250-µm particles.

The blasting procedure allows control of the size of microcavities. After the grit blasting procedure some particles may be encrusted on the implant surface, which is a contamination (figure 18). The particle must be removed with ultrasonic bath and acid etching.

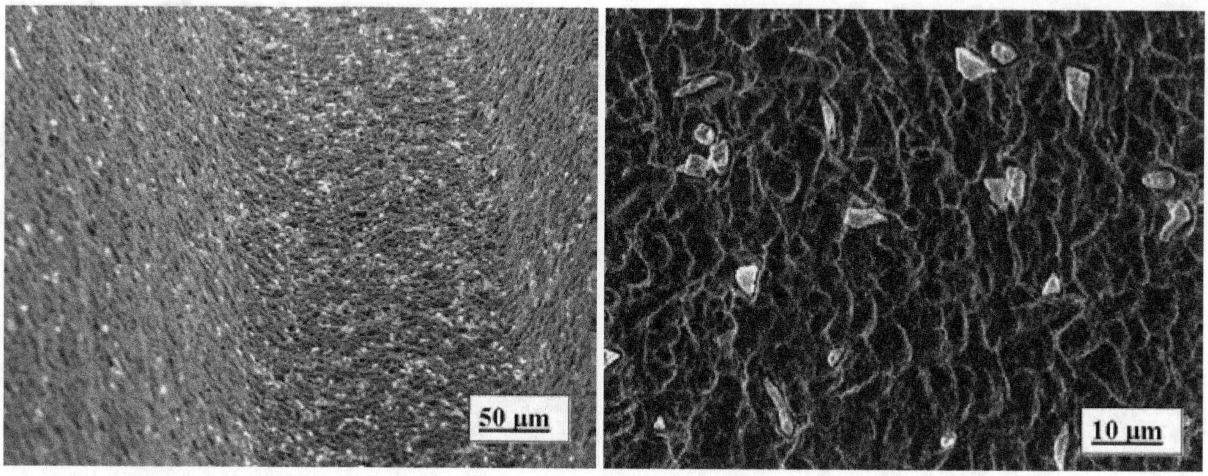

Fig. 18. Particles of alumina (left) and titanium oxide (right) encrusted on the sandblasted implant surface.

Sandblasting with TiO2 is also adopted in the production of implants Tioblast™ (Astra Tech Implant System, Sweden) and TitaniumFix BlackFix (TitaniumFix Implant, Brazil). Tioblast™ is gritblasted with 25-μm titanium oxide particles, which create small pits of predetermined size and shape. Another example of sandblasted implant is Bicon (Bicon LLC, Boston, MA) which is alumina-blasted/acid-etched titanium alloy substrate.

Wennerberg (Wennerbeg et al., 2003) evaluated the Tioblast™ implant. Their results showed this implant has S_a = 1.07 μm, S_{cx} = 10.11 μm and the surface parameter S_{dr} increased 29%.

Another procedure to implant surface treatment is acid etching after blasting. Acid treatment after blasting removes some atomic layers of the titanium surface deformed by the blasting procedure, but part of the residual strain remains at the implant surface.

Available implants SLA™ (Sand-blasted, Large grit, Acid-etched) from Straumann (Straumann ITI, Germany) are sandblasted and acid etched. Alumina particles in the size range 25–50 μm are used to sandblast the SLA™ implant. Sandblasting is followed by an acid etch in hot HCl/H2SO4 acid solution. These processes create micropits superimposed on the rough-blasted surface. Jarmar et al. measured the roughness on SLA™ and found it to be 1.98 ± 0.08 μm (Jarmar et al., 2008). Another way Wennerberg et al. (Wennerbeg et al., 2003) verified that SLA™ implant has Sa = 1.42 μm, waviness parameter S_{cx} = 16.60 μm and the surface parameter S_{dr} increased 33%.

14.5 Surface treatment with fluoride

It is known that fluoride ions have osteopromoting capacity leading to increased calcification of the bone. One of the characteristics of fluoride is its biphasic nature. Fluoride produces beneficial effects when used in low concentrations and toxic effects if used in high concentrations. In therapeutic doses, it is capable of causing mass increase of cortical and trabecular bone. If used in excessive doses, it can lead to bone deficient in collagen cross-links and with increased solubility. With high doses of fluoride, the tensile mechanical properties of the bone are reduced.

Fluoride increases proliferation and differentiation of osteoblasts (Cooper et al., 2006). Ion modification of the topographically enhanced c.p. titanium surface can affect bone formation by modulation of cellular activities at relatively early stages in wound healing at the implant surface. Fluoride increases the alkaline phosphatase activity and increases collagen synthesis.

According to Cooper et al. (Cooper et al., 2006) in vitro evaluation of hMSC (human mesenchymal stem cells) differentiation along the osteoblastic lineage demonstrated that fluoride ion modification of the TiO2 grit-blasted surface led to greater osteoblastic differentiation by adherent hMSCs. This conclusion is most strongly supported by the assessment of BSP expression showing greater expression on all fluoride ion-modified surfaces. The increased BSP expression observed in hMSCs cultured on fluoride ion-modified c.p. titanium was consistent. Whenever the fluoride surface ion content was greater than 5.0 ion % on the 25 μm grit-blasted surface, BSP expression increased (4 fold when compared to densitometric scanning versus Actin) and when fluoride surface ion content was greater than 1.0 ion%, BSP increased 1.6 fold. BSP expression is required for osteoblastic differentiation and mineralization in culture and is temporally associated with the onset of osteoid mineralization in vitro.

Human osteoblastic cells grown on the fluorapatite-collagen composites exhibited significantly higher proliferation and differentiation (according to alkaline phosphatase activity) than those on the hydroxyapatite-collagen composite and the investigators attributed this effect to fluoride release from the fluorapatite containing composite. In addition to direct effects of fluoride ions with osteoblastic cells or indirect fluoride ion effects on protein adsorption and subsequent cell adhesion, another possible indirect effect of fluoride at the c.p. titanium surface could be calcium phosphate precipitation that could influence local calcium concentrations and cell behavior. Ionic modification could alter the array of adhesive proteins adsorbed to the implant surface that could further affect cell and tissue interactions.

There is a relationship between cellular response and the concentration of F-ions (Cooper et al., 2006). For concentrations from 25 to 200 ngF-/mL, i.e., up to the threshold of toxicity, there is a linear increase of intracellular calcium. If the concentration is raised from 500 to 1000 ngF-/mL, the intracellular calcium falls to a level lower than for concentrations in the 100 ngF-/mL range. The cellular effects mentioned occur for short times of exposure to fluoride ions.

Berglundh et al. (Berglundh et al., 2007) studied the early stages of osseointegration to implants with a fluoride-modified surface. Six mongrel dogs, about 1-year old, were used. All mandibular premolars and the first mandibular molars were extracted. Three months later, mucoperiosteal flaps were elevated in one side of the mandible and six sites were identified for implant placement. The control implants (MicroThreadt) had a TiOblast™ surface, while the test implants (OsseoSpeed™) had a fluoride-modified TiOblast™ surface. The results showed that the amount of new bone that formed in the voids within the first 2 weeks of healing was larger at fluoride-modified implants (test) than at TiOblast™ (control) implants. It was further observed that the amount of bone-to-implant contact that had been established after 2 weeks in the macro-threaded portion of the implant was significantly larger at the test implants than at the controls. They suggested that the fluoride-modified implant surface promotes osseointegration in the early phase of healing following implant installation.

The OsseoSpeed™ (Astra Tech AB, Sweden) dental implant surface is fluoride-modified (hydrofluoric acid-treated surface). The implant surface is blasted and later etched with diluted hydrofluoric acid, which slightly reduces the high peaks. The final surface structure has an isotropic roughness – that is, there is no preferred direction of the surface irregularities (Ellingsen et al., 2004). During the blasting procedure, the surface roughness is increased. The OsseoSpeed surface has Sa = 0.91 ± 0.14 μm and the TiOblast™ surface has Sa = 1.12 ± 0.24 μm. The hydrofluoric acid treatment does not only change the microstructure, but also the surface chemistry. According to Ellingsen (Ellingsssen, 1995) the surface fluoride incorporated in the oxide acts as a precipitation site for calcium and phosphorus, and also allows covalent bonding to the phosphate to create fluoridated HA and fluorapatite.

14.6 Anodizing surface treatment and crystalline oxide structure

One of the methods used to treat the surface of implants is increasing the thickness and change the crystalline structure of the titanium oxide layer on the surface by anodizing.
Anodizing is an electrochemical process where the implant is immersed in an electrolyte while a current is applied, which will make the implant the anode in an electric cell. Commercial dental implants, such as TiUnite™ (NobelBiocare, Switzland) and Vulcano Actives™ (Conexão Sistemas de Prótese, Brazil), are anozided. The electrolyte and the current used in the implants treatment process create a porous surface structure (figure 19).

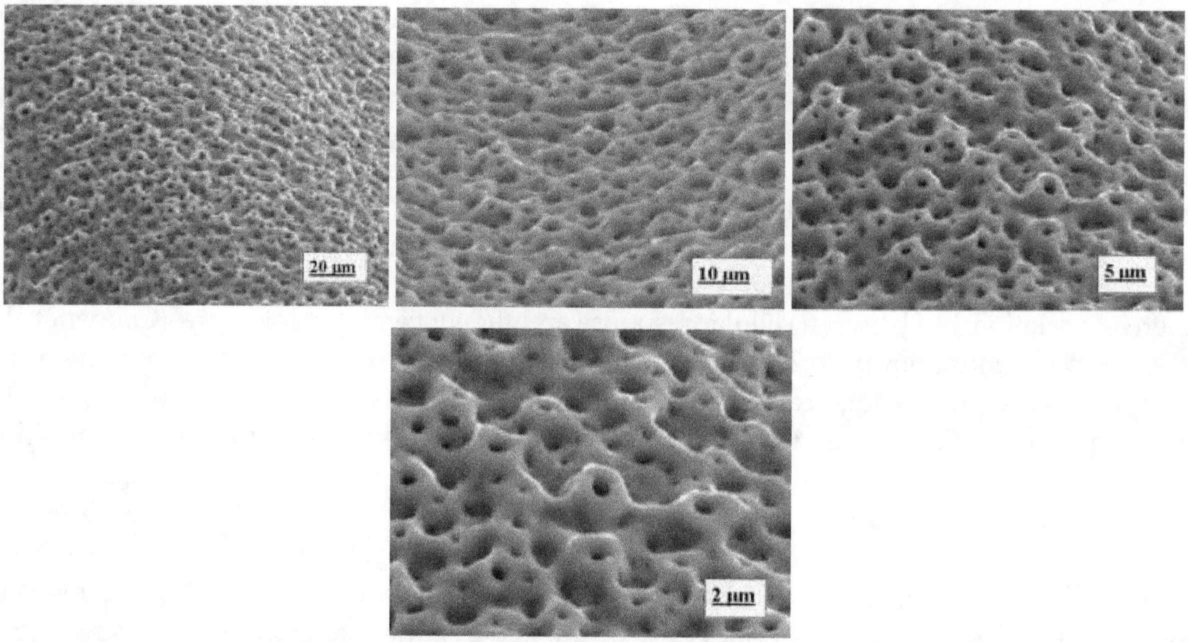

Fig. 19. Anodized dental implant surface, showing volcano shaped saliencies

As Oshida et al. (Oshida et al., 2010) oxides formed on Ti materials are varied with a general form; TiO_X ($1 < x < 2$). Depending on x values, there are five different crystalline oxides; i.e., (1) cubic TiO (ao = 4.24 Å), (2) hexagonal Ti2O3 (ao = 5.37 Å, α = 56°48′), (3) tetragonal TiO2 (anatase) (ao = 3.78Å, co = 9.50 Å), (4) tetragonal TiO2 (rutile) (ao = 4.58 Å, co = 2.98 Å), and (5) orthorhombic TiO2 (brookite) (ao = 9.17 Å, bo = 5.43 Å, co = 5.13 Å). Besides these, there are (6) non-stoichiometric oxide (when x is not integral), and (7) amorphous oxides. It is widely believed that, among these oxides, only rutile and anatase type oxides are stable at normal conditions. Of interest, choice for rutile formation or anatase formation depends on the acidity of used electrolyte. The rutile and anatase type oxides exibit different physical properties - interms of surface tension (Lim et al., 2001) prepared various surface conditions on pure titanium and measured surface contact angles, surface electrochemical potential and roughness. It was found that the surface covered with only rutile type TiO2 was hydrophobic, whereas that covered with a mixture of rutile and anatase type of oxides showed hydrophilicity.

Rutile and anatase titanium oxide are the most important oxide structures for osseointegration of implants. In addition to the increase in oxide layer thickness, the titanium oxide film obtained from electrochemical anodizing incorporates calcium and phosphorus as a heritage from the electrolyte. The surface has more than 7% phosphorus in the oxide layer, the highest percentage of amorphous hydroxides compared with other implants assessed by x-ray photoelectron spectroscopy (XPS). As a result, the titanium oxide existing on the implant surface shows changes in its morphology and crystal structure (Busquim et al., 2009).

Busquim et al. (Busquim et al., 2009) analyzed with x-ray diffraction, Raman and XPS the surface of anodized implant. They found that a predominance of anatase forms on anodized surfaces compared with MS, where the rutile crystal is predominant figure 20).

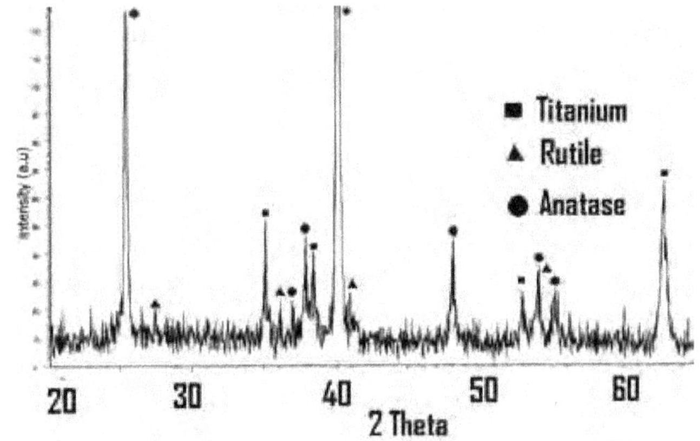

Fig. 20. X-ray diffraction pattern of the anodized titanium surface showing the presence of titanium oxides with crystalline structure in the form of rutile and anatase (dental implant Vulcano Actives™).

The anodized surface implant has a higher polarity compared with that of acid-treated samples, which causes adsorption of water and molecules. Adsorption of these molecules creates an electric field along the oxide thickness. This electric field induces titanium oxidation and, at the same time, the oxide layer thickness increases, thus decreasing both potential difference and the driving force for dissolution (Sul et al., 2006). In this way, taking into account that surface structure as well as morphology are correlated with wettability, changes in their properties affect adsorption of proteins needed for cell adhesion on the implant surface. Consequently, the performance of a given treated surface depends on the biological response of the implants used.

Depending on the anodizing parameters (potential, electrolyte chemical concentration, temperature), the solid oxide layer can be either compact or nanotubular (nanoporous). Figure 18 shows that the oxidized dental implant surface morphology has volcano shaped saliencies.

The TiO2 film obtained by electrochemical anodizing incorporates P and Ca ions from the electrolyte, which alters the final properties of titanium oxide (Elias & Meirelles, 2010). Experiments in cell cultures have shown that incorporated calcium ions on the implant surface increase the adhesion of human bone cells to the implant, when compared to unmodified titanium implants and implants with incorporated phosphate ions (Fröjd et al., 2008; Feng et al., 2004; Nayab et al., 2005). Also, the release of alkaline phosphatase from osteoblasts during bone formation has been found to be increased (Feng et al., 2004). The expected effect of the added calcium ions is a more rapid initiation of bone mineralization, because of the attraction of bone matrix proteins. The calcium ions may also function as binding sites for initial mineral crystal growth when they bond with phosphate ions in the extracellular body fluid (Ohtsu et al., 2007).

The characterization of the anodized implant surface by X-ray diffraction, Raman and XPS show that the surface of anodized implants shows a predominance of anatase. On machined implant surface the main oxide is rutile (Figure 11) with hydrophobicity. The sandblasted and acid etched implants surfaces OsseoSpeed™, Osseotite™, and SLA™ have rutile too, but their surface morphologies are different of machined implant. The anodized implant Vulcano Actives™ (Conexão Sistemas e Prótese, Brazil) and TiUnite™ (Nobel Biocare, Sweden) have rutile and anatase on the surface (figure 19).

The tissue healing process around anodized or acid etched implants, inserted in bone sites with and without defects, is quicker than in machined implants. Gurgel el al. (Gurgel et al., 2008) analyzed the efficiency of anodized implants. They used dog, and 3 months after teeth extraction, they produced defects measuring 5 mm high and 4 mm wide. After this they inserted the implants. The animals were sacrificed 3 months after the implant insertion. The researchers found that the percentages of bone-to-implant contact (BIC) and bone density (BD) of anodized implants were 57.03 ± 21.86% and 40.86 ± 22.73%, whereas machined implants had 37.39 ± 23.33% and 3.52 ± 4.87%, respectively.

Sul *et al.* (Sul et al., 2006) compared mechanical strength and osseous-conductivity of anodized implants containing magnesium, TiUnite™ (anodized) and Osseotite™ (double acid attack). The implants were inserted into rabbit tibia, and 3–6 weeks later removal torques and the percentage of bone-to-implant contact were measured. Figure 21 shows the experimental results. Magnesium implants demonstrated significantly greater removal torque values and more quantity of new bone formation than Osseotite™ at 3 and 6 weeks. Magnesium implants also showed higher removal torque values at 3 weeks and new bone formation at 6 weeks than TiUnite. The results indicate that surface chemistry facilitated more rapid and stronger osseointegration of the magnesium implants. This suggests potential advantages of magnesium implants for reducing high implant failure rates in the early post implantation stage and in compromised bone, making it possible to shorten bone healing time from surgery to functional loading, and enhancing the possibility of immediate/early loading.

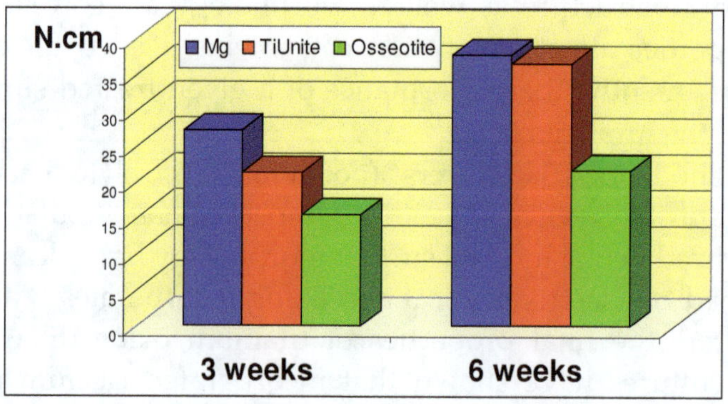

Fig. 21. Torque for removal (N.cm) and percentage of bone contact with implant surface Mg, TiUnite™ and Osseotite™. (Adapted from Sul et al. (Sul et al., 2006).

The anodized surface implant has a higher polarity compared with that of acid-treated samples, which causes adsorption of water and molecules. Adsorption of these molecules creates an electric field along the oxide thickness. This electric field induces titanium oxidation and, at the same time, the oxide layer thickness increases, thus decreasing both potential difference and the driving force for dissolution (Sul et al., 2006).

In this way, taking into account that surface structure as well as morphology are correlated with wettability, changes in their properties affect adsorption of proteins needed for cell adhesion on the implant surface. Consequently, the performance of a given treated surface depends on the biological response of the implants used.

Fröjd et al. (Fröjd et al., 20008) evaluated the bone response to an oxidized titanium implant (Ox) and a calcium-incorporated oxidized titanium implant (Ca). A blasted with 75 μm Al2O3 particles titanium implant (Bl) was used as control. The implants were topographically characterized using an optical interferometer and placed: one in each distal femoral metaphysis and two in each proximal tibial metaphysis in rabbits. The rabbits were killed 12 weeks after implant insertion. Topographical evaluation revealed three different surfaces: average height deviation (Sa, μm) values for Ca:Ox:Bl implants were 0.3:0.6:0.9, developed surface area ratios (%) 17:44:31. The Ca implants had a significantly denser surface, as represented by the parameter Sds, with 208 $\pm$ 24 sumsummits/μm^2; the Ox implants had a mean value of 136 $\pm$ 9 sumsummits/μm^{2}and the Bl implants 118 $\pm$ 9 sumsummits/μm^2. The core fluid retention index values were 1.33:1.33:1.38 in Ca, Ox and Bl implant, respectivaly. The mean percentages of bone contact to the implants placed in the tibia (Ca:Ox:Bl) were 47:30:34 and to the implants placed in the femur (Ca:Ox) 32:20. The mean percentages of surrounding bone area for the implants placed in the tibia were 40:47:37 and for the implants placed in the femur 43:46. A significant increase in bone contact was found for smooth (Sa <0.5 μm) but more densely peaked calcium-incorporated oxidized implants when compared to slightly rougher (Sa = 0.5-1.0 μm) oxidized or blasted implants.

14.7 Nanoroughness

Yang et al. (Yang et al., 2009) produced through the electrochemical anodizing treatment a mixed nano/submicron-scale TiO2 network layer (lateral pore size: 20–160 nm) on polished Ti surface. Results showed that a nano/submicron-scale TiO2 network layer with a lateral pore size of 20–160nm could be rapidly produced on Ti surface through electrochemical anodizing treatment. This TiO2 network layer significantly enhanced the whole blood coagulation and human bone marrow stem cell .

Webster *et al.* evaluated osteoblast adhesion *in vitro* on alumina and titania discs prepared by compacting powders with different sized particles onto the surface (Webster et al., 1999). The discs were sintered at different temperatures to obtain different nanoroughness parameters. Higher osteoblast adhesion was observed on both alumina and titania discs with increased mean root square deviation (Sq) and larger surface area. Additionally, discs prepared with an identical method consisting of Ti, Ti6Al4 and CoCrMo was tested. As previously reported on alumina and titania discs, increased osteoblast adhesion was found on the discs from the different groups with increased mean root square deviation (Webster & Ejiorf, 2004). Webster *et al.* investigated osteoblast adhesion and concentration of different proteins adsorbed on alumina, titania and HA, with different nanoroughnesses (Webster et al. 2000). Once again, the osteoblast adhesion was greater on the discs that exhibited increased nanoroughness, independently of the surface chemistry. Protein adsorption revealed a greater amount of vitronectin associated with increased osteoblast adhesion on the rougher discs. Osteoblast proliferation and alkaline phosphatase synthesis on these surfaces was evaluated in another study from the same group; alkaline phosphatase synthesis was higher after 21 and 28 days on the discs with increased nanoroughness values. De Oliveira and Nanci (Oliveira & Nanci, 2004) cultured bone rat calvaria cells on titanium discs etched with H2SO4 and H2O2. They observed that the acid-etched surface revealed nanopits, whereas the control failed to show such features, although the surface roughness was not numerically evaluated. The results indicated an overexpression of osteopontin and bone sialoprotein, both intra- and extra-cellularly, on cells seeded on the nano-modified group. In addition, a higher proportion of cells with peripheral cytoplasmic distribution of osteopontin were observed as early as 6 h.

Larlsson *et al.* evaluated turned plus anodized, electropolished, and electropolished plus anodized implants on a rabbit model after 1–6 weeks (Larsson et al., 1996). After 6 weeks, the electropolished implants showed decreased bone formation compared with the rougher implants. In an identical study, similar implants were investigated after 7–12 weeks of healing (Larsson et al., 1994 After 7 weeks, the results were similar to the previous study, which indicated higher bone formation to implants with increased surface roughness values (anodized) compared with the smooth implants (electropolished). After 12 weeks, the values for the rough implants were steady and the values for the electropolished implants increased to approximately the same level as that found for the rougher implants. Long-term evaluation of these implants for 1 year did not reveal any difference in bone formation (Larsson et al., 1997). It is concluded by *in vitro* and *in vivo* experiments that cell activity and bone healing may be optimized by modulating surface roughness on the nanometer level of resolution.

15. Conclusion

The success in implant dentistry depends on several parameters that may improve considering both biologic and mechanical criteria. Given below are some conclusions which show factors affecting the success of dental implants treatment.

- Although titanium is used extensively as a biomaterial, there are still doubts about the procedure to obtain the best biological response. Special relevance is the study of commercially pure titanium dental implant osseointegration.
- The strategy to improve dental implant osseointegration is to alter the biocompatibility of titanium implant surfaces, modifying the surgical technique and changing the implant design.
- The study of the interaction of cells with implant surface is a field of high topical interest and the detailed knowledge of these interactions can be used as the basis for the development of new surface treatments.
- Topographic characteristics, roughness, energy, and chemical composition modify cell growth and change cell function at the initial stages of osseointegration.
- Numerous surface modification approaches have been developed in order to improve commercially pure titanium dental implant osseointegration, to increase the primary stability and, in order to shorten the healing time.
- The surface properties of implants such as morphology, roughness, thickness of the oxide layer, chemical composition, impurity level and types of oxides depend on the surface treatment process.

- The titanium dental implant surface morphology was modified by chemical and electrochemical treatment. Most of these surfaces have been analyzed by *in vivo* and *in vitro* studies, showing that the surface characteristics of the dental implants influence cell activity, which modifies the differentiation, proliferation, differentiation, and formation of extracellular matrix.
- The results show that the acid etching, sandblasting and electrochemical implant surface treatments are better than plasma spray or laser treatment. But, there is not a consensus among researchers as to the best surface and even the shape of the implants.
- The dental implant primary stability depends on the shape and surface morphology. The secondary stability depends mainly on the implant surface. The torque to install a conical implant is larger than the torque to install a cylindrical implant.
- The implants submitted to a surface treatment have a higher roughness, higher friction coefficient and higher primary stability than the machined one.
- There is need for research to improve the description of the interaction of cells with the implant surfaces, as well as analysis of the influence of different parameters in the interaction with proteins, stimulation of bone formation, use of individualized therapy and able to submit response differentiated for patients considered critical.

16. Acknowledgments

This manuscript has been supported by grants, here gratefully acknowledged, from Brazilian Government Research Foundation (CNPq under the 472449/2004-4, 400603/2004-7, 500126/2003 and 6306343/2006-1 project and FAPERJ E_26/102.714/2008 project).

17. References

Albrektsson T, Brånemark PI, Hansson HA, and Jonsson U. Ultrastructural analysis of the interface zone of titanium and gold implants, in *Clinical Applications of Biomaterials* (Eds Lee AJC, Albrektsson T and Brånemark P.-l.), John Wiley, New York, USA, 1982. pp 167-l 77 Plenk. H. Pfklger, G. and Bohler. ISBN 0-86715-129-3.

Albrektsson T, Brånemark PI, Hansson, HA & Lindström J. (1981). Osseointegrated titanium implants. *Acta Orthopaedica Scandinavica*, 52, pp.155–179, ISSN 0001-6470.

Anitua E, Carda C, Andia I. (2007). A Novel Drilling Procedure and Subsequent Bone Autograft Preparation: A Technical Note. *International Journal of Oral Maxillofacial Implants*. Vol.22, pp.138–145, ISSN 0882-2786.

Anselme K, Bigerelle M. (2005). Topography effects of pure titanium substrates on human osteoblast long-term adhesion. *Acta Biomaterialia*. Vol.1, pp.211–222, ISSN 1742-7061.

Anselme K. (2000). Osteoblast adhesion on biomaterials. *Biomaterials*. Vol.21, pp.667-681, ISNN 0142-9612.

Askeland DR. (2006). *The Science and Engineering of Materials*. PWS-Kent Publishing Co, Canada.

Baier RE, Meyer AE. (1988). Implant surface preparation. *International Journal of Maxillofacial Implants*. Vol.3, pp.9-20, ISSN 0882-2786.

Beer A, Gahleitner A, Holm A, Tschabitscher M, Homolka P. (2003). Correlation of insertion torques with bone mineral density from dental quantitative CT in the mandible. *Clinical Oral Impl. Research.* Vol.14, pp.616–620, ISSN 0905-7161.

Berglundh T, Abrahamsson I, Albouy J-P, Lindhe J. (2007). Bone healing at implants with a fluoride-modified surface: an experimental study in dogs. *Clinical Oral Impant Research.* Vol.18, pp.147–152, ISSN 0905-7161.

Biesbrock AR, Edgerton M. Evaluation of the clinical predictability of hydroxyapatite-coated endosseous dental implants: a review of the literature. *International Journal of Oral Maxillofacial Implants.* 1995 Nov-Dec;10(6):712-20

Binon PP. (1998). Evaluation of the effectiveness of a technique to prevent screw loosening. *The Journal of Prosthetic Dentistry* Vol. 79, pp. 430-432, ISSN0022-3913.

Bogaerde LV, Pedretti G, Sennerby L, Meredith N. (2010). Immediate/Early Function of Neoss Implants Placed in Maxillas and Posterior Mandibles: An 18-Month Prospective Case Series Study. *Clinical Implant Dentistry and Related Research.* Vol.12, pp.83-94, ISSN 1523-0899.

Boyan BD et all. (2001). The titanium-bone cell interface in vitro: the role of structure of the surface in promoting osseointegration. In, Donald M Brunnette, Penti Tengvall, Marcus Textor, Peter Thomsen. *Titanium in medicine.* Springer-Verlag 2001. p564.

Braceras I, De Maeztu MA, Alava JI, Gay-Escoda C. (2009). In vivo low-density bone apposition on different implant surface materials. *International Journal of Oral Maxillofacial* Surgery. Vol.38, pp. 274–278, ISSN 0901-5027.

Branemark PI, Breine U, Johansson B, Roylance PJ. (1964). Regeneration on bone marrow. *Acta Anatomica.* Vol.59, pp.1-46, ISSN 0001-5180.

Brunette DM. (2001). Principles of cells behaviour on Ti surfaces. In: Brunette, et al. (Eds.), *Titanium in Medicine.* SpringerVerlag, Berlin, p.485.

Busquim TP, Elias CN, May JE, Kuri SE, Nascente PAP. (2009) Titanium Oxide Layer on the Surface of Anodized Dental Implants. In *Medical Device Materials V; Proceedings from the Materials & Processes for Medical Devices Conference* 2009 August 10–12, 2009, Minneapolis, Minnesota, USA, J. Gilbert, Ed., pp.60-65. ASM International, Metals Park, OH, USA. ISBN-13:978-1-61303-038-5.

Cho S-A and Jung S-K. (2003). A removal torque of the laser-treated titanium implants in rabbit tibia. *Biomaterials.*Vol. 24, pp. 4859–4863, ISSN 0142-9612.

Cochran DL, Schenk RK, Lussi A, Higginbottom FL, Buser D. (1998). Bone response to unloaded and loaded titanium implants with a sandblasted and acid-etched surface: a histometric study in the canine mandible. *Journal of Biomedical Material Research.* Vol.40, pp.1-11, ISSN 0021-9304.

Cooper LF, Zhou Y, Takebea J, Guo J, Abron A, Holme´n A, Ellingsen JE. (2006). Fluoride modification effects on osteoblast behavior and bone formation at TiO2 grit-blasted c.p. titanium endosseous implants. *Biomaterials.* Vol.27, pp.926–936, ISSN 0142-9612.

Cooper LF. (2003). Cellular interactions at cp Ti implants. In, *Bio-implant interface. Improving biomaterials and tissue reactions.* Jan Eirik Ellingsen and S. Petter Lyngstadaas. CRC Press 2003. pp.165-181.

Cordioli G, MajzoubZ, Piatelli A, Scarano A. (2000). Removal torque and histomorphometric investigation of 4 different titanium surfaces. *International Journal of Oral Maxillofacial Implants*. Vol.15, pp.668–74, ISSN 0882-2786.

Dee KC, Puleo DA, Bizios R. (2002a). *An introduction to tissue-biomaterials interactions*. John Wiley & Sons. p.192, ISBN: 978-0-471-25394-5.

Dee KC, Puleo DA, Bizios R. (2002b). *An introduction to tissue-biomaterials interactions*. John Wiley & Sons. p.49, ISBN: 978-0-471-25394-5.

Elias CN, Meirelles L. (2010). Improving osseointegration of dental implants. *Expert Review Medical Devices*. Vol.7, pp.241–256, ISSN 1743-4440.

Elias CN, Oshida Y, Limad JHC, Muller CA. (2008). Relationship between surface properties, roughness, wettability and morphology) of titanium and dental implant removal torque. *Journal of Mechanical Behavior of Biomedical Materials*. Vol.1, pp.234-242, ISSN 1751-6161.

Ellingsen JE, Johansson CB, Wennerberg A, Holmen A. (2004). Improved retention and bone to implant contact with fluoride modified titanium implants. *International Journal of Oral Maxillofacial Implants*. Vol.19, pp.659–666, ISSN 0882-2786.

Ellingsen JE. (1995). Pre-treatment of titanium implants with fluoride improves their retention in bone. *Journal of Materials Science: Materials in Medicine*. Vol.6, pp.749–753, ISSN 0957-4530.

Eriksson C, Lausmaa J, Nygren, H. (2001). Interactions between human whole blood and modified Ti-O2-surfaces: Influence of surface topography and titanium oxide thickness on leukocyte adhesion and activation. *Biomaterials*. Vol.22, pp.1987-1996, ISNN 0142-9612.

Faeda RS, Tavares HS, Sartori R, Guastaldi AC, Marcantonio E Jr. (2009). Biological performance of chemical hydroxyapatite coating associated with implant surface modification by laser beam: biomechanical study in rabbit tibias. *International Journal of Oral Maxillofacial Surgery*. Vol.67, pp.1706–1715, ISSN 0901-5027.

Feng B, Weng J, Yang BC, Qu SX, Zhang XD. (2004). Characterization of titanium surfaces with calcium and phosphate and osteoblast adhesion. *Biomaterials*. Vol.25, pp.3421–3428, ISNN 0142-9612.

Fröjd V, Franke-Stenport V, Meirelles L, Wennerberg A. (2008). Increased bone contact to a calcium-incorporated oxidized commercially pure titanium implant: an in-vivo study in rabbits. *International Journal of Oral Maxillofacial Surgery*. Vol.37, pp.561–566, ISSN 0901-5027.

Gaggl A, Schultes G, Muller WD, Karcher H. (2000). Scanning electron microscopical analysis of laser-treated titanium implants surfaces–a comparative study. *Biomaterials*. Vol.21, pp.1067-1073, ISSN 0142-9612.

Gurgel BC, Gonçalves PF, Pimentel SP, Nociti FH, Sallum EA, Sallum AW, Casati MZ. (2008). An oxidized implant surface may improve bone-to-implant contact in pristine bone and bone defects treated with guided bone regeneration: an experimental study in dogs. *Journal of Periodontology*. Vol.79, pp.1225–1231, ISSN 0022-3492.

Hayakawa T, Yoshinari M, Nemoto K, Wolke JGC, Jansen JA. (2000). Effect of surface roughness and calcium phosphate coating on the implant/bone response. *Clinical Oral Implant Research*. Vol. (11): 296-304, ISSN 0905-7161.

Hennessy KM, Pollot BE, Clem WC, Phipps MC, Sawyer AA, Culpepper BK, Bellis SL. (2009). The effect of collagen I mimetic peptides on mesenchymal stem cell adhesion and differentiation, and on bone formation at hydroxyapatite surfaces. *Biomaterials*. Vol.30, pp.1898-1909, ISSN 0142-9612.

Jarmar T, Palmquist A, Brånemark R, Hermansson L, Engqvist H, Thomsen P. (2008). Characterization of the surface properties of commercially available dental implants using scanning electron microscopy, focused ion beam, and high-resolution transmission electron microscopy. *Clinical Implant Dentistry Related Research*. Vol.10, pp.11–22, ISSN 1523-0899.

Javed F, Almas K, Crespi R, Romanos GE. (2011). Implant Surface Morphology and Primary Stability: Is There a Connection? *Implant Dentistry*. Vol. 20, pp. (1) 2011 40-46, ISSN 1056-6163.

Javed F, Romanos GE. (2010). The role of primary stability for successful immediate loading of dental implants. A literature review. *Journal of Dentistry*. Vol.38, pp.612-620, ISSN 0300-5712.

Jayaraman M, Meyer U, Buhner M, Joos U, Wiesmann HP. (2004). Influence of titanium surfaces on attachment of osteoblast-like cells in vitro. *Biomaterials*. Vol.25, pp.625–631, ISSN 0142-9612.

Johansson CB, Hamson BA and Albrektsson T. (1990) Quantive interfacial study bone and tantalum, niobium commerciallyp ure titanium. *Biomaterials*. Vol. 11, pp.277-280. ISSN 0142-9612

Kashiwagi K, Tsuji T, Shiba K. (2009). Directional BMP-2 for functionalization of titanium surfaces. *Biomaterials*. Vol.30, pp.1166-1175, ISSN 0142-9612.

Kikuchia L, Park JY, Victor C, Davies JE. (2005). Platelet interactions with calcium-phosphate-coated surfaces. *Biomaterials*. Vol.26, pp.5285–5295, ISSN 0142-9612.

Kokubo T, Kim HM, Kawashita M, Nakamura T. (1999). What kids of materials exhibit bone-bonding ? In JE Davies. *Bone Engineering* . Em Squared Incorporated, Toronto, Canada, pp.190-194.

Larsson C, Thomsen P, Aronsson B-O, Rodahl M, Lausmaa J, Kasemo B, Ericson LE.(1996). Bone response to surface-modified titanium implants: studies on the early tissue response to machined and electropolished implants with different oxide thicknesses. *Biomaterials*. Vol.17, pp.605-616, ISSN 0142-9612.

Larsson C, Emanuelsson L, Thomsen P et al. (1997). Bone response to surface modified titanium implants - studies on the tissue response after 1 year to machined and electropolished implants with different oxide thicknesses. Jornal of Materials Science: Materials in Medicine. Vol.8, pp.721–729, ISSN 0957-4530.

Larsson C, Thomsen P, Lausmaa J, Rodahl M, Kasemo B, Ericson LE. (1994). Bone response to surface modified titanium implants: studies on electropolished implants with different oxide thicknesses and morphology. *Biomaterials*. Vol.15, pp.1062–1074, ISSN 0142-9612.

Le Duc P, Wang Y. (2006).Protein adsortion at biomaterial-tissue interface. In *An Introduction to Biomaterials*, Edited Guelcher SA and Hollinger JO. Biomedical Materials Series. CRC Taylor &Francis Group 2006, p47.

Lekholm O, Zarb GA. (1985). Patient selection and preparation. In:Branemark PI et al. Editors: *Tissue integrated prostheses - Osseointegration in clinical dentistry.* Chicago, Quintessence, pp.199-209.

Li Y, Lee IS, Cui FZ, Choi SH. (2008). The biocompatibility of nanostructured calcium phosphate coated on micro-arc oxidized titanium. *Biomaterials.* Vol.29, pp.2025-2032, ISSN 0142-9612.

Lim JY, Liu X, Vogler EA, Donahue HJ. (2004). Systematic variation in osteoblast adhesion and phenotype with substratum surface characteristics. *Jorurnal of Biomedical Materials Research.* Vol.68A, pp.504–512, ISSN 1549-3296.

Lim YJ, Oshida Y, Andres CJ, Barco MT. (2001). Surface characterizations of variously treated titanium materials. *International Journal of Oral Maxillofacial Implants.* Vol.16, pp.333-342, ISSN 0882-2786.

Lincks J, Boyan BD, Blanchard CR, Lohmann CH, Liu Y, Cochran DL, Dean DD, Schwartz Z. (1998). Response of MG63 osteoblastlike cells to titanium and titanium alloy is dependent on surface roughness and composition. *Biomaterials.* Vol.19, pp.2219-2232, ISSN 0142-9612.

Menezes GC, Elias CN, Attias M, Silva-Filho FC. (2003). Osteoblast Adhesion onto Titanium Dental Implants. *Acta Microscopica.* Vol.12, pp.13-19, ISSN 1728-5917.

Misch CE. (2008). *Contemporary implant dentistry.* Mosby – St Louis 2008. 0801660734.

Morais LS, Serra GG, Palermo EFA, Andrade LR, Muller CA, Meyers MC, Elias CN. (2009). Systemic levels of metallic ions released from orthodontic mini-implants. *American Journal Orthodontics Dentofacial Orthopedics.* Vol.135, pp.:522-529. ISSN 0889-5406

Morton RK. Topography of Surfaces. (1994). In: ASM Handbook. *Surface Engineering.* Vol.5, ASM, Materials Park, OH, pp.136-138.

Nayab SN, Jones FH, Olsen I. (2005). Effects of calcium ion implantation on human bone cell interaction with titanium. *Biomaterials.* Vol.26, pp.4717–4727, ISSN 0142-9612.

Niinomi M. (2002). Recent Metallic Materials for Biomedical Applications. *Metallurgical and Materials Transaction A.* Vol.33A, pp.477-486, ISSN 1073-5623.

Novak MT, Bryers JD, Reichert WM. (2009). Biomimetic strategies based on viruses and bacteria for the development of immune evasive biomaterials. *Biomaterials.* Vol.30, pp.1989-2005, ISSN 0142-9612.

Ohtsu N, Sato K, Saito K, Asami K, Hanawa T. (2007). Calcium phosphates formation on CaTiO(3) coated titanium. Journal of *Materials Science: Materials in Medicine.* Vol.18, pp.1009–1016, ISSN 0957-4530.

Oliveira PT, Nanci A. (2004). Nanotexturing of titanium-based surfaces upregulates expression of bone sialoprotein and osteopontin by cultured osteogenic cells. *Biomaterials.* Vol.25, pp.403–413, ISNN 0142-9612.

Ong JL, andChan DCN. (2000). Hydroxyapatite and their use as coatings in dental implants: a review. *Critical Review in Biomedical Engineering.* Vol 28, pp.235-239. ISSN: 0278-940X.

Oshida Y, Tuna EB, Aktören O, Gençay K. (2010). Dental Implant Systems. *International Journal of Molecules Science.* Vol.11, pp.1580-1678, ISSN 1422-0067.

Owens DK and Wendt RC. (1969). Estimation of the surface free energy of polymers. *Journal of Applied Polymer Science*. Vol.13, pp1741-1747. ISSN 1097-4628.

Puleo DA, Bizios R. (1992). Mechanisms of fibronectin mediated attachment of osteoblasts to substrats in vitro. *Journal of Bone and Mineral Research*. Vol.18, pp.215-226, ISSN 0169-6009.

Richards RG. (1996). The effect of surface roughness on fibroblast adhesion in vitro. *Injury*. Vol.27, pp.S-C38-S-C43, ISSN 0020-1383.

Romanos GE, Toh CG, Siar CH, Swaminathan D. (2002). Histologic and histomorphometric evaluation of peri-implant bone subjected to immediate loading: an experimental study with Macaca fascicularis. *International Journal of Oral and Maxillofacial Implants*. Vol.17, pp.44–51, ISSN 0882-2786.

Santos MV, Elias CN, Cavalcanti Lima JH. The effects of superficial roughness and design on the primary stability of dental implants. *Clinical Implant Dental Related Research. In press*

Schuckert KH, Jopp S, Muller U. (2006). De Novo Grown Bone on Exposed Implant Surfaces Using Photodynamic Therapy and Recombinant Human Bone Morphogenetic Protein-2: *Case Report Implant Dentistry*. Vol.15, pp.361-365, ISSN 1056-6163.

Sener BC, Dergin G, Gursoy B, Kelesoglu E, Slih I. (2009). Effects of irrigation temperature on heat control in vitro at different drilling depths. *Clinical Oral Implant Research*. Vol.20, pp.294–298, ISSN ISSN 0905-7161.

Soballe K, Hansen ES, Brockstedt-Rasmussen H, Bunger C. (1993). Hydroxyapatite coating converts fibrous tissue to bone around loaded implants. *Journal of Bone and Joint Surgery* Br. Vol.75, pp.270–278, ISSN 0301-620X.

Stadlinger B, Pilling E, Huhle M, Mai R, Bierbaum S, Scharnweber D, Kuhlisch E, Loukota R, Eckelt U. (2008). Evaluation of osseointegration of dental implants coated with collagen, chondroitin sulphate and BMP-4: an animal study. *International Journal of Oral Maxillofacial Surgery*. Vol.37, pp.54-59, ISSN 0901-5027.

Sul YT, Johansson C, Albrektsson T. (2006). Which surface properties enhance bone response to implants? Comparison of oxidized magnesium, TiUnite, and Osseotite implant surfaces. *International Journal of Prosthodontics*. Vol.19, pp.319–328, ISSN 0893-2174.

Sun L, Berndt CC, Gross KA, Kucuk A. (2001). Material fundamentals and clinical performance of plasma-sprayed hydroxyapatite coatings: a review. *Journal of Biomedical Materials Research.* Vol.58, pp.570–592, ISSN 1549-3296.

Suzuki M, Guimaraes MV, Marin C, Granato R, Gil JN, Coelho PG. (2009). Histomorphometric Evaluation of Alumina-Blasted/Acid-Etched and Thin Ion Beam-Deposited Bioceramic Surfaces: An Experimental Study in Dogs. *International Journal of Oral Maxillofacial Surgery*. Vol.67, pp.602-607, ISSN 0278-2391.

Szmukler-Moncler S, Piattelli A, Favero GA, Dubruille JH. (2000). Considerations preliminary to the application of early and immediate loading protocols in dental implantology. *Clinical Oral Implants Research*. Vol.11, pp.12–25, ISSN 0905-7161.

Tang L and Hu W. (2005). Molecular determinants of biocompatibility. *Expert Review Medical Devices*. Vol. 2, pp.493-500, ISSN 1743-4440.

Tete S, Mastrangelo F, Traini T, Vinci R, Sammartino G, Marenzi G, Gherlone E. (2008). A Macro and Nanostructure Evaluation of a Novel Dental Implant. *Implant Dentistry*. Vol.17, pp.309-320, ISSN 1056-6163.

Thull R. (2002). Physicochemical principles of tissue material interactions. *Biomolecular Engineering*. Vol.19, pp.43-50, ISSN 1389-0344.

Vladkova TG. (2010). Surface Engineered Polymeric Biomaterials with Improved Biocontact Properties. *International Journal of Polymer Science*. Vol.2010, Article ID 296094, 22 pages, ISSN 1687-9422.

Togashi AY, Cirano FR, Lima LAPA. (2007). The role of implant surface chemistry in the biological bone response. *RPG Revista Pos Graduação*. Vol.13, pp.340-344.

Webster TJ, Ejiofor JU. (2004). Increased osteoblast adhesion on nanophase metals: Ti, Ti6Al4V, and CoCrMo. *Biomaterials*. Vol. 25, pp.4731–4739, ISSN 0142-9612.

Webster TJ, Ergun C, Doremus RH, Siegel RW, Bizios R. (2000). Enhanced functions of osteoblasts on nanophase ceramics. *Biomaterials*. Vol.21, pp.1803–1810, ISSN 0142-9612.

Webster TJ, Siegel RW, Bizios R. (1999). Osteoblast adhesion on nanophase ceramics. *Biomaterials*. Vol.20, pp.1221–1227, ISSN 0142-9612.

Wennerberg A, Albrektsson T, Andersson B. (1995). An animal study of cp titanium screws with different surface topographies. *Journal of Materials Science: Materials in M edicine*. Vol.6, pp.302–309, ISSN 0957-4530.

Wennerberg A, Albrektsson T, Lindhe J. (2003). Surface topography of titanium implants. pp.821-828. In Jan Lindhe, Thorkild Karring and Niklaus P. Lang Editor. *Clinical Periodontology and clinical dentistry*. Fourth edition 2003. Blackwell Munksgaard, a Blackwell Publishing Company. ISBN: 1-4051-0236-5. Oxford, UK.

Wennerberg A, Hallgren C, Johansson C, Danelli S. (1998). A histomorphometric evaluation of screw-shaped implants each prepared with two surface roughnesses. *Clinical Oral Implants Research*. Vol.9, pp.11–19, ISSN 0905-7161.

Wennerberg A. (1998). The importance of surface roughness for implant incorporation. *International Jornal of Machining and Tools Manufacturing*. Vol.38, pp.657-662, ISSN 0890-6955.

Wennerberg A. *On surface and implant incorporation*. Ph.D. Thesis. Goteborg University 1996.

Werner S, Huck O, Frisch B, Vautier D, Elkaim R, Voegel JC, Brunel G Tenenbaum H. (2009). The effect of microstructured surfaces and laminin-derived peptide coatings on soft tissue interactions with titanium dental implants. *Biomaterials*. Vol.30, pp.2291-2301, ISSN 0142-9612.

Verrier S, Pallu S, Bareille R, Jonczyk A, Meyer J, Dard M, Amédée J. (2002). Function of linear and cyclic RGD-containing peptides in osteoprogenitor cells adhesion process. *Biomaterials*. Vol.23, pp.585–596, ISSN 0142-9612.

Williams DF. (2008). On the mechanisms of biocompatibility. *Biomaterials*. Vol.29, pp. 2941–2953, ISSN 0142-9612.

Williams DF. Titanium and titanium alloys. In: Williams DF, editor. *Biocompatibility of clinical implant materials*, vol. I. Boca Raton, Florida: CRC Press, Inc.; 1981. p. 9–44.

Wolner C, Nauer GE, Trummer J, Putz V, Tschegg S. (2006). Possible reasons for the unexpected bad biocompatibility of metal-on-metal hip implants. *Materials Science and Engineering C*. Vol.26, pp.34-40, ISSN 0928-4931.

Yang W-E, Hsu M-L, Lin M-C, Chen Z-H, Chen L-K, Huang H-H. (2009). Nano/submicron-scale TiO2 network on titanium surface for dental implant application. *Journal of Alloys and Compounds*. Vol.479, pp.642–647, ISSN 0925-8388.

Zhu X, Chen J, Scheideler L, Reichl R, Geis-Gerstorfer J. (2004). Effects of topography and composition of titanium surface oxides on osteoblast responses. *Biomaterials*. Vol.25, pp.4087-4103, ISSN 0142-9612.

Permissions

All chapters in this book were first published in IDAREP, by InTech Open; hereby published with permission under the Creative Commons Attribution License or equivalent. Every chapter published in this book has been scrutinized by our experts. Their significance has been extensively debated. The topics covered herein carry significant findings which will fuel the growth of the discipline. They may even be implemented as practical applications or may be referred to as a beginning point for another development.

The contributors of this book come from diverse backgrounds, making this book a truly international effort. This book will bring forth new frontiers with its revolutionizing research information and detailed analysis of the nascent developments around the world.

We would like to thank all the contributing authors for lending their expertise to make the book truly unique. They have played a crucial role in the development of this book. Without their invaluable contributions this book wouldn't have been possible. They have made vital efforts to compile up to date information on the varied aspects of this subject to make this book a valuable addition to the collection of many professionals and students.

This book was conceptualized with the vision of imparting up-to-date information and advanced data in this field. To ensure the same, a matchless editorial board was set up. Every individual on the board went through rigorous rounds of assessment to prove their worth. After which they invested a large part of their time researching and compiling the most relevant data for our readers.

The editorial board has been involved in producing this book since its inception. They have spent rigorous hours researching and exploring the diverse topics which have resulted in the successful publishing of this book. They have passed on their knowledge of decades through this book. To expedite this challenging task, the publisher supported the team at every step. A small team of assistant editors was also appointed to further simplify the editing procedure and attain best results for the readers.

Apart from the editorial board, the designing team has also invested a significant amount of their time in understanding the subject and creating the most relevant covers. They scrutinized every image to scout for the most suitable representation of the subject and create an appropriate cover for the book.

The publishing team has been an ardent support to the editorial, designing and production team. Their endless efforts to recruit the best for this project, has resulted in the accomplishment of this book. They are a veteran in the field of academics and their pool of knowledge is as vast as their experience in printing. Their expertise and guidance has proved useful at every step. Their uncompromising quality standards have made this book an exceptional effort. Their encouragement from time to time has been an inspiration for everyone.

The publisher and the editorial board hope that this book will prove to be a valuable piece of knowledge for researchers, students, practitioners and scholars across the globe.

List of Contributors

Mustafa Ramazanoglu
Istanbul University/Department of Oral Surgery, Turkey

Yoshiki Oshida
Syracuse University/Department of Mechanical and Aerospace Engineering, USA

Ilser Turkyilmaz and Roxanna J. Nicoll
Department of Comprehensive Dentistry University of Texas, Health Science Center San Antonio, Texas, United States of America

Tatsuo Shirota, Masashi Hatori, Masanori Nakamura and Satoru Shintani
Showa University, Japan

Atsushi Nakamura
Yamato Tokushukai Hospital, Japan

Yoshiro Matsui
Kagawa University, Japan

Rogério Margonar,
Araraquara University Center - UNIARA, Araraquara, SP, Brazil

Cássia Bellotto Corrêa, Lúcia Roselino Ribeiro, Elcio Marcantonio and Luís Geraldo Vaz
São Paulo State University - UNESP, College of Dentistry, Araraquara, SP, Brazil

Erika Oliveira de Almeida
São Paulo State University - UNESP, College of Dentistry, Araçatuba, SP, Brazil
New York University-NYU, College of Dentistry, New York, NY, USA

Satoshi Yamaguchi, Shinji Ono, Yasufumi Yamanishi and Hirofumi Yatani
Graduate School of Dentistry, Osaka University, Japan

Takafumi Ohtani
Graduate Prosthodontics, University of Washington, USA

Taiji Sohmura
Bionic Inc., Japan

Chahine Gilbert and Kovacevic Radovan
Southern Methodist University, Dallas, Texas, USA

Smith Pauline
Army Research Lab, Aberdeen, Maryland, USA

Ajlouni Raed and Ajlouni Khaldoun
Baylor College of Dentistry, Dallas, Texas, USA

Laurence Evrard
Stomatology and Maxillo-facial Surgery Department, Hopital Erasme - ULB Brussels, Belgium

Yeung Stephen C H
Faculty of Dentistry, University of Sydney, Sydeny, Westmead Centre for Oral Health, Westmead Hospital, Westmead, Australia

Jeong Keun Lee
Ajou University School of Medicine, Republic of Korea

Su-Gwan Kim
Dept. of Oral and Maxillofacial Surgery, School of Dentistry, Chosun University, Republic of Korea

Carlos Nelson Elias
Instituto Militar de Engenharia, Biomaterials Laboratory Rio de Janeiro, RJ, Brazil

Index

R

S

T

V

Z

www.ingramcontent.com/pod-product-compliance
Lightning Source LLC
LaVergne TN
LVHW081018210926
848485LV00004B/893